T0293522

Introduction to Statistical Methods for Clinical Trials

CHAPMAN & HALL/CRC
Texts in Statistical Science Series

Series Editors

Bradley P. Carlin, *University of Minnesota, USA*
Julian J. Faraway, *University of Bath, UK*
Martin Tanner, *Northwestern University, USA*
Jim Zidek, *University of British Columbia, Canada*

Texts in Statistical Science

Introduction to Statistical Methods for Clinical Trials

Edited by

Thomas D. Cook
David L. DeMets

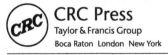

CRC Press
Taylor & Francis Group
Boca Raton London New York

CRC Press is an imprint of the
Taylor & Francis Group, an **informa** business

A CHAPMAN & HALL BOOK

Chapman & Hall/CRC
Taylor & Francis Group
6000 Broken Sound Parkway NW, Suite 300
Boca Raton, FL 33487-2742

© 2008 by Taylor & Francis Group, LLC
Chapman & Hall/CRC is an imprint of Taylor & Francis Group, an Informa business

No claim to original U.S. Government works

International Standard Book Number-13: 978-1-58488-027-1 (Hardcover)

Library of Congress Cataloging-in-Publication Data

Cook, Thomas D.
    Introduction to statistical methods for clinical trials / Thomas D. Cook, David L. DeMets.
       p. ; cm. -- (Interdisciplinary statistics series)
    "A CRC title."
    Includes bibliographical references and index.
    ISBN 978-1-58488-027-1 (hardback : alk. paper) 1. Clinical trials--Statistical methods. I. DeMets, David L., 1944- II. Title. III. Series: Interdisciplinary statistics.
    [DNLM: 1. Clinical Trials--methods. 2. Statistics--methods. 3. Data Collection--methods. 4. Research Design. WA 950 C771i 2007]

R853.C55C68 2007
615.5072'4--dc22
                                        2007036202

Visit the Taylor & Francis Web site at
http://www.taylorandfrancis.com

and the CRC Press Web site at
http://www.crcpress.com

Contents

List of figures

List of tables

Preface

This text is intended to be an introduction to statistical methods for clinical trials targeted to first- or second-year graduate students in statistics or biostatistics. It arose out of a very successful course taught at the University of Wisconsin in the joint statistics/biostatistics training program for the past 25 years. The structure is similar to a text by Friedman, Furberg, and DeMets entitled *Fundamentals of Clinical Trials* but with technical material included.

The topics are based on our collective experience in the design, conduct, and analysis of clinical trials in a variety of disease areas. The material is presented from a frequentist statistical perspective although some of the topics could also have a Bayesian presentation.

The chapters have been contributed by members of the Department of Biostatistics and Medical Informatics at the University of Wisconsin School of Medicine and Public Health. The editors, who are also chapter authors, have given organization to the text and provided extensive review and input to all the chapters as they have evolved. The authors of individual chapters have interest, experience, and expertise in the topics discussed and are identified on a separate authors page. The editors endorse and take full responsibility for all the material appearing in this book.

There is no ideal sequence to the topics we have selected but we have tried to follow the thought process used in the development of a protocol. Consequently, many of the chapters are interrelated and it may be necessary for the reader to occasionally "read ahead." For example, in order to understand some discussion in the sample size chapter, the reader may have to skip forward to chapters on survival analysis or repeated measures. Throughout the text, the authors have cross-referenced other chapters where further detail on a given topic may be found.

We have also tried throughout to remain consistent with three overarching philosophical approaches described in Chapter 2, *Defining the Question*. The first is our strong belief that the design, conduct, and analysis of randomized control trials (RCTs) should adhere, to the extent possible, to the *intent-to-treat* (ITT) principle. To our dismay, the use of "per-protocol" or "on-treatment" analyses is far too widespread. Recent events illustrate how departures from this principle can lead to confusing and misleading information. While valid alternatives to ITT may be available in a few very simple situations, it is our belief that, in the vast majority of cases, there are currently no valid, practical alternatives.

Our second overarching philosophical viewpoint is that RCTs are primarily hypothesis testing instruments. While inference beyond simple tests of the primary and secondary hypotheses is clearly essential for a complete understanding of the results, we note that virtually all design features of an RCT are formulated with hypothesis testing in mind. Some of the material, especially in Chapter 8, *Longitudinal Data*, and Chapter 9, *Quality of Life*, is unavoidably focused on complex model-based inference. Even in the simplest situations, however, estimation of a "treatment effect" is inherently model-based, dependent on implicit model assumptions, and the most well conducted trials are subject to biases that require that point estimates and confidence intervals be viewed cautiously. Inference beyond the population enrolled and treated under the circumstances of a carefully conducted trial is precarious—while it may be safe to infer that treatment A is superior to treatment B based on the result of RCTs (a conclusion based on a hypothesis test), it is less so to infer that the *size* of the effect seen in an RCT (even if could be known without error) would be realized once a treatment is adopted in common practice.

Thus, the third overarching philosophical perspective that we adopt is that the results of RCTs are best understood through the application of sound statistical principles, such as ITT, followed by interpretation rooted in clinical and scientific understanding. By this we mean that, while many scientific questions emerge in the analysis of trial data, a large proportion of these have no direct statistical answer. Nonetheless, countless "exploratory" analyses are performed, many of which deviate from sound statistical principles and either do not contribute to scientific understanding, or are in fact misleading. Our belief is that researchers, and especially statisticians, need to understand the inherent limitations of clinical studies and thoughtfully conduct analyses that best answer those questions for which RCTs are suited.

Chapter 1 introduces the clinical trial as a research method and many of the key issues that must be understood before the statistical methods can take on meaning. While this chapter contains very little technical material, many of the issues have implications for the trial statistician and are critical for statistical students to understand. Chapter 12, the last chapter, discusses the importance of the manner in which results of a trial are presented. In between, there are 10 chapters presenting various statistical topics relevant to the design, monitoring, and analysis of a clinical trial.

The material presented here is intended as an introductory course that should be accessible to masters degree students and of value to PhD graduate students. There is more material than might be covered in a one-semester course and so careful consideration regarding the amount of detail presented will likely be required.

The editors are grateful to our department colleagues for their contributions, and to a graduate student, Charlie Casper, who served as editorial assistant throughout the development of the text. His involvement was instrumental in its completion. In addition to the editors and contributors, we are grateful for helpful comments that have been received from Adin-Cristian Andrei, Murray Clayton, Mary Foulkes, Anastasia Ivanova, and Scott Diegel.

We also note that most of the data analysis and the generation of graphics in this book was conducted using R (R Development Core Team 2005) statistical software.

Thomas Cook
David DeMets

Madison, Wisconsin
July, 2007

Author Attribution

In preparing this text, the faculty listed below in the Department of Biostatistics and Medical Informatics took responsibility for early drafts of each chapter, based on their expertise and interest in statistical methodology and clinical trials. The editors, in addition to contributing to individual chapters, revised chapters as necessary to provide consistency across chapters and to mold the individual chapters into a uniform text. Without the contribution of these faculty to drafting these chapters, this text would not have been completed in a timely fashion, if at all.

Chapter				
1	Introduction to Clinical Trials	DeMets	Fisher	
2	Defining the Question	Cook	Casper	
3	Study Design	DeMets	Chappell	Casper
4	Sample Size	Cook		
5	Randomization	Casper	Chappell	
6	Data Collection and Quality Control	Bechhofer	Feyzi	Cook
7	Survival Analysis	Cook	Kim	
8	Longitudinal Data	Lindstrom	Cook	
9	Quality of Life	Eickhoff	Koscik	
10	Data Monitoring and Interim Analysis	Kim	Cook	DeMets
11	Selected Issues in the Analysis	DeMets	Cook	Roecker
12	Closeout and Reporting	DeMets	Casper	

Contributors

Robin Bechhofer, BA Researcher

T. Charles Casper, MS Research Assistant & Graduate Student

Richard Chappell, PhD Professor of Biostatistics and Statistics

Thomas Cook, PhD Senior Statistical Scientist

David DeMets, PhD Professor of Biostatistics and Statistics

Jens Eickhoff, PhD Statistical Scientist

Jan Feyzi, MS Researcher

Marian R. Fisher, PhD Research Professor

Kyungmann Kim, PhD Professor of Biostatistics

Rebecca Koscik, PhD Statistical Scientist

Mary Lindstrom, PhD Professor of Biostatistics

Ellen Roecker, PhD Senior Statistical Scientist

CHAPTER 1

Introduction to Clinical Trials

Clinical trials have become an essential research tool for the evaluation of the benefit and risk of new interventions for the treatment or prevention of disease. Clinical trials represent the experimental approach to clinical research. Take, for example, the modification of risk factors for cardiovascular disease. Large observational studies such as the Framingham Heart Study (Dawber et al. 1951) indicated a correlation between high cholesterol, high blood pressure, smoking, and diabetes with the incidence of cardiovascular disease. Focusing on high cholesterol, basic researchers sought interventions that would lower serum cholesterol. While interventions were discovered that lowered cholesterol, they did not demonstrate a significant reduction in cardiovascular mortality.[1] Finally, in 1994, a trial evaluating a member of the statin class of drugs demonstrated a reduction in mortality (Scandanavian Simvistatin Survival Study 1994). With data from well-controlled clinical trials, an effective and safe intervention was identified. Sometimes interventions can be adopted without good evidence and even become widely used. One case was the use of hormone replacement therapy (HRT) that is used to treat symptoms in postmenopausal women and is also known to reduce bone loss in these women, leading to reduced bone fracture rates. HRT also reduces serum cholesterol leading to the belief that it should also reduce cardiovascular mortality and morbidity. In addition, large observational studies have shown lower cardiovascular mortality for women using HRT than for those not using HRT (Barrett-Connor and Grady 1998). These observations led to a widespread use of HRT for the prevention of cardiovascular mortality and morbidity as well as the other indications. Subsequently, two trials evaluated the benefits of HRT in postmenopausal women: one trial in women with existing cardiovascular disease and a second without any evident disease. The first trial, known as HERS, demonstrated no benefit and suggested a possible risk of thrombosis (i.e., blood clots) (Grady et al. 1998). The second trial, known as the Women's Health Initiative, or WHI, demonstrated a harmful effect due to blood clotting and no cardiovascular benefit.[2] These trials contradicted evidence derived from non-randomized trials and led to a rapid decline in the use of HRT for purposes of reducing cardiovascular disease. HRT is still used when indicated for short-term symptom relief in postmenopausal women.

---

[1] The Coronary Drug Project Research Group (1975), The Lipid Research Clinics Program (1979)

[2] Writing Group for the Women's Health Initiative Randomized Controlled Trial (2002)

Incomplete understanding of the biological mechanism of action can sometimes limit the adoption of potentially effective drugs. A class of drugs known as *beta-blockers* was known to be effective for lowering blood pressure and reducing mortality in patients suffering a heart attack. Since these drugs lower blood pressure and lower heart rate, scientists believed these drugs should not be used in patients with heart failure. In these patients, the heart does not pump blood efficiently and it was believed that lowering the heart rate and blood pressure would make the problem worse. Nonetheless, a series of trials demonstrated convincingly an approximate 30% reduction in mortality.[3] An effective therapy was ignored for a decade or more because of belief in a mechanistic theory without clinical evidence. Thus, clinical trials play the critical role of sorting out effective and safe interventions from those that are not.

The fundamental principles of clinical trials are heavily based on statistical principles related to experimental design, quality control, and sound analysis. No analytical methods can rescue a trial with poor experimental design and the conclusions from a trial with proper design can be invalid if sound analytical principles are not adhered to. Of course, collection of appropriate and high quality data is essential. With this heavy reliance on statistical principles, a statistician must be involved in the design, conduct, and the final analyses phases of a trial. A statistician cannot wait until after the data have been collected to get involved with a clinical trial. The principles presented in this text are an introduction to important statistical concepts in design, conduct, and analysis.

In this chapter, we shall briefly describe the background and rationale for clinical trials, and their relationship to other clinical research designs as well as defining the questions that clinical trials can best address. For the purposes of this text, we shall define a clinical trial to be a prospective trial evaluating the effect of an intervention in humans. The intervention may be a drug, biologic (blood, vaccine, and tissue, or other products, derived from living sources such as humans, animals, and microorganisms), device, procedure, or genetic manipulation. The trial may evaluate screening, diagnostic, prevention, or therapeutic interventions. Many trials, especially those that attempt to establish the role of the intervention in the context of current medical practice, may have a control group. These and other concepts will be further discussed in this chapter and in more detail in subsequent chapters.

First, the historical evolution of the modern clinical trial is presented followed by a discussion of the ethical issues surrounding the conduct of clinical research. A brief review of various types of clinical research is presented emphasizing the unique role that clinical trials play. The rationale, need, and the timing of clinical trials are discussed. The organizational structure of a clinical trial is key to its success regardless of whether the trial is a single-center trial or a multicenter trial. All of the key design and conduct issues must be described in a research plan called a *trial protocol*.

---

[3] The International Steering Committee on Behalf of the MERIT-HF Study Group (1997), Krum et al. (2006), Packer et al. (2001)

1.1 History and Background

The era of the modern day clinical trial began in the post–World War II period, beginning with two trials in the United Kingdom sponsored by the Medical Research Council (1944). The first of these trials was conducted in 1944 and studied treatments for the common cold. The second trial, conducted in 1948, evaluated treatments for tuberculosis, comparing streptomycin to placebo. Hill (1971) incorporated many features of modern clinical trials such as randomization and a placebo-treated control group into this trial (Medical Research Council 1948).

In the United States, the era of the modern clinical trial probably began with the initiation of the Coronary Drug Project (CDP)[4] in 1965. The CDP was sponsored by the National Heart Institute (later expanded to be the National Heart, Lung, and Blood Institute or NHLBI), one of the major institutes in the National Institutes of Health (NIH). This trial compared five different lipid-lowering drugs to a placebo control in men who had survived a recent heart attack (myocardial infarction). In this study, all patients also received the best medical care known at that time. Eligible men were randomized to receive either one of the five drugs or a placebo. They were followed for the recurrence of a major cardiovascular event such as death or a second heart attack. Many of the operational principles developed for this trial are still in use. Shortly after the CDP began, the NHLBI initiated several other large clinical trials evaluating modifications of major cardiovascular risk factors such as blood pressure in the Hypertension Detection and Follow-up Program (HDFP Cooperative Group 1982), cholesterol in the Coronary Primary Prevention Trial (The Lipid Research Clinics Program 1979) and simultaneous reduction of blood pressure, cholesterol, and smoking in the Multiple Risk Factor Intervention Trial (Domanski et al. 2002). These trials, all initiated within a short period of time, established the clinical trial as an important tool in the development of treatments for cardiovascular diseases. During this same period, the NHLBI launched trials studying treatments for blood and lung diseases. The methods used in the cardiovascular trials were applied to these trials as well.

In 1973, the National Eye Institute (NEI) also began a landmark clinical trial, the Diabetic Retinopathy Study (DRS) (Diabetic Retinopathy Study Research Group 1976). Diabetes is a risk factor for several organ systems diseases including cardiovascular and eye diseases. Diabetes causes progressive stages of retinopathy (damage to the retina of the eye), ultimately leading to severe visual loss or blindness. This trial evaluated a new treatment of photocoagulation by means of a laser device. Many of the concepts of the CDP were brought to the DRS by NIH statistical staff. Several other trials were launched by the NEI using the principles established in the DRS (e.g., the Early Treatment Diabetic Retinopathy Study (Cusick et al. 2005)).

Other institutes such as the National Cancer Institute (NCI) of the NIH

---

[4] The Coronary Drug Project Research Group (1975)

aggressively used the clinical trial to evaluate new treatments. The NCI established several clinical trial networks, or cancer cooperative groups, organized by either geographic regions (e.g., the Eastern Cooperative Oncology Group, or ECOG, the South Western Oncology Group, or SWOG), disease areas (e.g., the Pediatric Oncology Group, or POG), or treatment modality (e.g., Radiation Treatment Oncology Group, or RTOG). By 1990, most disease areas were using clinical trials to evaluate new interventions. Perhaps, the most recent development was in the AIDS Clinical Trial Group (ACTG) which was rapidly formed in the late 1980s to evaluate new treatments to address a rapidly emerging epidemic of Acquired Immune Deficiency Syndrome (AIDS) (DeMets et al. 1995). Many of the fundamental principles of trial design and conduct developed in the preceding two decades were reexamined and at times challenged by scientific, medical, patient, and political interest groups. Needless to say, these principles withstood the scrutiny and challenge.

Most of the trials we have mentioned were sponsored by the NIH in the U.S. or the Medical Research Council (MRC) in the U.K. Industry-sponsored clinical trials, especially those investigating pharmaceutical agents, evolved during the same period of time. Large industry-sponsored phase III outcome trials were infrequent, however, until the late 1980s and early 1990s. Prior to 1990, most industry-sponsored trials were small dose-finding trials or trials evaluating a physiological or pharmacology outcome. Occasionally, trials were conducted and sponsored by industry with collaboration from academia. The the Anturane Reinfarction Trial (The Anturane Reinfarction Trial Research Group 1978) was one such trial comparing a platelet active drug, sulfinpyrazone (anturane), to placebo in men following a heart attack. Mortality and cause-specific mortality were the major outcome measures. By 1990 many clinical trials in cardiology, for example, were being sponsored and conducted by the pharmaceutical industry. By 2000, the pharmaceutical industry was spending $2.5 billion dollars on clinical trials compared to $1.5 billion by the NIH. In addition, standards for the evaluation of medical devices as well as medical procedures are increasingly requiring clinical trials as a component in the assessment of effectiveness and safety.

Thus, the clinical trial has been the primary tool for the evaluation of a new drug, biologic, device, procedure, nutritional supplement, or behavioral modification. The success of the trial in providing an unbiased and efficient evaluation depends on fundamental statistical principles that we shall discuss in this and following chapters. The development of statistical methods for clinical trials has been a major research activity for biostatisticians. This text provides an introduction to these statistical methods but is by no means comprehensive.

Some of the most basic principles now used in clinical trial design and analysis can be traced to earlier research efforts. For example, an unplanned natural experiment to examine the effect of lemon juice on scurvy for sailors was conducted by Lancaster in 1600 as a captain of a ship for the East Indian Shipping Company (Bull 1959). The sailors on the ships with lemons on board were free of scurvy in contrast to those on the other ships without lemons. In 1721, a smallpox experiment was planned and conducted. Smallpox was an epidemic that caused suffering and death. The sentences of inmates at the Newgate prison in Great Britain were commuted if they volunteered for inoculation. All of those inoculated remained free of smallpox. (We note that this experiment could not have been conducted today on ethical grounds.) In 1747, Lind (1753) conducted a planned experiment on the treatment of scurvy with a concurrent control group while on board ship. Of 12 patients with scurvy, ten patients were given five different treatments, two patients per treatment, and the other two served as a control with no treatment. The two sailors given fruit (lemons and oranges) recovered. In 1834, Louis (1834) described the process of keeping track of outcomes for clinical studies of treatment effect, and the need to take into consideration the patients' circumstances (i.e., risk factors) and the natural history of the disease.

While Fisher (1926) introduced the concept of randomization for agricultural experiments, randomization was first used for clinical research in 1931 by Amberson Jr., McMahon, and Pinner (1931) to study treatments for tuberculosis. As already described, Bradford Hill used randomization in the 1948 MRC tuberculosis trial (Hill 1971).

1.2 Ethics of Clinical Research

Clinical research in general and clinical trials in particular must be conducted in a manner that meets current ethical standards. Ethical standards change over time and can vary by geographical regions, societies, and even between individuals making the formulation of ethical standards complex and challenging. The ethical imperative for the establishment of ethical standards was starkly demonstrated by the discovery of Nazi atrocities carried out using concentration camp prisoners during World War II. As a result, the Nuremburg Code was established in 1947 and set standards for physicians and scientists conducting medical research (U.S. Government 1949). Two of the main tenants of the Nuremburg Code (summarized by Table 1.1) were that medical research must have patient consent and all unnecessary physical and mental suffering and injury should be avoided. The degree of risk should not exceed the potential benefit and a volunteer should be able to stop whenever they choose. The Declaration of Helsinki, first set forth in 1964 with later revisions (World Medical Association 1989), gives further guidance on the conduct of human research with specific reference to informed consent. The Belmont Report, summarized in Table 1.2, was issued in 1979 by the NIH as a guide establishing the need for *respect for persons*, especially those with diminished autonomy such as children and prisoners, the concept of *beneficence* to maximize the benefits while minimizing the risks, and the need for *justice* in the distribution of new experimental treatments.[5] The U.S. Department of Health

---

[5] National Commission for the Protection of Human Subjects of Biomedical and Behavioral Research (1979)

Table 1.1 *Nuremberg Code Principles*.

1. Voluntary consent
2. Experiment to yield results for good of society
3. Experiment based on current knowledge
4. Experiment to avoid all unnecessary suffering
5. No *a priori* reason to expect death
6. Risk not exceed importance of problem
7. Protect against remote injury possibilities
8. Conduct by scientifically qualified persons
9. Subject free to end experiment at any time
10. Scientist free to end experiment

*U.S. DHHS Institutional Review Board Guidebook Appendix 6 The Nuremberg Code, Declaration of Helsinki, and Belmont Report. www.hhs.gov/ohrp/irb/irb_appendices.htm

Table 1.2 *Principles established in the Belmont Report.*

1. Boundaries between practice and research
2. Basic ethical principles

   Respect for persons: recognition of the personal dignity and autonomy (i.e., self governance) of individuals and special protection of those with diminished autonomy (e.g., children, prisoners)

   Beneficence: obligation to protect persons from harm by maximizing potential benefits and minimizing potential risks of harm

   Justice: benefits and burdens of research be distributed fairly

3. Applications (parallels each basic ethical principle)

   Application of respect for persons: informed consent that contains information, comprehension, and voluntariness

   Application of beneficence: risk/benefit assessment is carefully considered in study design and implementation

   Application of justice: selection of research subjects must be the result of fair selection procedures

and Human Services (DHHS) through both the NIH[6] and the U.S. Food and Drug Administration (FDA)[7] also provide clinical research guidelines. In addition, NIH and FDA guidelines for monitoring trials will be discussed in detail in Chapter 10.

These federal documents discuss issues related to the experimental design, data management, and data analysis. The experimental design must be sound and not expose subjects to unnecessary risks while providing an adequate and fair test of the new experimental treatment. Studies must be sufficiently large to ensure reliable conclusions and the outcome assessed in an unbiased manner. Furthermore, adequate provisions must be made to protect the privacy of patients and the confidentiality of the data collected. The research plan must include provisions for monitoring of the data collected to ensure patient safety and to avoid prolonging an experiment beyond what is necessary to assess safety and effectiveness. All institutions that conduct federally sponsored research or research that is under federal regulation must have a body that reviews all proposed research to be conducted in their facility. These bodies are typically called Human Subjects Committees (HSC) or Institutional Review Boards (IRB). IRBs must comply with federal regulations or guidance documents as well as the local guidelines and ethical standards. An institution that fails to comply with these federal mandates may be sanctioned and have all federal funds for research terminated or put on hold until compliance is established. In addition, all federally regulated trials, including those sponsored by pharmaceutical companies and medical device companies, must comply with these IRB regulations. Thus these regulations, including those relevant to statistical design, data management, data monitoring, and data analysis, must be adhered to.

One of the key aspects of research studies in humans is the requirement for informed consent. Trial participants must be fully informed about the nature of the research, the goals, the potential benefits, and possible risks. The basic elements of the informed consent are given in Table 1.3. Participants must know that there may be alternatives to the treatment options in the study, and that their participation is entirely voluntary. Furthermore, even if they decide to start the trial, they may stop participation at any time. These issues have implications for the design, monitoring, and analysis of clinical trials discussed throughout this book.

Ethical concerns do not end with the local IRB. Journals that publish results of clinical trials are also establishing ethical standards. For example, the New England Journal of Medicine (Angell 1997) stated that they "will not publish unethical research regardless of scientific merit ... [T]he approval of the IRB in and informed consent of the research subjects are necessary but not sufficient conditions." One area of dispute is the conduct of clinical trials in developing countries in which many citizens do not have access to mod-

---

[6] http://grants.nih.gov/grants/guide/notice-files/not98-084.html
[7] http://www.fda.gov/cber/guidelines.htm

Table 1.3 *Eight basic elements of informed consent (45 CFR 46.116).*

---

1. A statement that the study involves research, an explanation of the purpose(s) of the research, the expected duration of the subject's participation, and a description of the research procedures (e.g., interview, observation, survey research).

2. A description of any reasonably foreseeable risks or discomforts for the subjects. Risks should be explained to subjects in language they can understand and be related to everyday life.

3. A description of any benefits to the subject and/or to others that may reasonably be expected from the research.

4. A disclosure of appropriate alternative procedures or courses of treatment, if any, that might be advantageous to the subject.

5. A statement describing the extent, if any, to which the confidentiality of records identifying the subject will be maintained.

6. For research involving more than minimal risk, a statement whether compensation is available if injury occurs and, if it is, what it consists of and from whom further information may be obtained.

7. An explanation of whom to contact for answers to pertinent questions about the research and research subject's rights. The name and phone number of the responsible faculty member as well as contact information for an IRB must be included for these purposes. In addition, if the project involves student research, the name and phone number of the student's adviser/mentor must also be included.

8. A statement that research participation is voluntary and the subject may withdraw from participation at any time without penalty or loss of benefits to which the subject is otherwise entitled. If the subject is a patient or client receiving medical, psychological, counseling, or other treatment services, there should be a statement that withdrawal will not jeopardize or affect any treatment or services the subject is currently receiving or may receive in the future. If the subject is a prisoner, there should be a statement that participation or non-participation in the research will have no effect on the subject's current or future status in the prison. If a survey instrument or interview questions are used and some questions deal with sensitive issues (including but not limited to illegal behavior, mental status, sexuality, or sexual abuse, drug use, or alcohol use) the subjects should be told they may refuse to answer individual questions.

---

ern western medicine. The control therapies used in trials must be consistent with the best that particular country can afford or deliver, yet these therapies are likely to be inferior to the standard of care in the United States or Europe. If such trials cannot be performed, the medical treatments in these countries will not advance through direct and rigorous evaluation of alternative treatments, perhaps those that are more affordable or more practical. Love and Fost (2003) comment on a trial in Vietnam that compared a simple and affordable treatment for breast cancer to the local standard of care, even though the new treatment is viewed as far inferior to that provided to women in the United States. In fact, Love and Fost (1997) report that this simple therapy, that involves removing the patient's ovaries and providing tamoxifen, a drug affordable by these patients, was clinically superior to the local traditional standard of care. Thus, this trial provided a substantial advance for the women of Vietnam while answering fundamental scientific questions. The ethical issues are non-trivial, however, and must be given careful consideration. Regardless of the outcome of this debate, it is clear that the standard for statistical conduct in all trials must be the highest possible in order to meet ethical criteria, a responsibility borne largely by the trial biostatistician.

1.3 Types of Research Design and Types of Trials

Medical research makes progress using a variety of research designs and each contributes to the base of knowledge regardless of their limitations. The most common types of clinical research designs are summarized in Table 1.4. The simplest type, and which is often used, is the case report or anecdote—a physician or scientist makes an astute observation of a single event or a single patient and gains insight into the nature or the cause of a disease. An example might be the observation that the interaction of two drugs causes a life threatening toxicity. It is often difficult, however, to distinguish the effects of a treatment from those of the natural history of the disease or many other confounding factors. Nevertheless, this unplanned anecdotal observation remains a useful tool. A particularly important example is a case report that linked a weight reduction drug with the presence of heart valve problems (Mark et al. 1997).

Epidemiologists seek associations between possible causes or risk factors and disease. This process is necessary if new therapies are to be developed. To this end, observational studies are typically conducted using a larger number of individuals than in the small case report series. Identifying potential risk factors through observational studies can be challenging, however, and the scope of such studies is necessarily limited (Taubes 1995).

Observational studies can be grouped roughly into three categories (Table 1.4), referred to as *retrospective, cross-sectional*, and *prospective*. A *case-control* study is a retrospective study in which the researcher collects retrospective information on *cases*, individuals with a disease, and *controls*, individuals without the disease. For example, the association between lung cancer

Table 1.4 *Types of research.*

Case Report An astute clinician or scientist observes an event or situation indicating a potential problem that is unusual or never before noted.

Observational A class of studies that are characterized by data collection on a cohort of individuals with the intent of correlating potential risk factors with clinical outcomes.

  Retrospective This design observes individuals or cases who have an event or disease diagnosis and then collects data on prior medical history or exposure to environmental, behavior, and other factors. A control group without the event or disease is also identified. The goal is to identify specific exposures that are more frequent in cases than control individuals.

  Cross-Sectional A cohort of individuals is observed and data collected at a single point in time. The cohort will have a mixture of individuals with disease and without. The goal is to find associations between exposure and the presence of the disease.

  Prospective A cohort of individuals is identified and followed prospectively, or forward in time. Exposure variables measured at the beginning are correlated with incident or new events. The goal is to identify disease risk factors.

Clinical Trial An experiment in which a group of individuals is given an intervention and subsequent outcome measures are taken. Results of intervention are compared to individuals not given the intervention. Selection of control group is a key issue.

  Historical Historical controls are obtained by using data from previous individuals not given the experimental intervention.

  Concurrent Data from individuals who are not being given the intervention are collected during the same period of time as from the intervention group.

  Randomized The assignment of intervention or control to individuals is through a randomization process.

Table 1.5 *Research biases.*

Selection Bias Bias affecting the interventions that a patient may receive or which individuals are entered into the study.

Publication Bias Studies that have significant (e.g., $p < 0.05$) results are more likely to be published than those that are not. Thus, knowledge of literature results gives a biased view of the effect of an intervention.

Recall Bias Individuals in a retrospective study are asked to recall prior behavior and exposure. Their memory may be more acute after having been diagnosed with a disease than the control individuals who do not have the disease.

Ascertainment Bias Bias that comes from a process where one group of individuals (e.g., intervention group) is measured more frequently or carefully than the other group (e.g., control).

---

and smoking was established primarily through a number of large case-control studies (Shopland (ed) 1982). A large number of patients with lung cancer were interviewed and information was obtained on their medical history and behavior. The same information was obtained on individuals not having the diagnosis of lung cancer. Comparisons are typically made between the frequency of factors in medical history or lifestyle. In the case of lung cancer, it became apparent, and overwhelmingly convincing, that there was a substantially higher frequency of a history of smoking in those individuals who developed lung cancer compared to those individuals free of lung cancer. The case-control design has proven to be quite useful, especially for relatively rare diseases such as lung cancer. As with all observational studies, however, the case control design has limitations and is vulnerable to bias. For example, associations do not imply causation, but rather that the proposed risk factor and the disease occur together, either by chance or because of a third, possibly unknown, factor. The choice of a control group is also critical and bias can be introduced if it is not chosen properly. Control groups selected from the literature or from previous cohorts are subject to publication bias or selection bias. Furthermore, both case and control groups are vulnerable to recall bias (see Table 1.5).

The *cross-sectional* design compares individuals in a defined population at a particular moment in time, again looking for associations between potential risk factors and disease frequency. In this design, some of the biases present in the case control design can be minimized or eliminated. Publication bias and recall bias are eliminated. This design, however, can only evaluate those who are alive at the time of the evaluation and therefore a degree of bias is inherent. Again, associations that are identified are not necessarily causative factors, but rather factors that coexist with the disease under investigation. Examples of cross-sectional studies are the Wisconsin Epidemiologic Study of Diabetic Retinopathy (WESDR) (Klein et al. 1985) and the Beaver Dam Eye Study (Klein et al. 1991). These studies initially were established as cross sectional studies to identify possible risk factors for eye diseases. WESDR, for example, identified serum levels of glycosylated hemoglobin as a risk factor for the incidence and progression of diabetic retinopathy.

A third observational design is the *prospective cohort* study in which a cohort of individuals is identified and followed forward in time, observing either the incidence of various diseases of interest or survival. At the beginning, extensive information is collected on individuals including, for example, medical history, blood and urine chemistry, physiologic measurements, and perhaps genetic material. Associations are sought between all of these baseline data and the occurrence of the disease. One of the earliest and best known prospective studies was the Framingham Heart Study (FHS) (Dawber et al. 1951). Several hundred individuals in the town of Framingham, Massachusetts were identified in 1950 and followed for the next three decades. Initially, a large amount of information based on medical history and physical examination was collected. The FHS was primarily interested in heart disease and from this study, researchers identified high cholesterol and other elevated lipids, high blood pressure, smoking, and diabetes as possible risk factors for heart disease. Again, these associations did not establish causation. Clinical trials conducted later, and described later, examined the impact of modification of these possible risk factors and the reduction of disease incidence. Nonetheless, the FHS was essential in the identification of these risk factors and played a landmark role.

Because of the potential for bias, observational studies have led to many false positive associations (Taubes 1995) that could not be replicated. Examples include the association of high cholesterol and rectal cancer, smoking and breast cancer, vasectomy and prostate cancer, red meat and either breast or colon cancer, and excessive water consumption and bladder cancer. Despite these false positive associations, the observational design is an important component of the research cycle. While replication of results are an essential to ensure credibility of the results, this may not be sufficient. For example, observational studies have suggested that low serum beta-carotene is associated with an increase in lung cancer. A synthetic beta-carotene tablet was developed and three trials were conducted to test whether increasing the level of serum beta-carotene through dietary supplementation resulted in a lower incidence of either lung cancer, or cancer in general. The Alpha-Tocopheral Beta-Carotene trial (ATBC)[8] was a trial in a cohort of Finnish male heavy smokers. Contrary to the observational studies, the incidence of lung cancer increased in those given beta-carotene supplements despite the documented increase in serum beta-carotene. This result was repeated in a U.S. based trial

---

[8] The Alpha-Tocopherol, Beta-Carotene Cancer Prevention Study Group (1994)

in smokers and asbestos workers, referred to as CARET (Omenn et al. 1994). A third trial, the Physicians Health Study (PHS) (Hennekens et al. 1996), evaluated beta-carotene supplementation in a cohort of U.S. male physicians. Again, while serum beta-carotene was increased, the incidence of lung cancer and all cancers did not change. Remarkably, the observation of an association between the baseline level of beta-carotene and the incidence of lung cancer was found in all three trials, confirming the previous observational studies. Still, increasing the level with a beta-carotene supplement did not reduce the incidence of lung cancer. Replication did not guarantee that the association is causal.

Thus, whether case-control studies, cross-sectional studies, or prospective studies are used, the role of the observational studies is critical in identifying factors to be further studied as possible risk factors for disease progression or occurrence. The next step is to attempt to modify the proposed risk factor and determine if the incidence can be lowered. Laboratory research and small clinical studies are conducted to identify safe and effective drugs, biologics, or devices that can modify the risk factor. This process can take months or years. For cholesterol and blood pressure, drugs were eventually developed that modified blood pressure and cholesterol levels. Later, trials using these drugs established that changes in these risk factors resulted in a reduction in heart disease progression and death. For example, the Hypertension Detection Follow-up Program (HDFP) (HDFP Cooperative Group 1982) demonstrated the positive benefits of lowering blood pressure in patients with mild to moderate hypertension. The Scandinavian Study of Simvistatin (Scandanavian Simvistatin Survival Study 1994) established that treatments that lower cholesterol may also lower the risk of death and heart attacks. This text is focused on the statistical issues in the design, conduct, and analysis of such trials. These trials are essential in the completion of the research process.

In fact, the research process is a dynamic interaction between observation, laboratory results, and clinical trials illustrated by Figure 1.1. All three elements are essential and may be conducted simultaneously as researchers probe all aspects of a medical problem.

Clinical trials are categorized into 4 phases, summarized in Table 1.6. These clinical trial phases will be described in more detail in Chapter 3. Briefly, although the precise goals and designs may vary between disease areas, the goal in phase I is usually to determine the maximum dose that can be tolerated without excessive adverse effects. Typically, phase I trials are conducted either in healthy volunteers or in patients who have failed all regular treatments. phase II trials are usually conducted to evaluate the biological activity of the new drug to determine if it evokes the response that was expected and warrants further development. Phase III trials are comparative trials that evaluate the effectiveness of the new treatment relative to the current standard of care. These trials may add the new treatment to the standard of care and compare that to the standard of care alone. Some trials compare two known active agents to determine which is superior, or in some cases, to determine if the

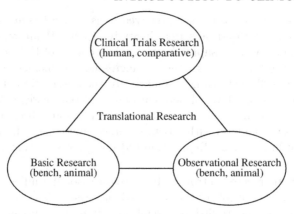

Figure 1.1 *The research triangle.*

Table 1.6 *Clinical trial phases.*

Preclinical Once a risk factor is identified, laboratory research is conducted
to identify a means to modify the risk factor, testing it in the laboratory
and often in animal models.

Phase I With a new intervention available from laboratory research, the first
step is to determine if the intervention can be given to humans, by what
method, and in what dose.

Phase II Trials in the second phase typically measure how active the new
intervention is, and learn more about side effects.

Phase III Trials in the third phase compare whether the new intervention is
more effective than a standard control intervention.

---

two have similar effectiveness. Phase IV trials usually follow patients who
have completed phase III trials to determine if there are long term adverse
consequences.

Phase III trials are also classified according to the process by which a control
arm is selected. *Randomized control trials* assign patients to either the new
treatment or the standard by a randomization method, described in Chapter 5.
Non-randomized phase III trials can be of two general types. The *historical
control* trial compares a group of patients treated with the new drug or device
to a group of patients previously treated with the current standard of care. A
concurrent control trial, by contrast, compares patients treated with the new
treatment to another group of patients treated in the standard manner at the
same time, for example, those treated at another medical facility or clinic. As
will be discussed in Chapter 5, the randomized control trial is considered to be

the gold standard, minimizing or controlling for many of the biases to which other designs are subject. Trials may be single center or multiple center, and many phase III trials are now multinational.

Trials may also be classified by the nature of the disease process the experimental intervention is addressing. Screening trials are used to assess whether screening individuals to identify those at high risk for a disease is beneficial, taking into account the expense and efforts of the screening process. For example, a large cancer screening trial is evaluating the benefits of screening for prostate, lung, colon, and ovarian cancer (Prorok et al. 2000). These trials must, by nature, be long term to ascertain disease incidence in the screened and unscreened populations. Screening trials are conducted under the belief that there is a beneficial intervention available to at-risk individuals once they are identified. Primary prevention trials assess whether an intervention strategy in a relatively healthy but at risk population can reduce the incidence to the disease. Secondary prevention trials are designed to determine whether a new intervention reduces the recurrence of the disease in a cohort that has already been diagnosed with the disease or has experienced an event (e.g., heart attack). Therapeutic or acute trials are designed to evaluate an intervention in a patient population where the disease is acute or life threatening. An example would be a trial that uses a new drug or device that may improve the function of a heart that has serious irregular rhythms.

1.4 The Need for Clinical Trials

Since the introduction of the modern clinical trial in 1950, a great deal of medical research has been conducted into the causes and possible treatments of numerous diseases. Diagnostic methods have improved so that disease or disease progression can be detected earlier and more accurately. During this time, the number of approaches to the treatment or prevention of disease has increased dramatically and these must be evaluated to establish their effectiveness and proper role. Since the clinical course of many diseases is complicated, determining if a new therapy is effective or superior to existing treatments is not an easy task. It often requires a systematic evaluation using large numbers of patients and astute clinical observation.

The clinical trial has become a standard tool because it is the most definitive and efficient method for determining if a new treatment is more effective than the current standard or has any effectiveness at all. Observational studies have potential for bias and one cannot conclusively determine from an uncontrolled study whether differences in outcomes (or lack of differences) can be directly attributed to the new intervention. As discussed previously, many potential risk factors have been identified through uncontrolled studies and later shown to be spurious (Taubes 1995).

Controlled clinical trials are also an effective mechanism to distinguish incidence of side effects and adverse effects due to the therapy from those caused by the disease process itself. For example, in the Coronary Drug Project, cardiac arrhythmias were observed in 33% of the patients on either Niacin or Clofibrate, two of the drugs being tested.[9] On the other hand, 38% of the patients on the placebo arm had cardiac arrhythmias as well. Without the control arm, one might have associated the adverse effect with the drugs instead of recognizing that it is a consequence of the underlying disease. As another example, 7.5% of the patients on clofibrate experienced nausea, but 6.2% of the placebo patients did as well. Again, the nausea is not attributable to the drug, but this might not have been realized without the control comparison.

One of the most compelling reasons for the use of clinical trials is that if they are not conducted, new, but ineffective or even harmful, treatments or interventions can become part of medical practice. Many ineffective or harmful interventions have been in use for a long time before their effects were understood. One of the classic examples is the use of high dose oxygen in infants born prematurely.

Children born prematurely typically have lungs that are not fully developed and thus have difficulty breathing. As described by Silverman (1979), the practice of giving premature infants high doses of oxygen began in the 1940s and eventually became established as the standard of care. During the same time period, an epidemic of retrolental fibroplasia, which often leads to blindness in premature infants, began. A careful review of case records indicated that these affected premature infants received the "state of the art" medical care, including high dose oxygen. In the early 1950s, some researchers began to suspect the high dose oxygen but the evidence was not convincing. Furthermore, a careful study of the use of oxygen was ethically challenging since this was the accepted standard of care. One trial attempted to examine this question by randomizing premature infants to receive either high (standard) or low dose oxygen. Because of the belief that high dose was the ethical treatment, nurses turned up the oxygen levels at night in those infants randomized to the low dose oxygen group. Later, in 1953, another randomized clinical trial was launched in 800 premature infants. Results indicated that 23% of the infants receiving the high dose oxygen were blinded compared to 7% in those receiving a low dose (50% of standard) oxygen when needed. This trial confirmed earlier suspicions and, when the results were published in 1954, the practice diminished. It was estimated that perhaps 10,000 infants had been blinded by the practice of high dose oxygen administration. A widely used but untested intervention was ultimately shown to be harmful.

The high dose oxygen story is not the only case of untested interventions being ineffective or harmful but in widespread use. Many common, accepted treatments have never been formally tested. The FDA regulatory laws were not in effect prior to 1968 so that drugs developed prior to that time were "grandfathered." Medical devices are regulated by the FDA as well but as a result of different legislation having different requirements. Many devices may have been tested to assess functionality but not necessarily clinical effective-

---

[9] The Coronary Drug Project Research Group (1975)

ness. Surgical and other procedures do not fall under FDA regulation and thus many have not been rigorously tested. The same is true of many behavioral modifications or nutritional supplements.

The Intermittent Positive Pressure Breathing (IPPB) trial[10] is an example in which a device used for patients with advanced pulmonary obstructive disease became an established, expensive practice but was later shown to have no clinical benefit. The IPPB delivered bronchodilator drugs deep into the lung under pressure based on the hypothesis that distributing the drug throughout the entire lung would be beneficial. The treatment using IPPB requires an expensive device and technical staff trained in the use of this device. When IPPB was compared to a inexpensive hand held nebulizer that also delivered the drug, the clinical effect was the same, as measured by standard pulmonary function tests. Over time, the use of this expensive but ineffective therapy has diminished.

The treatment of cardiac arrhythmias provides another convincing example. Cardiac arrhythmias are associated with a higher incidence of sudden death and drugs developed to suppress arrhythmias were approved by the FDA for use in high risk patients. Cardiologists, however, began using these drugs more broadly in lower risk patients. The Cardiac Arrhythmia Suppression Trial (CAST)[11] was designed to test whether the use of these new drugs would in fact reduce the risk of sudden death and total mortality. CAST was a well designed, randomized placebo controlled trial. Shortly after the trial began, when approximately 15% of the mortality information had accrued, the trial was terminated with a statistically significant increase in both sudden death and total mortality among subjects receiving anti-arrhythmic agents. A class of drugs that was rapidly becoming part of medical practice was discovered to be harmful to patients with cardiac arrhythmias.

Finally, the use of an effective intervention can be delayed because trials were not conducted in a timely fashion. Chronic heart failure (CHF) is a disease of a failing heart that is not able to pump efficiently, and the risk of mortality increases with the progression of the disease. The efficiency of the heart is measured by the ejection fraction—how much of the heart chamber is emptied with contraction relative to when it has been filled. A class of drugs known as beta-blockers were known to be effective in lowering blood pressure in individuals with high blood pressure and in slowing or controlling the heart rhythm following a heart attack. Since CHF patients already are having trouble with an inefficient heart, treating them with a drug that would slow down the heart rhythm and lower blood pressure seemed like the wrong approach. For several years, using beta-blockers in CHF patients was discouraged or proscribed even though there was research suggesting that beta-blockers may in fact be beneficial to CHF patients. Three trials were conducted in CHF

---

[10] The Intermittent Positive Pressure Breathing Trial Group (1983)
[11] The Cardiac Arrhythmia Suppression Trial (CAST) Investigators (1989)

patients, using different beta-blocking drugs, and all three demonstrated significant and substantial reduction in mortality, contrary to common belief.[12]

While we cannot afford to study every new medical intervention with a carefully controlled clinical trial, we must study those for which the outcome is serious and with the potential for serious adverse effects. Regulatory agencies world-wide require that most new drugs and biologics must be rigorously tested. Devices are increasingly being tested in a similar manner. It not clear, however, when the new use of an existing drug or device must receive the same rigorous evaluation. Regulatory requirements address many but not all of these circumstances. No requirements exist for procedures and behavioral modifications. Thus, society and the medical profession together must make judgments, realizing that a degree of risk is assumed when an intervention is not tested by a clinical trial. In some cases, that risk may be justified, but those circumstances should be rare.

1.5 The Randomization Principle

As discussed in Chapters 2, 3, and 5, the process of randomization has three primary benefits. The first is that randomization guarantees that assigned treatment is stochastically independent of outcome. In non-controlled studies, confounding occurs when *exposure* to the agent of interest is associated with or the result of the disease in question, often resulting in spurious conclusions regarding causality. Randomization ensures that this cannot happen—any observed association is either causal or the result of chance, and the latter can be well controlled. Second, randomization tends to produce comparable groups with regard to measured and unmeasured risk factors, thus making the comparison between the experimental and standard or control groups more credible (Byar et al. 1976). Finally, randomization justifies the analysis typically conducted without depending on external distribution assumptions. That is, common tests such as t-tests and chi-square tests are approximations to the randomization test associated with the randomization procedure. This principle has been discussed generally by Kempthorne (1977), for example, and specifically for clinical trials by Lachin (1988b). This principle will be discussed in more detail in Chapter 5.

1.6 Timing of a Clinical Trial

Often there is a relative narrow window of time during which a trial can be conducted. As previously indicated, if an intervention becomes part of the established standard of care without rigorous safety and efficacy assessments, it can become ethically challenging to rigorously test its safety and effectiveness. Thus, it is important to evaluate a new intervention before it becomes part of clinical practice. We have already discussed several examples where

---

[12] The International Steering Committee on Behalf of the MERIT-HF Study Group (1997), Krum et al. (2006), Packer et al. (2001)

interventions become part of practice before a trial has been conducted. These examples include the use of high dose oxygen in premature infants (Silverman 1979), intermittent positive pressure breathing device in chronic obstructive pulmonary patients[13] and a class of arrhythmia drugs in patients with cardiac arrhythmias.[14] Other examples include the use of hormone replacement therapy (HRT) for reducing the risk of heart disease in post menopausal women,[15] and the use of coronary artery bypass graft (CABG) surgery to treat patients who were experiencing symptoms such as angina (heart pain) due to the occlusion (narrowing) of coronary vessels from atherosclerosis (Healy et al. 1989).

CABG is a surgical procedure that takes healthy vessels from other parts of the body and grafts them onto the heart to bypass the occluded segments of the coronary vessels. CABG became a rapidly accepted surgery procedure before being evaluated in randomized clinical trials. When the Coronary Artery Surgery Study (CASS) was conducted, there was a reluctance on the part of many cardiac surgeons to randomize their patients to either medical therapy or CABG. As a result, a registry of patients who were to undergo CABG was a part of CASS (CASS Principal Investigators and their Associates 1983). Many more patients were entered into the registry than were entered into the randomized trial. The randomized portion of CASS demonstrated that CABG did not reduce mortality relative to medical therapy in the less advanced cases—those with fewer occluded coronary vessels—in spite of its increasingly widespread use.

Conversely, large phase III confirmatory trials should be designed and conducted only after sufficient background information regarding the population and the new intervention is available. Information about the level of risk or disease incidence in the population of interest is required before the entry criteria and sample size can be determined. Researchers also must have knowledge about the safety of the intervention, the dosing schedule, and the stability of the treatment formulation. In the trial design, the clinical outcomes of interest must be determined as well as the expected size of the effect of the intervention. Financial resources and patient availability must also be determined.

Launching a trial prematurely, before adequate knowledge is available for proper design, may lead to operational problems. For example, researchers may find the entry criteria too strict and the number of patients eligible is much less than required, making recruitment goals unattainable, or, the risk level of the trial population may be less than expected resulting in recruitment goals that are too small. If insufficient information is available, the trial may have to be suspended until the design can be corrected, or if that is not possible, the trial may have to be terminated wasting time and resources before the trial can begin again or another trial designed.

---

[13] The Intermittent Positive Pressure Breathing Trial Group (1983)
[14] The Cardiac Arrhythmia Suppression Trial (CAST) Investigators (1989)
[15] Writing Group for the Women's Health Initiative Randomized Controlled Trial (2002)

1.7 Trial Organization

In the mid 1960s, when the National Heart Institute was planning a series of risk factor intervention trials, beginning with the CDP, they planned for the organizational structure of such trials. A task force was commissioned, chaired by Dr Bernie Greenberg, that issued a 1967 report that became known as the Greenberg Report. This report was formally published in 1988, long after its impact on the early NIH trials (Heart Special Project Committee 1998). As

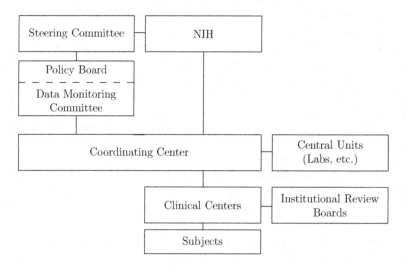

Figure 1.2 *NIH model. Reprinted with permission from Fisher, Roecker, and DeMets (2001). Copyright © 2001, Drug Information Association.*

shown in Figure 1.2, there are several key functional components. All trials must have a *sponsor* or *funding agency* to pay for the costs of the intervention, data collection, and analysis. Funding agencies often delegate the management of the trial to a *steering committee* or *executive committee*, a small group composed of individuals from the sponsor and the scientific investigators. The steering committee is responsible for providing scientific direction and to monitor the conduct of the trial. The steering committee may appoint working committees to focus on particular tasks such as recruitment, intervention details, compliance to intervention, outcome assessment, as well as analysis and publication plans. Steering committees usually have a chair who serves as the spokesperson for the trial. A network of investigators and clinics is typically needed to recruit patients, apply the intervention and other required patient care, and to assess patient outcomes. Clinical sites usually will have a small staff who dedicate a portion of their time to recruit patients, deliver the intervention, assess patient responses, and complete data collection forms. For some trials, one or more central laboratories are needed to measure blood chemistries in a uniform manner or to evaluate electrocardiograms, x-rays, eye photographs, or tumor specimens. Figure 1.3 depicts a modification of the NIH clinical trial model that is often used for industry sponsored trials (Fisher et al. 2001). The major difference is that the data coordinating center operation depicted in Figure 1.2 has been divided into a data management center and a statistical analysis center. The data management center may be internal to the sponsor or contracted to an outside organization. The statistical analysis center may also be internal or contracted to an external group, often an academic-based biostatistics group. As described in Chapter 10, careful mon-

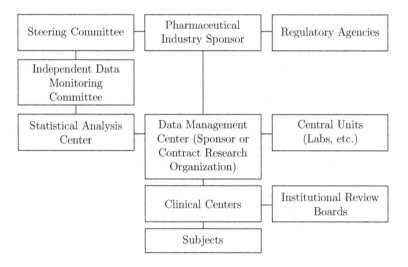

Figure 1.3 *Industry-modified NIH model. Reprinted with permission from Fisher, Roecker, and DeMets (2001). Copyright © 2001, Drug Information Association.*

itoring of trials is ethically and scientifically mandated. This responsibility is largely the task of the Data Monitoring Committee (DMC), also referred to as the Data and Safety Monitoring Board (DSMB). The DMC is made up of experts in the clinical condition of the patient or participant, the intervention being studied, epidemiology of the disease, statistics, and clinical trials. Their role is to monitor the accumulating data and to terminate a trial early if there is convincing evidence of harm, if the intervention has shown overwhelming benefit earlier than expected, or has no chance of being successfully completed. In some circumstances, the DMC may recommend modifications to the trial.

A statistical and data management center is also necessary and is where much of the day to day trial activity takes place. In the original NHLBI model, these two functions are performed in one center, referred to as a trial coordinating center, although these functions can be separated into two centers, a statistical analysis center and a data management center. These centers design and implement the data collection process, including processes for data entry, data editing, and data quality control. The statistical analysis of safety and efficacy data are provided to the DMC periodically. Reports on trial progress are also submitted regularly to the Steering Committee.

The process set forth by the Greenberg Report and implemented by the NHLBI focused on the multicenter clinical trial. The process has been widely adopted by most federally sponsored trials and trials that come under regulatory review. On a smaller scale, this model can also be useful for single center trials, since the same functions must be performed.

1.8 Protocol and Manual of Operations

In order for a trial to be successful, a careful design and plan must be developed. The details of this plan are described in two documents. First, the overall rationale and features of the trial are described in a trial *protocol*. An outline of a typical protocol is shown in Table 1.7. The protocol must describe the study rationale, and include a statement of the hypothesis being tested, the measurements to be made, the fundamental experimental design, the size of the trial, the intervention delivered, patient eligibility, and the general analysis plan.

The *Manual of Operations* is a much more detailed document. While the protocol is similar to a general blueprint for a house, the Manual of Operations is similar to a construction document. Details are provided, for example, of how to deliver the intervention, how to make the specified measurements, how to complete the data collection forms, and standard definitions of terms and procedures.

1.9 Regulatory Issues

Statisticians as well as other clinical trial investigators must understand and follow clinical trial regulations; failure to comply can lead to serious consequences for themselves, their employer, and the research sponsor (i.e., the agency, institution, or organization, if any, that sponsored the research; the research sponsor can be governmental, private, or non-profit in nature). Many clinical trial regulations are mandated by the federal government and others are imposed by the local medical research institution or research sponsor.

1.9.1 Institutional Review Board

The section of the U.S. Code of Federal Regulations (CFR) known as 45 CFR 46 specifies the Institutional Review Board (IRB) as one mechanism through which human subjects are protected. The IRB is a body of experts appointed by the local institution, university, or medical facility that conducts research on humans. Before a study can be initiated, the IRB must review and approve a protocol for human research including the process of informed consent. The IRB must approve all proposed protocol modifications and conduct an annual review of the trial progress. The IRB is responsible for monitoring the

Table 1.7 *Protocol outline.*

---

1. Background of the study
2. Objectives
   (a) Primary question and response variable
   (b) Secondary question and response variable
   (c) Subgroups hypotheses
   (d) Adverse effects
3. Design of the study
   (a) Study population
       i. Inclusion criteria
       ii. Exclusion criteria
   (b) Sample size assumptions and estimates
   (c) Enrollment of participants
       i. Informed consent
       ii. Assessment of eligibility
       iii. Baseline examination
       iv. Intervention allocation (e.g., randomization method)
   (d) Intervention
       i. Description and schedule
       ii. Measures of compliance
   (e) Follow-up visit and description and schedule
   (f) Ascertainment of response variables
       i. Training
       ii. Data collection
       iii. Quality control
   (g) Data analysis
       i. Interim monitoring
       ii. Final analysis
   (h) Termination policy
4. Organization
   (a) Participating investigators
   (b) Statistical unit or data coordinating center
       i. Laboratories and other special units
       ii. Clinical center(s)
   (c) Study administration
       i. Steering committees and subcommittees
       ii. Data monitoring committee
       iii. Funding organization
   Appendix
   Definitions of eligibility criteria
   Definitions of response variables

---

safety of trial participants, either directly or by delegating this to a properly constituted Data Monitoring Committee (DMC), as described in Chapter 10. Failure to comply with these IRB requirements can result in the suspension or permanent termination of all research at an institution if the violations are serious and not subject to remediation.

1.9.2 Informed Consent Process Guidelines

The Informed Consent document is, in essence, a contract between the investigators and a subject with the provision that the subject can withdraw at any time. Once IRB approval of the protocol has been obtained, the research question cannot be modified without revision and approval of the Informed Consent document that should allow subjects to be aware of these changes and, ideally, then consent again to continue in the clinical trial. As a minimum requirement before analyzing the data collected, the statistician should read the Informed Consent document and any subsequent revisions. Mandatory contents of the Informed Consent document are summarized in Table 1.3.

1.9.3 Food and Drug Administration & Other Regulatory Agencies

Many trials are conducted to obtain evidence of drug or device effectiveness and as assessment of potential risks. In order to market a drug or a device in the United States and in most parts of the world, governmental regulatory agencies must review the data to assess whether the benefits outweigh the risks. In the United States, that federal agency is the Food and Drug Administration (FDA). The FDA was created in 1906 to address food safety but had its responsibilities expanded in the subsequent decades. In 1962, the Kefauver-Harris Amendments to the Food and Drug Act introduced major changes in the process for approval of drugs in the U.S. The amendment requires evidence of adequate and well-controlled studies, including clinical investigations, by qualified experts with scientific training and experience to evaluate the effectiveness of a drug prior to FDA approval. One effect of the amendment is to generally require at least two trials demonstrating benefit. In 1970, further legislation recommended that appropriate statistical methods be used in the evaluation process. These two legislative actions are particularly important in promoting good statistical science in the design, conduct, and analysis of clinical trials.

The FDA is now a large complex organization with many responsibilities and several functional centers but the three centers of special interest for clinical trials are the Center for Drug Evaluation and Research (CDER), the Center for Biologics Evaluation and Research (CBER), and the Center for Device and Radiation Health (CDRH). In the European Union (EU), the European Medicines Agency (EMEA) provides similar review through the Committee for Medical Products for Human Use (CHMP).

The regulatory agencies of Europe, Japan, and the United States have collaborated to bring a degree of consistency to drug and device guidelines. The project is called the International Conference on Harmonization (ICH). The purpose of the ICH is to make the recommendations regarding standards for achieving greater harmonization in the interpretation and requirements for product registration and approval. The guidelines can be found on the internet.[16] The topics covered by ICH are summarized in Table 1.8. Among

Table 1.8 *ICH7 efficacy guidance documents.*

E1A The Extent of Population Exposure to Assess Clinical Safety For Drugs Intended for Long-Term Treatment of Non-Life-Threatening Conditions

E2A Clinical Safety Data Management: Definitions and Standards for Expedited Reporting (continues through E2E)

E3 Structure and Content of Clinical Study Reports

E4 Dose-Response Information to Support Drug Registration

E5 Ethnic Factors in the Acceptability of Foreign Clinical Data

E6 Good Clinical Practice: Consolidated Guidance

E7 Studies in Support of Special Populations: Geriatrics

E8 General Considerations for Clinical Trials

E9 Statistical Principles for Clinical Trials

E10 Choice of Control Group and Related Issues in Clinical Trials

E11 Clinical Investigations of Medicinal Products in the Pediatric Population

E14 Clinical Evaluation of QT/QTc Interval Prolongation and Proarrhythmic Potential for Non-Antiarrhythmic Drugs

---

these guidelines is ICH-E9 covering statistical principles for clinical trials. The guidelines in this document must be considered by statisticians working for either the pharmaceutical, biologic, or medical device industry, as well as those in academia. The documents may change over time and so they should be consulted with some regularity. There are other statistical guidelines provided by the FDA which can also be found on the FDA web site and should be consulted. The statistical principles presented in this text are largely consistent with those in the ICH documents.

We point out one area of particular interest. As described in Chapter 10, all trials under the jurisdiction of the FDA must have a monitoring plan. For some trials involving subjects with a serious disease or a new innovative intervention, an external data monitoring committee may be either required or highly recommended. An FDA document entitled *Guidance for Clinical Trial*

---

[16] http://www.fda.gov/cber/ich/ichguid.htm

Sponsors on the Establishment and Operation of Clinical Trial Data Monitoring Committees[17] contends that the integrity of the trial is best protected when the statisticians preparing unblinded data for the DMC are external to the sponsor and uninvolved in discussions regarding potential changes in trial design while the trial is ongoing. This is an especially important consideration for critical studies intended to provide definitive evidence of effectiveness. There are many other guidelines regarding the design, conduct, and analysis of clinical trials.[18]

1.10 Overview of the Book

In the chapters that follow, many statistical issues pertinent to the development of the protocol will be examined in great detail including basic experimental design, sample size, randomization procedures, interim analyses, survival, and longitudinal methods for clinical trials along with other analysis issues. While critical to the conduct and analysis of the trial, these components depend on having a carefully defined question that the trial is intended to answer, a carefully selected study population and outcome variables that appropriately measure the effects of interest. Failure to adequately address these issues can seriously jeopardize the ultimate success of the trial. Thus, Chapter 2 provides guidelines for formulating the primary and secondary questions and translating the clinical questions into statistical ones. In Chapter 3, we examine designs used in clinical trials, especially for comparative trials.

While the size of early phase studies is important, the success of phase III or comparative trials relies critically on their sample size. These trials are intended to enable definitive conclusions to be drawn about the benefits and risks of an intervention. Claiming a benefit when none exists, a *false positive*, would not be desirable since an ineffective therapy might become widely used. Thus, the false positive claims must be kept to a minimum. Equally important is that a trial be sensitive enough to find clinically relevant treatment effects if they exist. This kind of sensitivity is referred to as the *power* of the trial. Failure to find a true effect is referred to as a *false negative*. Statisticians refer to the false positive as the *type I* error and the false negative as the *type II* error. Chapter 4 will present methods for determining the sample size for a trial to meet prespecified criteria for both false positive and false negative rates.

Given that the randomized control clinical trial is the gold standard, the process of randomization must be done properly. For example, a randomization process that mimics the simple tossing of a fair coin is certainly a valid process but may have undesirable properties. Thus, constrained randomization procedures are commonly used in order to ensure balance. Some of these methods produce balance on the number of participants in each arm through-

---

[17] www.fda.gov/cber/gdlns/clintrialdmc.htm, issued March 2006, accessed June 9, 2006
[18] www.FDA.gov

out the course of enrollment, while others also produce balance relative to prespecified risk factors. These methods will be introduced in Chapter 5.

As we describe in Chapter 6, a variety of types of data must be collected in order to answer key questions in the trial. Baseline data help to establish the type of participant enrolled in the trial and determine whether the treatment arms are balanced. Data must be collected regarding key outcome variables and adverse events as well as information on how well participants comply with their assigned intervention. It is common for more data to be collected than the protocol requires, thus increasing effort and the cost of the trial. Moreover, data that is collected needs quality control. In order to conserve effort and cost, the data must be prioritized for quality control. Some common methods for evaluating data quality are also presented.

Chapters 7, 8, and 9 provide an introduction to common analysis methods used in clinical trials. Chapter 7 introduces methods for *survival analysis* (or failure time analysis), a term used generally to mean analysis of data involving the timing of a particular kind of event (failure). Methods described in the chapter include the estimation of event time distributions, also referred to as *survival curves*, of which the Kaplan-Meier estimate is the most commonly used, methods comparing two such survival curves, including the commonly used log-rank test, and the Cox proportional hazards model which allows for baseline factors to be adjusted for in a regression like manner. Chapter 8 presents basic methods for the analysis of repeated measures data, the simplest of which might be to fit a straight line to each group and compare the slopes to assess the intervention effect. Chapter 9 introduces concepts and methods commonly used with quality of life measures.

In typical clinical trials, trial participants are enrolled over a period of time. Likewise, data accumulate over time and participants pass through various stages of the trial. An ethical obligation to the participant is that a trial not continue longer than necessary to determine benefits and risks of an intervention compared to a standard or control. In fact, all trials must have a monitoring plan. Some trials involving high risk patients or a novel therapy may need an independent group of experts, called a data monitoring committee, to review the accumulating data and make a judgment. Repeatedly analyzing a single variable or several variables raises statistical issues, including an increased type I error rate. Chapter 10 describes statistical methods, along with examples, that provide guidance for determining when an emerging trend represents a true effect of treatment or simply data variability.

While the trial design and conduct may be successful in producing a trial with minimal bias and maximum sensitivity, there are principles in the analysis of data that must be recognized or serious bias can inadvertently be introduced. Several such issues in the analysis of the data are presented in Chapter 11. These include the concept of accounting for all patients randomized or enrolled, described later as the "intent-to-treat" principle. Also, the danger of dividing or subgrouping the data too finely is discussed.

Finally, the results of a trial must be reported accurately and clearly. Chapter 12 presents recommendations for reporting trial results, consistent with universal guidelines recommended by medical journals. Essential information includes baseline data, primary, and secondary outcome data, compliance data, adverse events and toxicity, plus selected predefined subsets. Accurate reporting of trials is important since the results may be used by other researchers and health care providers to assess how these results should be interpreted and utilized in their practices or used in the design of future trials.

CHAPTER 2

Defining the Question

A clinical trial is the culmination of what is typically many years of preliminary research spent developing compounds, devices, or other interventions intended to provide health benefits to humans. Generally an intervention is developed that targets a specific disease process such as atherosclerosis in heart disease or retinopathy in individuals suffering from diabetes, although occasionally a compound developed for a particular disease finds utility in another seemingly unrelated disease area. The ultimate goal of a clinical trial is to establish the safety and effectiveness of the intervention in the target population. Evidence of safety is generally obtained considering a broad range of standard assessments including laboratory tests and reports of adverse events. Evidence of efficacy, on the other hand, is often more difficult to define. Therapeutic efficacy ultimately must have a direct observable effect on the health status of the individual, either by prolonging life, curing a nonfatal disease, or reducing the effect of disease symptoms on quality of life.

For life threatening diseases, improved survival is the frequent target of the intervention. For less severe disease, the target is likely to be symptomatic improvement. For example, treatments for arthritis are expected to reduce joint pain and improve mobility; treatments for asthma would be expected to reduce the incidence of asthmatic episodes or reduce their severity and improve respiratory function. Some diseases, such as hypertension (high blood pressure) or hyperlipidemia (high cholesterol), are asymptomatic in that the disease can only be detected by clinical tests. These diseases render the individual at increased risk of certain adverse events such as heart attacks and strokes, which can be both debilitating and ultimately life-threatening. Often, however, particular laboratory measures that are predictive of adverse outcomes are simply associated with or consequences of the disease process and interventions that directly target them have no effect on the underlying disease process. For example, increased glycosylated hemoglobin (Hb_{A1C}) is an indicator of sustained elevations of serum glucose among diabetics, but an intervention that directly targets Hb_{A1C} without altering the underlying glucose levels themselves will have little or no long term benefit. For many diseases, progression is assessed using non-invasive scans such as CT, PET, or MRI. Trained readers can often make qualitative judgments regarding the nature of the disease but it may be difficult to quantify these assessments in a way that is useful for statistical analysis.

Consequently, great care must to taken in formulating the primary efficacy question of a trial; ensuring that the outcomes are clinically relevant, measurable, and that a valid statistical comparison can be performed. Clinical relevance requires that the appropriate population be targeted and that effects of the intervention on the primary outcome reflect true benefit to the subjects. Measurability requires that we can ascertain the outcome in a clinically relevant and unbiased manner. Finally, we must ensure that the statistical procedures that are employed make comparisons that answer the clinical question in an unbiased way without requiring untestable assumptions.

We begin this chapter with a discussion of the statistical framework in which trials are conducted. First, randomized clinical trials are fundamentally hypothesis testing instruments and while estimation of treatment effects is an important component of the analysis, most of the statistical design elements of a clinical trial—randomization, sample size, interim monitoring strategies, etc.—are formulated with hypothesis tests in mind and the primary questions in a trial are framed as tests of specific hypotheses. Second, since the goal of a trial is to establish a causal link between the interventions employed and the outcome, inference must be based on well established principles of causal inference. This discussion provides a foundation for understanding the kinds of causal questions that RCTs are able to directly answer.

Next, while a trial should be designed to have a single primary question, invariably there are secondary questions of interest. Specifically, beyond the primary outcome, there are likely to be a number of secondary questions of interest ranging from the effect on clinical outcomes such as symptom relief and adverse events, to quality of life, and possibly economic factors such as length of hospital stay or requirement for concomitant therapies. In addition, there is typically a set of clearly defined subgroups in which the primary, and possibly some of the secondary, outcomes will be assessed. Ultimately, even when there is clear evidence of benefit as measured by the effect on the primary outcome, these secondary analyses provide supporting evidence that can either strengthen or weaken the interpretation of the primary result. They may also be used to formulate hypotheses for future trials.

Implicit in any trial are assessments of safety. Because many toxic effects cannot be predicted, a comprehensive set of safety criteria cannot be specified in advance, and safety assessments necessarily include both prespecified and accidental findings.

Lastly, we outline the principles used in formulating the clinical questions that the trial is intended to answer in a sound statistical framework, followed by a discussion of the kinds of clinical outcomes that are commonly used for evaluating efficacy. Included in this section we outline the statistical theory for the validity of surrogate outcomes. Once the clinical outcome is defined, the result must be quantified in a manner that is suitable for statistical analysis. This may be as simple as creating a dichotomous variable indicating clinical improvement or the occurrence of an adverse event such as death, or it may be a complex composite of several distinct components. Finally, we must specify an analysis of the quantitative outcome variables that enables the clinical question to be effectively answered.

2.1 Statistical Framework

We introduce the statistical framework for randomized trial through the detailed discussion of an example. While randomized clinical trials are the best available tools for the evaluation of the safety and efficacy of medical interventions, they are limited by one critical element in particular—they are conducted in human beings. This fact introduces two complications; humans are inherently complex, responding to interventions in unpredictable and varied ways and, in the context of medical research, unlike laboratory animals, there is an ethical obligation to grant them personal autonomy. Consequently, there are many factors that experimenters cannot control and that can introduce complications into the analysis and interpretation of trial results. Some of these complications are illustrated by the following example.

Example 2.1. *Low density lipoprotein* (LDL) is a particle containing fatty acids that circulates in the blood and is produced in the liver. High levels of LDL are associated with increased risk of cardiovascular disease which leads to heart attacks, strokes, and other adverse consequences. A class of drugs known as *statins* have been shown to lower LDL levels in the blood and reduce the incidence of certain adverse cardiovascular events. The TNT ("Treating to New Targets") trial was a double-blind randomized trial conducted to determine if lowering LDL beyond the commonly accepted levels using a high daily dose (80mg) of atorvastatin results in fewer major cardiovascular events than that achieved with a lower daily dose (10mg) of atorvastatin.

Prior to randomization, all subjects meeting inclusion criteria received 10mg of atorvastatin for eight weeks, after which subjects meeting the screening criteria were randomized to either continue with the 10mg dose or receive the 80mg dose. There were a total of 4995 and 5006 subjects enrolled in the 80mg and 10mg groups respectively. Table 2.1 shows the means of both treatment groups at baseline and three-months for subjects with LDL measurements at both times. In this example, *baseline* is defined to be the time of randomization so baseline LDL is expected to reflect the subject response to the 10mg dose. For this example, we consider only the effect of treatment on LDL levels rather than clinical events.   □

Table 2.1 *Baseline and three-month LDL levels in TNT for subjects with values at both time points.*

| Dose | N | Mean LDL (mg/dL) | |
		Baseline	3-Month
80mg	4868	97.3	72.5
10mg	4898	97.6	99.0
Difference		0.3	26.5

p-value for difference < 0.0001

First, from the hypothesis test Table 2.1, for which the p-value is extremely small, it is clear that the $80mg$ dose results in highly statistically significant additional LDL lowering relative to the $10mg$ dose. Given that the sample size is very large, however, differences that are statistically significant may not be clinically relevant, especially since a possible increase in the risk of serious adverse side-effects with the higher dose might offset the potential benefit. It is important, therefore, that the difference be quantified in order to assess the risk/benefit ratio. The mean difference of $26.5mg/dL$ is, in fact, a large, clinically meaningful change, although, as will be discussed later in this chapter, it should be considered a *surrogate* outcome and this effect is only meaningful if it results in a decrease in the risk of adverse outcomes associated with the progression of cardiovascular disease.

The observed mean difference may have other uses beyond characterizing risk and benefit. It may be used to compare the effect of the treatment to that observed in other trials that use other drugs or other doses, or differences observed in other trials with the same doses but conducted in a different population. It may also be used by treating physicians to select a dose for a particular subject or by public health officials who are developing policies and need to compare the cost effectiveness of various interventions. Thus it is important not only that we test the hypothesis of interest, but that we produce a summary measure representing the magnitude of the observed difference, typically with a corresponding confidence interval. What must be kept in mind, however, is that a test of the null hypothesis that there is no effect of treatment is always valid (provided that we have complete data), while an estimate of the *size* of the benefit can be problematic for reasons that we outline below. These drawbacks must be kept in mind when interpreting the results.

To elaborate on the significance of the observed treatment difference, we first note that the mean difference of $26.5mg/dL$ is only one simple summary measure among a number of possible measures of the effect of the $80mg$ dose on three month LDL. To what extent, then, can we say make the following claim?

The *effect* of the $80mg$ dose relative to the $10mg$ dose is to lower LDL an additional $26.5mg/dL$ at three months.

Implicit in this claim is that a patient who has been receiving the $10mg$ dose for a period of time will be expected to experience an additional lowering of LDL by $26.5mg/dL$ when the dose is increased to $80mg$. Mathematically, this claim is based on a particular model for association between dose and LDL. Specifically,

$$\text{Three-month LDL} = \beta_0 + \beta_1 z + \epsilon \tag{2.1}$$

where β_0 and β_1 are coefficients to be estimated, z is zero for a subject receiving the $10mg$ dose and 1 for a subject receiving the $80mg$ dose, and ϵ is a random error term. Note that the effect of treatment is captured by the parameter β_1. The validity of the claim relies upon several factors:

1. the new patient is comparable to the typical subject enrolled in the trial,

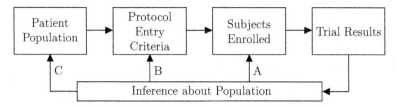

Figure 2.1 *Populations for which clinical trial inference is conducted.*

2. an unbiased estimate of the parameter β_1 (the "treatment effect") can be obtained from the data, and

3. the model in equation (2.1) adequately describes the effect of treatment.

It is important to understand that each of these conditions is likely to fail and, therefore, that we must use caution in interpreting the overall mean difference. We consider each in turn.

First, a new patient would be comparable to the typical subject enrolled in the trial provided that the study sample can be considered representative of the overall population to which the model, and ultimately the claim, applies. Unfortunately, the sample from which the estimate is obtained may be far removed from population of interest, as illustrated by Figure 2.1. The leftmost box on the top of Figure 2.1 represents the population of patients for whom an approved intervention will be medically indicated. Ideally the study would be conducted in a random sample from this population. Unfortunately, study protocols necessarily must specify inclusion and exclusion criteria that precisely define the population of subjects who are allowed to enroll in a trial and for a variety of reasons these criteria will likely exclude certain kinds of subjects from the target population. Individuals meeting these criteria are shown in the second box. The third box represents the subjects actually enrolled and it is likely that these subjects do not represent a random sample from the population meeting the enrollment criteria. For example, enrollment will only be available to subjects with access to a participating center, the local investigator can further select which eligible patients to recommended for enrollment, and finally the patient must consent to the treatments, procedures, and visit schedule required for participation in the trial. Patients for whom trial procedures constitute a potential burden may refuse participation. While we might expect that inference based on trial data can reasonably be made at point A of Figure 2.1, there are additional potential difficulties at this point. For example, it is widely believed that the patient care is generally superior in controlled trials than in the common practice. Physicians in research settings tend to keep abreast of the best clinical practice guidelines and have access to superior facilities and technology. Subjects in clinical trials are generally seen more frequently in the clinic and subject to more extensive diagnostic tests than other patients. Thus the outcomes observed in clinical trials may not reflect the outcomes that might be observed in other settings.

Especially in light of the difficulties at point A, inferences at points B and C regarding the broader populations becomes increasingly tenuous. Thus, at best, estimates of the benefit of a new intervention obtained in a clinical trial may bear little resemblance to what will be observed in general practice.

The second factor underlying the validity of the claim above is whether or not unbiased estimates of the parameters of the model can be obtained from the data. We consider two reasons why observed differences in outcomes may not reflect the actual effect of treatment. We first note that 235 subjects had missing values of LDL at the three-month visit. It is likely that the reason that these data are missing is related to the condition of the subject, and hence that the expected responses among these subjects would be different than the expected responses among subjects with non-missing values. Thus, even if the model were to hold for the population under study, the sample for whom data are available is not necessarily representative of the population of enrolled subjects. A great deal of methodological research has been undertaken, and much is still being done, to account for missing data so that unbiased estimates can be obtained. All methods for accounting for missing data make untestable assumptions and, therefore, while they may provide reasonable guesses regarding the effect of treatment, it is impossible to quantify the degree to which bias has been introduced. This topic will be discussed in greater detail in Chapter 11, *Issues in the Analysis*.

The second reason that the true treatment difference may not be estimable from the data is that subjects fail to adhere to their assigned treatment regimen. In TNT, 246 subjects discontinued their assigned study medication before the three-month visit. Because these subjects received only a fraction of their assigned medication, it is likely that they received only a fraction of the benefit. Thus, the observations from these subjects may not reflect the full effect of treatment, and the observed treatment difference will not represent the effect of treatment had full adherence to treatment been strictly enforced. Nor does adherence to assigned treatment in a controlled trial necessarily reflect adherence in practice—it may in fact be better, and, therefore, the observed difference may actually overestimate the expected benefit. Of course, participation is voluntary and adherence cannot be ethically compelled so that in most trials the treatment effect under full adherence can never be obtained. As with issues regarding missing data, the issue of full adherence is discussed in more detail in Chapter 11.

Finally, we address the question of the adequacy of the model in equation (2.1). There are two ways in which this equation can be inadequate. First, while it may seem self evident, equation (2.1) requires that the quantities in question exist. Specifically, 8 subjects in the $80mg$ group and 7 subjects in the $10mg$ group died before the three month visit. While admittedly these represent a small number of subjects given the large sample size in TNT, they raise the issue of how the outcome of three-month LDL is meaningfully defined. In particular, the quantity of interest can only be defined for living subjects, and the model can only be applied to a subset of subjects. Obviously, one could restrict the application of equation (2.1) to only living subjects; however, if there is an association between treatment, the outcome of interest (LDL in this case), and mortality, one cannot rule out the possibility that death confounds the association between the outcome and treatment. For example, if subjects assigned to the high dose group were more likely to die if they had high LDL, and subjects assigned to the low dose group were more likely to die if they had low LDL, an apparent association between LDL and treatment could be induced even if there was no effect by the treatment on LDL. Thus, restricting the model to only survivors may cast doubt on whether observed associations are causal or simply artifacts of more complex interrelationships between the outcome, treatment, and mortality. In the TNT example, since mortality is small and the differences in LDL large, an argument that the apparent association is induced solely in this way is untenable. We note, however, that in general this *cannot* be demonstrated on purely statistical grounds, but rather requires the combination of statistical analysis and informed clinical judgment. Nonetheless, it is conceivable that mortality may introduce a small bias into the estimation of the underlying effect of treatment on LDL.

Next, ignoring the problem of mortality, the model in equation (2.1) may not capture the effect of treatment observed in TNT in a way that allows the estimate to be meaningfully applied. Consider Table 2.2 in which the TNT population is divided into approximately equal sized groups (quartiles) by baseline LDL. The differences in LDL between treatment groups vary as

Table 2.2 *Differences in three-month LDL levels in TNT as a function of baseline LDL. Note that the standard errors are sufficiently small that the overall trends are highly statistically significant.*

Baseline	Mean Difference in Three-month LDL (mg/dL)	% change in LDL 3-Month
LDL $\leq$ 85	23.2	30.7
85 $<$ LDL $\leq$ 97	25.1	27.4
97 $<$ LDL $\leq$ 110	27.1	26.2
110 $<$ LDL	29.4	24.6

a function of baseline value, implying that there is an interaction between change in LDL and the baseline level. Because the overall treatment difference is the average difference over the range of baseline LDL values in the study population and the effect of treatment (as measured by β_1 in the model) varies with baseline value, the expected difference in mean response between groups in a particular trial depends on the distribution of subjects enrolled in the trial. For example, if a second trial were undertaken in the same population from which the TNT subjects were drawn, but with a different distribution of baseline LDL values, the expected overall observed mean difference at three months would likely be different than that observed in TNT, even though the underlying effect of the treatment is exactly the same. Hence, the results from the two trials would not be directly comparable.

Since the type of interaction we have observed is considered *removable* (it can be removed by transforming the response), we might consider the alternative model

$$\text{\% Change in Three-month LDL} = \beta_0 + \beta_1 z + \epsilon \qquad (2.2)$$

from Table 2.2; however, this model may fail as well, and the same difficulties in interpretation would apply. The "correct" model is probably too complex to provide a useful, easily interpretable summary measure.

As we will see in later chapters, while the goal of providing a meaningful summary of the magnitude of the treatments effects is desirable, clinical trials are fundamentally hypothesis testing instruments. Trial design from the randomization, sample size to interim monitoring plans are generally all approached from a hypothesis testing perspective.

Ultimately, the questions that clinical trials can answer concern the extent to which a trial provides evidence that a treatment is effective. Questions concerning the magnitude of the effect are inherently problematic and while estimates of treatment effect are important, one must interpret them cautiously. The principle espoused by George Box that "all models are wrong, some are useful" (Box and Draper 1987) should always be kept in mind when interpreting trial results.

2.1.1 Causal Inference

Ultimately, the goal of a clinical trial is to establish a causal link between the treatments employed and the outcomes that are measured. Before discussing the principles involved with defining the question to be addressed by a clinical trial, it is helpful to understand some fundamental principles of causal inference.

Controlled clinical trials are unique among tools available for research involving human subjects in the sense that they are the only kinds of studies that directly address causation via experimentation. While observational studies have historically played a key role in identifying both risk factors for disease and potential therapeutic agents, they only indirectly address issues of causation. Hill (1965) suggested nine criteria useful for distinguishing association from causation in the study of environment and disease. Briefly, Hill's criteria are *strength, consistency, specificity, temporality, biological gradient, plausibility, coherence, experiment,* and *analogy.* Following is a brief summary of each of these criteria.

1. *Strength.* If the incidence or severity of disease is substantially larger among exposed individuals than among unexposed individuals, the exposure may be more likely to be a direct cause than the association induced by a third factor.

2. *Consistency.* A causal relationship should be consistently observed by different persons, in different places, circumstances, and times.

3. *Specificity.* If a particular exposure is associated with a single, or small number of, adverse outcome(s), it is less likely to be due to a third factor.

4. *Temporality.* Clearly, a cause must precede the result in time.

5. *Biological Gradient.* The term *biological gradient* refers to the expectation that factors that affect outcomes tend to do so *monotonically*; as exposure increases, there should be an accompanying increase (or decrease) in adverse outcomes.

6. *Plausibility.* Biological plausibility is helpful, but Hill acknowledges that it is limited by current biological understanding, and cannot be a strict requirement.

7. *Coherence.* A potential causal relationship should not conflict with well established knowledge.

8. *Experiment.* Is there experimental evidence supporting causation?

9. *Analogy.* Are there prior experiences that are generally similar to the present association?

Hill's criteria are intended for use in observational studies—settings in which the investigator cannot control the assignment of treatments or other interventions to subjects. Fortunately, randomized controlled trials provide a more direct method of establishing causality. The approach that is taken in this book can be set within the framework formulated by Rubin (1974) and often referred to as the *Rubin causal model.*

Our discussion of this model is taken primarily from Holland (1986). To describe the Rubin causal model, we suppose that there is a population consisting of units (subjects), U, that there are two treatments of interest, denoted t (experimental treatment) and c (control treatment) and that each subject is exposed to either t or c. Denote by $Y_s(u)$ the response that would be observed for subject $u \in U$ were they to be exposed to treatment s. Thus, $Y_t(u)$ and $Y_c(u)$ are the *potential outcomes* were subject u to be exposed to t and c respectively. At least one of these outcomes will never be observed (hence the term *potential*), depending on the treatment to which a subject is exposed. We consider the *causal effect* of treatment for subject u to be $Y_t(u) - Y_c(u)$, the difference between the potential outcomes. It is also important to note that there is no expectation that $Y_t(u) - Y_c(u)$ is the same for all subjects.[1]

Central to the idea of a causal effect is that the subject could have been exposed to *either* of t and c. Thus, under this model, subject characteristics such as age and race cannot be causes since they cannot be different (at least at a given, fixed time). Clearly these characteristics can be *risk factors* for

---

[1] Holland (1986) discusses a disagreement between Sir Ronald Fisher and Jerzy Neyman regarding whether the appropriate null hypothesis is that $Y_t(u) - Y_c(u) = 0$ for *all* units (in this case agricultural plots), or only in expectation. This argument is largely philosophical, however, because in general the former is untestable.

diseases so here we are distinguishing between causes, which can be manip-
ulated, and other types of risk factors. (See Holland (1986) for an engaging
discussion of several historical alternative viewpoints.)

Furthermore, in the expression for the causal effect $Y_t(u) - Y_c(u)$, we require
that all conditions other than exposure to treatment be identical. In particular, $Y_t(u)$ and $Y_c(u)$ refer to the subject response at the *same point in time*.
Strictly speaking, this definition excludes crossover studies in which a subject
is exposed sequentially to two or more treatments because the responses to
each treatment are observed at different times, and, therefore, under different
conditions (e.g., the subject is older at the second time). This observation leads
to what Holland (1986) calls the *Fundamental Problem of Causal Inference:*

> It is impossible to *observe* the value of $Y_t(u)$ and $Y_c(u)$ on the same unit and,
> therefore, it is impossible to *observe* the effect of t on u.

A consequence of this principle is that inference in clinical trials must necessarily be restricted to populations, by which we mean a set of individuals
meeting prospectively defined criteria, and not individual subjects. Hence, all
questions addressed by clinical trials must be formulated as population level
questions. Thus, at best, a controlled clinical trial can provide an estimate of
population average causal effect,

$$E[Y_t(u) - Y_c(u)] \qquad (2.3)$$

where the expectation is taken over the population in question.

In practice, obtaining an estimate of $E[Y_t(u) - Y_c(u)]$ requires an additional
condition. Specifically, we have that $E[Y_t(u) - Y_c(u)] = E[Y_t(u)] - E[Y_c(u)]$,
and, because of the fundamental problem of causal inference, we necessarily must estimate $E[Y_t(u)]$ and $E[Y_c(u)]$ in two separate sets of subjects (or
possibly the same subjects, but at different times, raising another set of potential difficulties that are described in Chapter 3). Letting $S(u)$ denote the
treatment to which unit u is exposed, unbiased estimation of the causal effect
requires that

$$E[Y_t(u) - Y_c(u)] = E[Y_t(u)|S(u) = t] - E[Y_c(u)|S(u) = c]. \qquad (2.4)$$

The right hand side of equation (2.4) is the difference in mean responses for
subjects receiving t and c and follows automatically if the exposure to treatment τ is independent of the response $Y_\tau(u)$ for $\tau = t, c$. In observational
studies it is impossible to confirm independence. In fact it can usually be
refuted by identifying *confounding* factors—factors that are associated with
both exposure and response. In observational studies, one hopes that conditional on a set of observed potential confounding factors, the response is
independent of exposure, so the independent (causal) effect of exposure can
be estimated via sophisticated models adjusting for confounding factors. In
randomized studies (provided the randomization is correctly performed), *assignment* to treatment τ is guaranteed to be independent of response, so (2.4)
is also guaranteed to hold if we consider $S(u)$ to be assigned treatment. Thus,

in principle, the causal effect of assignment to treatment can be estimated using the relation $E[Y_t(u) - Y_c(u)] = E[Y_t(u)|S(u) = t] - E[Y_c(u)|S(u) = c]$.

To illustrate how (2.4) can break down, recall that elevated serum LDL has been shown to be a risk factor for coronary artery disease, often resulting in heart attacks and death. Various classes of drugs have been developed that lower serum LDL. Some of these, statins, for example, have also been shown to reduce the incidence of coronary heart disease (CHD) events (Scandanavian Simvistatin Survival Study 1994). Using the principles of causal inference that we outlined above, we can only infer from these studies that statins have two effects: lowering LDL, and reducing incidence of CHD events. It is commonly inferred, therefore, that lowering LDL has the beneficial effect of reducing the risk of CHD events. We note that this conclusion is *not* based on direct statistical inference, but statistical inference combined with informed scientific judgment. If could also be wrong, if, for example, the mechanism by which statins reduce CHD events is independent of its effect on LDL. To put this question into the Rubin causal model framework, for simplicity (and unrealistically) suppose that LDL has two levels and let h be the state of having high LDL and l be the state of having low LDL. The "causal effect" of LDL level would then be $E[Y_h(u) - Y_l(u)]$, under the assumption that all other conditions are identical, which requires that we could directly manipulate LDL without any other direct effects. In the case in which LDL is lowered by treatment with a statin, this certainly fails because in state l, not only does the subject have low LDL, but they have also been exposed to a statin, unlike state h.

An additional complication in the estimation of $Y_h(u) - Y_l(u)$ is that there may be subjects for whom a particular statin does not have the desired effect on LDL. In this case $Y_l(u)$ cannot be defined because the level l is unattainable. If we let $R(u)$ be the achieved LDL level (h or l), the temptation at the conclusion of a statin trial may be to estimate the effect of LDL level using $E[Y_h(u) - Y_l(u)] = E[Y_h(u)|R(u) = h] - E[Y_l(u)|R(u) = l]$. This estimate requires that $E[Y_h(u)|R(u) = h] = E[Y_h(u)]$ which is impossible to verify, and may be meaningless since the $E[Y_h(u)]$ only makes sense if we can directly manipulate LDL.

Thus, while randomized trials are the "gold standard" for the assessment of therapeutic effects, direct inference of causation is limited to those factors that we can directly manipulate—the therapeutic agents or interventions to which subjects can be assigned. The identification of more general causal relationships requires the assimilation of trial results with scientific understanding obtained from other research areas including animal and mechanistic laboratory studies.

2.1.2 The Intent-To-Treat Principle

An immediate consequence of the condition in equation (2.4) is the "intent-to-treat" (ITT) principle. According to the ITT principle, "all subjects meeting admission criteria and subsequently randomized should be counted in their

originally assigned treatment groups without regard to deviations from assigned treatment" (Fisher et al. 1990). This principle implies, for example,
that all primary events observed during the follow-up period must be reported and included in the analysis. Violations of the ITT principle include
elimination of subjects because they did not comply fully with the experimental intervention, or that the event occurred some time after the intervention
was discontinued. In each of these cases, the exclusion of subjects or events
from the analysis induces dependence between those observed to be on a particular treatment and the outcome. For example, in "on-treatment" analyses
in which follow-up ends at the point that subjects (prematurely) discontinue
therapy, sicker, higher risk subjects are more likely to be excluded, and discontinuation is also likely to be related to treatment. Using the notation from
the previous section, the "on-treatment" estimand is the difference

$$E[Y_t(u)|S(u) = t, \text{"on-treatment"}] - E[Y_t(u)|S(u) = c, \text{"on-treatment"}].$$
(2.5)

First, this comparison is problematic because it further restricts the population to the subgroup of those who remain on treatment and second, and most
important, it does so in a potentially treatment-dependent way—subjects assigned treatment t who remain on treatment may not have done so had they
been assigned treatment c and vice versa. Only under stringent (and unverifiable) conditions does the equation (2.5) equal the quantity of interest given
in equation (2.3).

   The ITT principle forms the basis for the material presented in Chapters 3,
4, and 5, and is discussed greater detail in Chapter 11 (analysis).

2.2 Elements of Study Question

Most randomized controlled clinical trials are designed to answer a broad
clinical question such as "Is the intervention X safe and effective in individuals
with (or at risk for) disease Y?" Implicit in this question is that, first, that
there is a population of interest—those with, or at risk for, the disease of
interest—and second, that both safety and effectiveness are of interest. Each
of these components must be more precisely specified for a particular trial. In
this section, we outline the major elements that constitute the primary and
secondary questions of a trial. We begin with a brief discussion of the study
population.

2.2.1 The Population

The study population is precisely defined by the eligibility criteria for a trial
and which are clearly specified in the study protocol. Protocol eligibility criteria are generally divided into inclusion and exclusion criteria. The inclusion
criteria define the target population for the intervention while the exclusion
criteria specify subjects within the target population for whom the treatment
is contraindicated or those whose inclusion would complicate interpretation

of the results or require unacceptably large sample size. The nature of the inclusion criteria will be determined by whether the trial is primary prevention, secondary prevention, or therapeutic. In a primary prevention trial, subjects would not have a history of the target disease, but may be chosen to have risk factors that increase their likelihood of developing the disease. For example, the Physicians Health Study (Steering Committee of the Physicians' Health Study Research Group 1989; Hennekens et al. 1996; Ridker et al. 1997) investigated the potential cardiovascular benefit of aspirin and beta-carotene in healthy men. In a secondary prevention trial, the target population comprises those with a history of the disease in question but who are not presently symptomatic or are in remission. The population in therapeutic trials includes individuals with acute or life threatening disease for whom the intervention is intended to alleviate symptoms, delay progression or death, or in some cases, cure the disease.

Typically subjects for whom the intervention might pose excessive risk, such as pregnant or lactating women, are excluded. Subjects for whom evaluation of the outcomes of interest may be difficult or who have comorbid conditions that independently influence the outcome may be excluded. For example, in a heart failure trial, subjects who are on a heart transplant waiting list may be excluded because a compatible heart could become available at any time, rendering data from the subject difficult to interpret. Subjects who are likely to die within a few months, or years in a long term trial, may be excluded because their death is not likely to be related to treatment. These deaths increase the variance of test statistics without a corresponding increase in the signal, thereby reducing the power of the study to detect a treatment related mortality difference.

The eligibility criteria are critical because they have an impact on the generalizability of the result and the ease of subject recruitment. Typically, less restrictive criteria allow for more generalizable results and potentially easier of subject recruitment at the expense of the requirement for a larger sample size. Conversely, if more restrictive criteria are used, the results are less generalizable and recruitment may be more difficult; however, because the population is more homogeneous, variability is reduced and a smaller sample size may be possible.

Those who volunteer for a trial are also a selected population, sometimes exhibiting what is referred to as the "healthy volunteer effect", since these individuals are at often at lower risk than the general population of subjects (see Figure 2.1). For trials with survival outcomes in particular, this can result in under-powered trials (Ederer et al. 1993).

2.2.2 Primary and Secondary Questions

Because there are invariably multiple questions of interest in a clinical trial, they are usually divided into primary, secondary, and sometimes, tertiary questions. Because of the comparative nature of randomized trials, the questions of interest generally involve direct treatment comparisons. Other kinds of questions, such as those related to the natural history of the disease or the effect of baseline covariates, may be of interest; however, since these do not involve comparisons between treatment groups, they are usually not included with the prespecified questions specified in the protocol.

Corresponding to each clinical question is one or more outcomes[2] of interest and a single statistical analysis, usually in the form of an hypothesis test. Except in equivalence or non-inferiority trials, the *null hypothesis* usually states that there is no effect of treatment on the (distribution of) the primary outcome. For example, the primary question might be "Is there a greater reduction in three month serum LDL in subjects with elevated baseline LDL taking $80mg$ atorvastatin than in subjects taking $10mg$ atorvastatin?" The outcome of interest is reduction in three month serum LDL, and the analysis consists of a test of the null hypothesis that there is no difference between doses in three-month LDL. Because there is generally a one-to-one correspondence between the question and the outcome, in what follows, we often use the question and the outcome interchangeably.

There are two broad categories of outcomes, *clinical outcomes* and *surrogate outcomes*. *Clinical outcomes*, or *clinically relevant* outcomes, are outcomes that reflect the survival or symptomatic status of the subject. *Surrogate outcomes* are responses that have been shown to be associated with clinical outcomes but do not in themselves directly reflect survival or the clinical status of the subject. Examples of surrogate outcomes include blood pressure, cholesterol, and tumor size. In early phase trials in which the goal is to identify treatments with potential benefit, non-clinical surrogate outcomes play an important role. Generally trials using surrogate outcomes require fewer subjects and follow-up time, and therefore can often be conducted more quickly and efficiently than trials using clinical outcomes. Thus, surrogate outcomes can be ideal for early phase trials that are not intended to definitively establish efficacy. In phase III confirmatory trials, however, it is essential that clinical benefit be established and the use of surrogate outcomes may be problematic. There are numerous examples of treatments that have been shown to have a positive effect on a surrogate outcome that did not translate into clinical benefit. It is important, therefore, that the primary outcome be appropriate to the goals of the trial. A detailed discussion of surrogate outcomes appears in Section 2.4.

The chief reason for having a single primary question is that if there are multiple primary analyses, the control of the overall type I error rate of the trial requires that a multiple comparison procedure (usually the Bonferroni procedure) be use to adjust the significance levels for each hypothesis test (multiple comparison procedures are discussed in detail in Chapter 11). With each additional hypothesis test, power for any one hypothesis will generally decrease unless the sample size is increased accordingly. There are also diffi-

---

[2] Many authors use *endpoint* to refer to the outcome in a trial. Because of the potential for confusion with the use of this term we prefer to use *outcome* (Meinert 1996)

culties with interpretation if benefit is demonstrated for only one of a number
of outcomes, especially if there are others for which benefit would have greater
clinical significance. Therefore, the primary question should be the question
with the greatest clinical importance.

Once the primary question is specified, there are invariably additional, secondary questions of interest. Secondary questions are generally other important clinical questions that either add support to the primary question, or are
of interest in their own right. In either case, secondary questions should also
be limited in number and stated in advance in the protocol. For example, the
primary outcome might be total mortality and a secondary outcome might be
the composite outcome of first occurrence of either death or hospitalization
(see Section 2.5 later in this chapter for a detailed discussion of composite outcomes). Alternatively, death or hospitalization might be the primary outcome
and death alone may be a secondary outcome. For many diseases, all-cause
mortality may be the preferred outcome, but because mortality rates are relatively low, a very large sample size might be required. In this case, if treatment
would be expected to reduce both mortality and a nonfatal clinical outcome
such as hospitalization, the composite outcome may allow a smaller trial to
be conducted. All-cause mortality would likely be a secondary outcome. This
strategy, however, can still lead to confusion when results are inconsistent.
For example, in the TNT trial (LaRosa et al. 2005), the primary outcome was
the composite of coronary heart disease death, nonfatal myocardial infarction,
resuscitated cardiac arrest, and fatal and nonfatal stroke. This observed incidence rate for the primary outcome was 20% lower in the high dose arm
than in the low dose arm, yet the rates of all-cause mortality were virtually
identical. This result led to concerns regarding the benefit of the higher dose
(Pitt 2005).

Cancer trials often use disease free survival (alive without disease recurrence) as the primary outcome and total mortality as the leading secondary
outcome. A lung study might have a pulmonary test such as FEV1 (forced
expiratory volume in one second) as the primary and quality of life as a secondary outcome. If there are a number of secondary outcomes, they should
be either grouped or ordered by clinical importance.

2.2.3 Subgroup Questions

Another category of secondary questions concern the effect of treatment in
specific baseline subgroups of subjects. Generally these are defined by cohort
by demographic factors, disease categories, or known risk factors. For example, a clinician may want to know if the therapy is effective equally in men
and women, across race and age groups, and by prior history of the disease or
treatment. Subgroups may be used to confirm a result from a previous trial.
Subgroup analyses can also be used to generate new hypotheses. The primary
purpose of subgroup analyses, however, is to assess the consistency of an intervention's effect across groups defined by a variety of baseline characteristics.

Similar to the primary and secondary questions, the subgroup questions must be stated in advance in the protocol and limited in number. A detailed discussion of subgroup analyses appears in Chapter 11.

2.2.4 Safety Questions

The primary, secondary, and subgroup questions are generally aimed at assessing efficacy, the goal being to establish that the intervention is therapeutically effective for one or more outcome measures and subpopulations. In order to fully evaluate the benefit to risk ratio, it is equally important that the safety profile of the intervention be established. While the efficacy questions can be limited—many treatments target a specific component of the disease and are not expected to show benefit for all possible disease-related outcomes— the safety evaluation must be comprehensive. Safety questions usually involve a combination of outcomes including *adverse events*, comprising all undesirable experiences potentially associated with the treatment, *serious adverse events* (SAEs), which are adverse events meeting specific criteria for seriousness (see Section 6.1.2), and laboratory measures including analyses of blood or urine samples or other diagnostic procedures such as CT or MRI scans and electrocardiograms (ECGs). Reports of AEs and SAEs are direct evidence of symptomatic safety problems, whereas laboratory tests assess problems that are associated with internal organ abnormalities or other problems that may not exhibit external symptoms for some time.

For trials under regulatory agency review, SAEs must be reported to the IRB and the FDA within a 24 hour period if judged by a medical review to be related to the intervention. Specific AEs or SAEs may have been identified in earlier phase I and phase II trials and these can be pre-defined as being of special interest in a phase III trial. Because SAEs occurring with a low frequency may not have been identified in earlier trials it may be difficult in a larger phase III trial to determine whether an unexpected difference by treatment in the frequency of a particular adverse event is a result of treatment or is a chance occurrence. Because the number of possible adverse events and lab abnormalities is both potentially quite large and unpredictable *a priori*, formal adjustments for multiple comparisons become impractical. The evaluation of the analyses of adverse events requires both statistical and clinical judgment, and many safety questions may not be resolved for many years, if ever.

2.3 Outcome or Response Measures

Once the population and the questions of interest have been defined, the investigators must precisely specify the outcome measures that will be used to answer the questions. For many questions the outcome will be clear. If the primary question addresses the effect of treatment on all-cause mortality, the outcome is the dichotomous variable indicating whether or not death has occurred, and possibly the date or time of death. If the question involves an assessment such as the respiratory function, the difficulty arises when subjects are unable to perform the assessment. While this can be considered a type of missing data, it is likely that the inability to perform the assessment is indicative of poor function and this situation can potentially be handled in the analysis (see Section 2.3.1, page 54).

A more complex situation is one in which, for example, rescue therapy is available that can interfere with the assessment. For example, if a therapy is intended to lessen the frequency or severity of asthma attacks in asthmatic subjects, subjects may have access to inhaled bronchodilators that can be used at the time of the attack to also lessen its severity. For this question, assessments of respiratory function at the time of the attack may not reflect the severity of the attack were the rescue medication not available. In this case it may be useful to include the requirement for rescue medication as a component of the outcome. Approaches for combining outcomes are discussed in more detail in Section 2.5.

The outcome variables will, in general, be one of the following types.

Binary Binary outcome variables take one of two values, usually either the presence or absence of a condition, or the occurrence of an adverse event such as death or disease recurrence.

Ordered categorical An ordered categorical variable (often called an *ordinal* variable) has three or more levels that have a natural ordering from best to worst or vice versa. An example is New York Heart Association class which measures severity of heart failure and ranges from I (no symptoms) to IV (severe symptoms). Note that an unordered categorical variable with three or more levels is usually not a suitable outcome measure because there is no clear way to decide if one treatment is superior to another.

Continuous Continuous variables are those that, theoretically, can take all possible values within an interval on the real line. Examples include blood pressure and blood chemistries such as LDL. Often ordinal variables taking more than a few values are considered continuous. For example, a pain scale taking integer values between 0 (no pain) and 10 (worst pain imaginable) may be considered to be a continuous variable.

Failure time A failure time outcome is a combination of binary and continuous variables, consisting of an event indicator (0 if the event did not occur, 1 if the event did occur) and a failure time (either the time of the failure, or the maximum follow-up time if the failure did not occur). If lengths of follow-up differ among subjects, those with more follow-up have higher probabilities of failure and simple binary outcome analyses may not be appropriate. The use of a failure time outcome enables the differing lengths of follow-up to be correctly accounted for in the analysis. (See Chapter 7, *Survival Analysis*.)

Because continuous outcomes usually require an assessment by trained personnel, they generally correspond to subject status at specific times. Binary and ordinal outcomes may also be assessed at specific times or they may reflect subject status during all or a portion of the follow-up period. A binary variable representing 28-day mortality, for example, indicates whether or not a subject died sometime within the first 28 days of follow-up. Subjects with a particular disease may experience episodes of worsening that are categorized on an ordinal scale. A possible summary outcome may be the severity of the worst episode during follow-up.

In some trials, outcomes, particularly ordinal or continuous measures, are assessed at each of a series of follow-up visits. The primary outcome of interest may be the value at a particular visit, or the values at all visits may be combined using model-based approaches, nonparametric analyses, or a combination. For progressive diseases, the rate of change of the outcome may be of interest. For chronic or acute conditions, either the average or the area under the curve may be used to capture the total experience of the subject over the follow-up period. Model-based approaches may employ standard longitudinal data approaches and are discussed in detail in Chapter 8.

Following are some general principles for formulation of outcome variables.

- It is helpful for outcome variables to be well known and measured using standard techniques so that the results can be more easily interpreted by the clinical community. The use of standardized outcomes also enables the results to be more readily compared to those of other trials.

- Response variables must be able to be ascertained in all subjects. An outcome that can be obtained in only a small percentage of subjects is of little value. For example, a cardiovascular trial might use a radionuclide imaging technique to determine the size of a heart attack. If this technique requires a delay in the subject's care, then not all subjects will be able to be assessed, data will be missing, and treatment comparisons are likely to be biased.

- Outcome variables must be reproducible and specific to the question. For many trials involving serious diseases, death, hospitalization, disease recurrence, or some other event may be the natural outcome variable. Heart function, pulmonary function, visual impairment, or quality of life, while often of interest, can be more challenging to precisely define.

2.3.1 Analysis of Outcome Variables

The analysis of the outcome variables typically has two components: a test of the hypotheses of interest, and a summary measure of the observed effect size, usually in the form of a parameter estimate and an accompanying confidence interval. As we have indicated in Section 2.1, provided that we have complete ascertainment of the outcomes of interest, the test of the null hypothesis that there is no effect of assignment to treatment is unbiased (see Section 11.1 for a discussion of bias in hypothesis testing) regardless of subject compliance to the protocol. Summary measures, on the other hand, are subject to the difficulties also described in Section 2.1 and must be interpreted cautiously. Here we briefly highlight commonly used analyses for binary, ordinal, and continuous outcomes. Analyses of failure time outcomes are discussed in detail in Chapter 7. Here, unless otherwise noted, we assume that there are two treatment groups.

Binary outcomes

For binary data, we assume that the probability of the event in question is π_j where $j = 1, 2$ is the treatment group. Therefore, if the number of subjects in group j is n_j, then the number of events in group j, x_j, has a binomial distribution with size n_j and probability π_j. The null hypothesis is $H_0 \colon \pi_1 = \pi_2$. The observed outcomes for binary data can be summarized as a 2×2 table as follows.

	Event		
	Yes	No	Total
Group 1	x_1	$n_1 - x_1$	n_1
Group 2	x_2	$n_2 - x_2$	n_2
Total	m_1	m_2	N

There are several choices of tests of H_0 for this summary table. The most commonly used are the *Fisher's exact test*, and *Pearson chi-square test*.

Fisher's exact test is based on the conditional distribution of x_1 under H_0 given the marginal totals, m_1, m_2, n_1, and n_2. Conditionally, x_1 has a hypergeometric distribution,

$$\Pr\{x_1 \mid n_1, n_2, m_1, m_2\} = P_{x_1} = \frac{\dbinom{n_1}{x_1}\dbinom{n_2}{x_2}}{\dbinom{N}{m_1}} \qquad (2.6)$$

independent of the common (unknown) probability $\pi_1 = \pi_2$. Using Fisher's exact test we reject $H_0 \colon \pi_1 \leq \pi_2$ if

$$\sum_{P_l \leq P_{x_j}} P_l < \alpha. \qquad (2.7)$$

Note that the sum is over all values of x_1 for which the probability in (2.6) is smaller than that for the observed value. This test is "exact" in the sense that, because the conditional distribution does not depend on the unknown parameters, the tail probability in equation (2.7) can be computed exactly. Because equation (2.7) uses the exact conditional distribution of x_1, the type I error is guaranteed to be at most α. For tables with at least one small marginal total, Fisher's exact test is conservative, and often extremely so. The actual type 1 error for $\alpha = .05$ is often on the order of 0.01 (D'Agostino 1990) with a corresponding reduction in power.

The Pearson chi-square test uses the test statistic

$$X^2 = \frac{(x_1 N - n_1 m_1)^2 N}{m_1 m_2 n_1 n_2} = \frac{(x_1 - n_1 m_1 / N)^2 N^3}{m_1 m_2 n_1 n_2}.$$

Note that X^2 is the score test statistic based on the binomial likelihood (See Appendix A.3), which, in multi-way tables, has form $\sum (E-O)^2/E$ where the sum is over all cells in the summary table, E is the expected count under H_0, and O is the observed cell count. Under H_0, the conditional expectation of x_1 given the total number of events, m_1, is $m_1 n_1/N$, so X^2 measures how far x_1 is from its conditional expectation. Asymptotically, X^2 has a chi-square distribution with one degree of freedom (χ_1^2). At level $\alpha = 0.05$, for example, we would reject H_0 if $X^2 > 3.84$, the 95th percentile of the χ_1^2 distribution. In small samples X^2 no longer has a chi-square distribution and conventional wisdom suggests that because of this, the Pearson chi-square test should only be used when the expected counts in each cell of the table are at least 5 under H_0. This belief has been shown to be incorrect, however (see, for example, Fienberg (1980), Appendix IV and Upton (1982)). Fienberg suggests that the type I error is reasonably well controlled for expected cell counts as low as 1. For some values of π_1, n_1, and n_2 the actual type I error can exceed the nominal level, but usually only by a small amount. The *continuity corrected* Pearson chi-square test (sometimes referred to as *Yate's* continuity correction) has the form

$$X_C^2 = \frac{(|x_1 - n_1 m_1/N| - 0.5)^2 N^3}{m_1 m_2 n_1 n_2}.$$

Using the continuity corrected chi-square test approximates the Fisher's exact test quite well. An alternative discussed by Upton (1982) is

$$X_U^2 = \frac{(x_1 N - n_1 m_1)^2 (N - 1)}{m_1 m_2 n_1 n_2}.$$

While Upton recommends X_U^2, it is not commonly used and many software packages do not produce it. In moderate to large trials X_U^2 and X^2 will be virtually identical. Our belief is that the X^2 is the preferred test statistic for 2×2 tables.

While the 2×2 table is a useful summary for binary outcomes, it does not provide a single summary of the effect of treatment.

There are three commonly used summary statistics for binary outcomes.

Risk Difference The *risk difference* is the difference in estimates of the event probabilities,

$$\hat{\Delta} = \hat{\pi}_2 - \hat{\pi}_1 = x_2/n_2 - x_1/n_1.$$

Risk Ratio The *risk ratio* (sometimes referred to as the *relative risk*) is the ratio of the estimated probabilities,

$$\hat{r} = \frac{\hat{\pi}_2}{\hat{\pi}_1} = \frac{x_2/n_2}{x_1/n_1}.$$

Odds Ratio The *odds ratio* is the ratio of the observed *odds*,

$$\hat{\psi} = \frac{\hat{\pi}_2/(1 - \hat{\pi}_2)}{\hat{\pi}_1/(1 - \hat{\pi}_1)} = \frac{x_2/(n_2 - x_2)}{x_1/(n_1 - x_1)}.$$

There is extensive discussion in the literature regarding the preferred summary measure.[3] Our belief is that the preferred summary measure is the one most adequately fits the observed data. This view is summarized by Breslow and Day (1988), "From a purely empirical viewpoint, the most important properties of a model are simplicity and goodness of fit to the observed data. The aim is to be able to describe the main features of the data as succinctly as possible" (page 58). To illustrate this principle, if baseline variables are available that predict outcome, then the best summary measure is the one for which there is the least evidence of interaction between treatment and baseline risk. For example, suppose that the risk ratio $r = \pi_2/\pi_1$ is independent of baseline predictors, then, the risk difference is $\Delta = \pi_2 - \pi_1 = (r - 1)\pi_1$. For subjects with low baseline risk, i.e., small π_1, then the risk difference is small, and for subjects with large baseline risk, the risk difference is large. In this situation, the risk difference fails to adequately fit the observed data.

Similarly, in this situation, the odds ratio will fail to capture the observed effect of treatment. Here

$$\psi = \frac{r\pi_1/(1 - r\pi_1)}{\pi_1/(1 - \pi_1)} = r\frac{1 - \pi_1}{1 - r\pi_1}.$$

For small π_1, $\psi \approx r$, whereas for large π_1, ψ will be further from 1 ($\psi > r$ if $r > 1$ and $\psi < r$ if $r < 1$) Because $r \approx \psi$ for small π_1 (some authors suggest $\pi_1 < 0.1$), $\hat{\psi}$ is often used as an approximation to $\hat{r}$ when $\hat{r}$ cannot be calculated directly, such as in case-control studies, or when logistic regression models are used to account for potential confounding variables. When π_1 is large, ψ and r can be quite different and statisticians should always be sure to report the one that is most suitable, making it clear that they are different summary measures. If π_1 is large, because $\pi_2 \leq 1$, there is an upper limit on the risk difference δ and the risk ratio r; $\Delta \leq 1 - \pi_1$ and $r < 1/\pi_1$. Because of this limitation, Cook (2002b) suggests that the constant odds ratio model is more likely to hold, and the odds ratio may be preferred in this setting, contrary the belief of many authors.[3]

Ordinal outcomes

Ordinal outcomes may be viewed as multinomial observations, y, taking values $0, 1, 2, \ldots, K$, where $K \geq 2$, with $\Pr\{y = k\} = \pi_{jk}$ where j is the assigned treatment group, and $\sum_k \pi_{jk} = 1$. The null hypothesis that there is no effect of treatment is $H_0: \pi_{1k} = \pi_{2k}$ for each k. Without loss of generality, we will assume that higher levels represent better outcomes.

The data can be summarized by a $2 \times (K + 1)$ table.

---

[3] See, for example, Davies et al. (1998), Bracken and Sinclair (1998), Deeks (1998), Altman et al. (1998), Taeger et al. (1998), Sackett et al. (1996), Zhang and Yu (1998), Senn (1999), Cook (2002b) among many others for discussions of risk ratios versus odds ratios

	Response Level					
	0	1	2	$\cdots$	K	Total
Group 1	x_{10}	x_{11}	x_{12}	$\cdots$	x_{1K}	n_1
Group 2	x_{20}	x_{21}	x_{22}	$\cdots$	x_{2K}	n_2
Total	m_0	m_1	m_2	$\cdots$	m_K	N

A general test of H_0 is the score statistic $\sum_{j,k}(x_{jk}-E_{jk})^2/E_{jk}$ where, as with the Pearson chi-square test, the sum is over the $2(K+1)$ cells of the table and $E_{jk}=n_jm_k/N$ is the expected count in cell j,k under H_0, given the margins of the table. The difficulty with this general test is that it is not necessarily sensitive to alternative hypotheses of interest, and the result may be difficult to interpret. Suppose $K=2$ and consider the alternative hypothesis given by $\pi_{10}=.3$, $\pi_{11}=.4$, $\pi_{12}=.3$, $\pi_{20}=.2$, $\pi_{21}=.6$, and $\pi_{22}=.2$. If treatment 2 is the experimental treatment, then the effect of treatment is to reduce the number of responses in the best and worst categories, but there is no net benefit, and this hypothesis is of little interest. We are usually willing to sacrifice power for this kind of hypothesis in favor of tests with power for alternatives in which there is clear evidence of benefit.

The alternative hypotheses of greatest interest are those for which, for an arbitrary level, k, subjects in the experimental group have at lower probability than control subjects of achieving a response no higher than level k; that is, alternative hypotheses of the form

$$H_1: \Pr\{y_2 \le k\} < \Pr\{y_1 \le k\}, \ k = 0, 1, 2, \ldots, K-1, \qquad (2.8)$$

where y_1 and y_2 are subjects randomly selected from groups 1 and 2, respectively.[4]

One commonly used family of alternative distributions satisfying conditions such as (2.8) is defined by

$$\frac{\Pr\{y_2 \le k\}}{1-\Pr\{y_2 \le k\}} = \psi\frac{\Pr\{y_1 \le k\}}{1-\Pr\{y_1 \le k\}} \qquad (2.9)$$

for some $\psi > 0$. The model implied by this condition is sometimes called the *proportional odds* model. The binary case we have already discussed can be considered a special case in which $K=1$, and ψ is the odds ratio. Under this model, all 2×2 tables derived by dichotomizing the response based on $y_j \le k$ versus $y_j > k$ have a common odds ratio ψ. The null hypothesis under this model is $H_0: \psi = 1$. It can be shown that the score test for this hypothesis is the well known *Wilcoxon rank-sum* test (or *Mann-Whitney U*-test), which is available in most statistical analysis software packages. A more detailed discussion of this test follows under *continuous outcomes*.

Alternatively, one could use the Student t-test which is a test of $H_0: E[y_1] = E[y_2]$. Since the normality assumption is clearly violated, especially if K is small, the t-test may be less powerful than the Wilcoxon rank-sum test. Furthermore, the t-test is based on a location shift model that, again, does not

---

[4] This condition is called (strict) *stochastic ordering*; the cumulative distribution in one group is (strictly) either above of below that of the other.

hold because the scale is discrete and the range is likely to be the same in both groups.

It is less clear which statistic summarizing treatment differences is most meaningful for ordinal data. The common odds ratio ψ in (2.9) may be a mathematically natural summary measure; however, the clinical interpretation of this parameter may not be clear. Because the nonparametric Wilcoxon rank-sum test is equivalent to the score test, a logical choice might be the difference in group medians; however, the medians could be the same in both groups if K is small. The difference in means, while not derived from a natural model for the effect of treatment, may be the most interpretable summary statistic.

Continuous Outcomes

When outcome measures are known to be normally distributed (Gaussian), hypothesis tests based on normal data (Student t-tests or analysis of variance (ANOVA)) are optimal and test hypotheses regarding the effect of treatment on mean responses. If outcomes are not normal, we may rely on the central limit theorem which ensures the validity of these tests if sample sizes are sufficiently large. In the non-normal case, however, tests based on ANOVA are no longer optimal and other kinds of test statistics may be preferred. Occasionally the statistical analysis specified in a trial protocol will indicate that a test for normality should be performed and the test statistic used for the analysis be based on the results of the test of normality. Given the imperative that hypothesis tests be prespecified, it is preferable that a clearly defined test that relies on few assumptions is preferred.

An alternative class of tests are *nonparametric* or *distribution free* tests. The most commonly used nonparametric test for testing the null hypothesis of no difference between two of groups is the *Wilcoxon rank-sum* test which is also equivalent to the *Mann-Whitney U-test*. The Wilcoxon rank-sum test is computed by sorting all subjects by their response, irrespective of treatment group, and assigning to each a *rank* that is simply an integer indicating their position in the sort order. For example, the subject with the lowest response receives a rank of one, the second lowest a rank of two and so on. Because in practice data are always discrete (outcomes are rarely measured with more than three or four significant digits), there are likely to be tied observations for which the sort order is ambiguous. For these observations, the usual convention is to assign to each the average of the ranks that would have been assigned to all observations with the same value had the ties been arbitrarily broken. Specifically, the rank for subject i in group j is

$$r_{ij} = \sum_{p,q} I(x_{pq} < x_{ij}) + \frac{I(x_{pq} = x_{ij}) + 1}{2}, \qquad (2.10)$$

where the sum is over all observations in both groups and $I(\cdot)$ is the indicator function (taking a value of one if its argument is true, zero otherwise). The original responses are discarded and the mean ranks are compared. The test statistic is the sum of the ranks in one group, say $j = 1$, minus its expectation,

$$S = \sum_i r_{i1} - \frac{n_1(n_1 + n_2 + 1)}{2}. \tag{2.11}$$

We reject H_0 if

$$\frac{S^2}{\text{Var}(S)} > \chi_{1,\alpha}^2,$$

where $\chi_{1,\alpha}^2$ is the $100 \times \alpha$-percentage point of the chi-square distribution with 1 degree of freedom. In large samples this is essentially equivalent to performing a t-test using the ranks. In small samples, the variance that is used has a slightly different form. If samples are sufficiently small, the mean difference in ranks can be compared to the *permutation distribution* which is the distribution obtained by considering all possible permutations of the treatment labels. Permutation tests of this form are discussed in more detail in Chapter 5, *Randomization*. We note that if responses are normally distributed, so that the t-test is optimal, the relative efficiency of the Wilcoxon test is approximately 95% of that of the t-test, so the Wilcoxon test can be used in the normal case with little loss of power.

As noted above, if responses are *ordinal*, the Wilcoxon rank-sum test is derived from the score test for proportional odds logistic regression models. If the response has two levels, the Wilcoxon rank-sum test reduces to the Pearson chi-square test, and thus is appropriate for nearly all univariate responses, continuous or otherwise.

It can also be shown that the Wilcoxon rank-sum test is equivalent to the following formulation of the Mann-Whitney U-statistic. Suppose that we have n_1 observations in treatment group 1 and n_2 in treatment group 2, and form all $n_1 n_2$ possible pairs of observations (x, y) where x is an observation from group 1 and y is an observation from group 2. Assign each pair a score, $h(x, y)$, of 1 if $x > y$, -1 if $x < y$, and 0 if $x = y$. The Mann-Whitney U-statistic is the mean of these scores:

$$U = \frac{1}{n_1 n_2} \sum_{\text{all pairs } (x,y)} h(x, y).$$

The theory of U-statistics allows a variance to be calculated (since each observation occurs in multiple terms of the sum, the terms are correlated, and the variance formula is somewhat complicated).

The appeal of this formulation is that it results in a somewhat intuitive interpretation of the U-statistic that is not readily apparent in the rank-sum formulation. We note that

$$Eh(x, y) = \Pr\{X > Y\} - \Pr\{X < Y\}$$

where X and Y are random observations from groups 1 and 2 respectively. Hence, if the distributions of X and Y are identical, we have that $Eh(x, y) = 0$. The null hypothesis, therefore, is $H_0: Eh(x, y) = 0$ which is equivalent to

H_0: $\Pr\{X > Y\} = \Pr\{X < Y\}$. Thus, the Mann-Whitney U-test (and, therefore, the Wilcoxon rank-sum test) tests the null hypothesis that a random observation from group 1 is as likely to be greater than as less than a random observation from group 2. This formulation has an attractive clinical interpretation—if the null hypothesis is rejected in favor of group 1, then a subject is more likely to have a better outcome if treated with treatment 1 than with treatment 2. This differs from the interpretation of the t-test. If the null hypothesis is rejected using the t-test in favor of group 1, we conclude that the *expected* outcome (measured on the original scale of the observations) is greater on treatment 1 than on treatment 2. If the distributions of outcomes are skewed, the conclusions of the two tests could, in fact, be opposite. That is, mathematically, we could have $\Pr\{X > Y\} > \Pr\{X < Y\}$ yet have $EX < EY$.

For normal data, the two null hypothesis are mathematically equivalent and under an alternative hypothesis in which the variances are equal, the t-test has more power; however, if the variances are unequal, the t-test is no longer optimal, and the Wilcoxon rank-sum test can be more powerful.

The properties of the two tests are summarized below.

- The t-test

  - is most powerful when data are known to be normal with equal variances,
  - is not optimal when responses are not normal or have unequal variances,
  - tests the differences in mean responses, and mean difference can be summarized in the original response units with a confidence interval if desired.

- The Wilcoxon rank-sum test (Mann-Whitney U-test)

  - has power near that of the t-test when responses are normal,
  - can have greater power when responses are not normal,
  - has a natural interpretation in terms of the probability that a subject will have a better response on one treatment versus another.

While we recommend that the nonparametric test be used in most circumstances, there may be situations in which there are compelling reasons to prefer the t-test.

One context in which the t-test is not appropriate is as follows. Suppose that a continuous outcome measure such as respiratory or cardiac function is obtained after a specific period of follow-up, but some subjects are unable to perform the test either because they have died or the disease has progressed to the point that they are not physically capable of performing the test. Because the lack of response is informative regarding the condition of the subject, removing them from the analysis, or using naive imputation based on earlier observed values is not appropriate. Rather, it may be sensible to consider these responses to be worse than responses for subjects for whom measurements are available. If, for example, the response is such that all measured values are positive and larger values correspond to better function, then imputing zero for subjects unable to be measured indicates that the responses for these subjects are worse than the actual measurements. Because the Wilcoxon rank-sum test only takes the ordering into account, the choice of imputed value is immaterial provided that it is smaller than all observed responses. Multiple imputed values can also be used; for example, zero for subjects alive but unable to perform the test, and -1 for subjects who have died. This strategy requires that the nonparametric Wilcoxon rank-sum test be used. In some cases, if there is a significant difference in mortality between groups, the difference may be driven primarily by differences in mortality rather than differences in the outcome of interest. While this may seem to be a drawback of the method, since the goal is to assess the effect of treatment on the measure response, in this case a complete case analysis (based solely on directly observed responses) of the outcome of interest is meaningless because it compares responses between quite different subpopulations—those who survived on their respective treatments. There is no obvious, simple solution to the problem of unmeasurable subjects.

Treatment differences for continuous data can be summarized in several ways. The most natural may be simply the difference in means along with an appropriate measure of variability (standard error or confidence interval). Alternatively, depending on the clinical question, it may be more appropriate to use the difference in medians, although the variance for the difference in medians is difficult to derive. (One can use the formula for the variance of the median derived from the bootstrap by Efron (1982).) The Hodges-Lehmann estimator (Hodges and Lehmann 1963) can be used for estimates of location shift based on the Wilcoxon rank-sum tests; however, in some situations the location shift model is not appropriate.

One situation in which the difference in medians may be the most meaningful is when worst scores are imputed for subjects who have died or are physically unable to be tested. If subjects with imputed low scores make up less than half of each group, the median scores will not depend on the choice of imputed value and the group medians will represent the values such that half the subjects have better responses and half have worse responses. In this setting, the location shift model on which the Hodges-Lehmann estimate is based is not appropriate because the imputed low scores are the same for the two groups—only the proportion of subjects assuming these values is subject to change.

Example 2.2. Returning to the TNT example from Section 2.1, Figure 2.2 shows normal probability plots (also known as "Q-Q" plots, see, for example, Venables and Ripley (1999)) of the 3-month changes in LDL for the two treatment groups. Normal probability plots are useful for detecting deviations from normality in observed data. If the underlying distribution is normal, then we expect that the points in the normal probability plot will fall on a diagonal straight line with positive slope. In both treatment groups, the observations clearly fail to fall on straight lines which is strong evidence of a lack of nor-

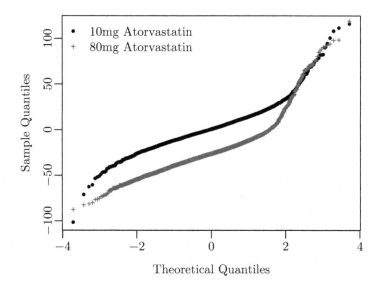

Figure 2.2 *Normal probability (Q-Q) plot of change in LDL at 3 months by treatment in the TNT study.*

mality. In fact, the upper tails of the two distributions (changes above about 37mg/DL) are essentially identical, and in greater numbers than would be expected if the distributions were normal.

The differences by treatment are large enough that samples of size 15 have good power to detect the treatment difference at conventional significance levels. For the sake of this example, we will imagine that the distributions shown in Figure 2.2 represent the underlying population. Table 2.3 shows

Table 2.3 *Power for Wilcoxon rank-sum test and Student's t-test for change in 3-month LDL in TNT. Power is estimated using 10,000 samples with 15 subjects per group.*

	Significance Level		
	0.05	0.01	0.005
Student t-test	94.0%	86.2%	82.4%
Wilcoxon rank-sum test	99.2%	96.0%	92.9%

power for samples drawn from the TNT population with 15 subjects per group. The distributions in each treatment group are sufficiently non-normal, that the Wilcoxon rank-sum test has greater power than the Student t-test for this population. The t-test requires between 30% and 50% greater sample size

to achieve the same power as the Wilcoxon rank-sum test, depending on the
desired significance level.   □

Failure Time Outcomes

The analysis of failure time outcomes is discussed in detail in Chapter 7. A
discussion of the construction of composite failure time outcomes appears in
Section 2.5.

Stratification

In multi-center, and especially in international, studies, one might expect differences in the baseline characteristics of subjects enrolled in different centers
or geographic regions. It can be helpful to conduct *stratified* analyses that
account for these differences, to both ensure that confounding resulting from
chance imbalances do not arise, and account for the increased variability arising from these differences, thereby increasing study power.

Any of the hypothesis tests discussed for binary, ordinal, and continuous
data have a stratified counterpart. For continuous data, the counterpart to
the Student t-test is simply a 2-way analysis of variance with treatment and
stratum as factors. The hypothesis test of interest is based on the F-test for
treatment.

Both the Pearson chi-square test and Wilcoxon rank-sum test are based
on statistics of the form $O - E$ where O is the observed result and E is the
expected result under the null hypothesis. For each there is an accompanying
variance, V. The alternative hypothesis of interest is that the nonzero effect
of treatment is the same in all strata, and in particular that we expect all
$O - E$ to be positive or negative. If we let O_i, E_i, and V_i be the values of O,
E, and V within the ith stratum, assuming that strata are independent, we
can construct stratified test statistics of the form

$$\frac{(\sum O_i - E_i)^2}{\sum V_i},\tag{2.12}$$

that, under H_0, have a chi-square distribution with 1 degree of freedom.

For binary data, using O, E, and V from the Pearson chi-square test, equation (2.12) is known as the *Cochran-Mantel-Haenszel* test (or sometimes just
Mantel-Haenszel test). For the Wilcoxon rank-sum test, O is the observed
rank-sum in either the treatment or control group, E is the expected rank
sum for the corresponding group. The stratified version of the Wilcoxon rank-
sum test is usually referred to as the *Van Elteren* test (Van Elteren 1960).

2.4 The Surrogate Outcome

We have already noted (Section 2.2.2) that the choice of outcome variable can
have a significant impact on the size and length of a trial. While most clini-

cians and patients would prefer to base treatment decisions on the effect that a new intervention might be expected to have on clinical outcomes such as survival or quality of life, the assessment of effects on these outcome variables may require larger trials. *Surrogate outcomes* have been proposed as alternatives, and because they can often be both ascertained more quickly and more sensitive to the direct effect of treatment, their use can result in trials that are smaller and of shorter duration (Prentice 1989; Fleming and DeMets 1996).

The medical community has, on occasion, accepted evidence for the effectiveness of interventions based on surrogate outcomes. Examples include treatments for hypertension that are shown to lower blood pressure, treatments for osteoporosis that increase bone density, treatments that improve heart function for patients with congestive heart failure, treatments that elevate immune cell counts in patients with AIDS, and treatments that suppress arrhythmias in patients at risk for sudden death.

2.4.1 Criteria for Surrogacy

Prentice (1989) identified two criteria that must be satisfied if a particular outcome is to be considered a valid surrogate for a particular clinical outcome:

1. the proposed surrogate must be predictive of the clinical outcome and

2. the proposed surrogate must fully capture the effect of the intervention on the clinical outcome.

The first criterion is usually straightforward to demonstrate while the second is far more difficult, if not impossible, to establish. Figure 2.3 illustrates a simple causal pathway in which the effect of treatment on the clinical outcome results from the effect of treatment on the surrogate outcome. The surrogate outcome is predictive of the clinical outcome (condition 1) and because the adverse clinical outcome results directly from the effect of disease on the surrogate outcome, an intervention that disrupts the effect of disease on the surrogate will also disrupt the effect of disease on the clinical outcome. Hence, under this model, the evidence for a either a beneficial or harmful effect of treatment on the surrogate is sufficient to establish the same effect on the clinical outcome (Fleming and DeMets 1996). On the other hand, the causal pathway is more likely to be similar to one of those shown in Figure 2.4. In each of these scenarios, condition 1 holds because the surrogate outcome and the clinical outcome are both driven by the common underlying disease. On the other hand, condition 2 fails to be satisfied by each. In scenario A, the surrogate has no direct effect on the clinical outcome so a treatment that simply disrupts the effect of disease on the surrogate will have no effect on the clinical outcome. In scenario B, while interfering with the effect of disease on the surrogate has an effect on the clinical outcome, the surrogate will not capture the entire effect. In scenario C, the intervention disrupts the effect of disease on the clinical outcome, but has no effect on the surrogate. Finally, in scenario D the treatment has a direct effect on the clinical outcome inde-

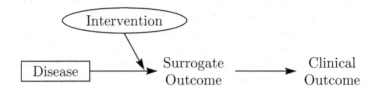

Figure 2.3 *Causal pathway diagram for valid surrogate outcome. (Figure adapted from Fleming and DeMets (1996))*

pendent of the disease processes, possibly in addition to effects on the disease process.

These criteria were mathematically formalized by Prentice (1989) and summarized and generalized by Fleming (1992). The following is based on Fleming's formulation. Let T and S be the true clinical outcome of interest and the proposed surrogate, respectively, and let Z indicate treatment (lower case letters represent values of each). Let f be used to represent the probability density function (p.d.f.) of its arguments. For example, $f(t)$ is the p.d.f. of T and $f(t|z)$ is the conditional p.d.f. of T given Z. A valid surrogate, S, should satisfy

$$f(s|z) = f(s) \iff f(t|z) = f(t). \tag{2.13}$$

That is, the null hypotheses of no treatment effect is true for the surrogate if and only if it is true for the clinical outcome. The criteria described by Prentice are sufficient in most cases to establish (2.13). Symbolically, conditions 1 and 2 can be written

$$f(t|s) \neq f(t) \text{ and} \tag{2.14}$$
$$f(t|s, z) = f(t|s). \tag{2.15}$$

To see that (2.15) is sufficient for ($\Rightarrow$) in (2.13), we use properties of conditional densities to give

$$f(t|z) = \int f(t, s|z) \, ds = \int f(t|s, z) f(s|z) \, ds.$$

Now, assuming the left side of (2.13) holds,

$$f(t|z) = \int f(t|s, z) f(s) \, ds$$

and combined with (2.15) gives

$$f(t|z) = \int f(t|s) f(s) \, ds = \int f(t, s) \, ds = f(t),$$

which is the right hand side of (2.13). Additional restrictions are needed along with (2.14) to give ($\Leftarrow$), but in many cases such restrictions are reasonable.

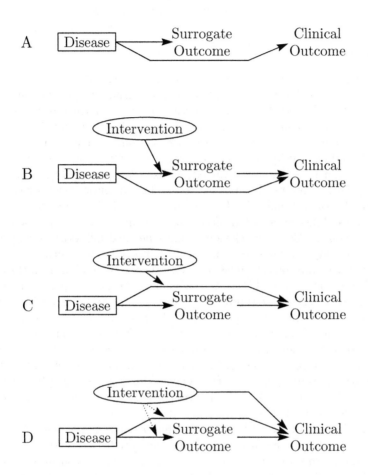

Figure 2.4 *Reasons for failure of surrogate endpoints. A. The surrogate is not in the causal pathway of the disease process. B. Of several causal pathways of disease, the intervention affects only the pathway mediated through the surrogate. C. The surrogate is not in the pathway of the effect of the intervention or is insensitive to its effect. D. The intervention has mechanisms for action independent of the disease process. (Dotted lines indicate mechanisms of action that might exist. Figure adapted from Fleming and DeMets (1996))*

The preceding derivations have all assumed that the variables T and S are continuous, but the same arguments apply when one or both are discrete. In fact, in the case of a binary surrogate outcome, ($\Leftarrow$) can be shown to hold when (2.14) and (2.15) are true (Burzykowski et al. 2005).

2.4.2 Examples

We now describe several cases for which criterion (2.15) was not met. The Nocturnal Oxygen Therapy Trial (NOTT) (Nocturnal Oxygen Therapy Trial Group 1980) evaluated the effect of nocturnal versus continuous oxygen supplementation in 203 subjects with advanced chronic obstructive lung disease (COPD). The primary outcomes were a series of pulmonary function tests including forced expiratory volume in one second (FEV_1), forced vital capacity (FVC) and functional residual capacity (FRC), and quality of life measures including the Minnesota Multiphasic Personality Inventory (Dahlstrom et al. 1972), the Sickness Impact Profile (Bergner et al. 1976), and the Profile of Mood States (Waskow and Parloff 1975). Mortality was one of several secondary outcomes. At the conclusion of the scheduled follow-up period, none of the pulmonary function tests demonstrated a difference between the two oxygen supplementation schedules, nor were there any differences in the quality of life outcomes. Nonetheless, the mortality rate in the nocturnal oxygen group was twice that of the continuous oxygen group (Figure 2.5) and statistically significant at the 0.01 level. While each of the pulmonary function tests could be potential surrogate outcomes for the clinical outcome of survival, none captured the beneficial effect of continuous oxygen. If the pulmonary function had been the sole outcome, then one might have concluded that both doses of oxygen were equally effective. Obviously, those suffering from COPD would have been ill served by such a conclusion. Fortunately, the mortality outcome was also available.

Another important example is the Cardiac Arrhythmia Suppression Trial (CAST).[5] Recall that cardiac arrhythmias are predictive of sudden death. Drugs were approved on the basis of arrhythmia suppression in a high risk group of subjects. CAST was conducted on a less severe group of subjects using mortality as the primary outcome. Prior to randomization, subjects were required to complete a *run-in* period and demonstrate that their arrhythmia could be suppressed by one of the drugs. At the conclusion of the run-in, subjects responding to the drug were randomized to either an active drug or a corresponding placebo. Surprisingly, CAST was terminated early because of a statistically significant increase in mortality for subjects on the active arrhythmia suppressing drugs. Arrhythmia suppression failed to capture the effect of the drug on the clinical outcome of all-cause mortality. If CAST had not used mortality as a primary outcome, many thousands of patients may have been treated with this class of drugs.

---

[5] The Cardiac Arrhythmia Suppression Trial (CAST) Investigators (1989)

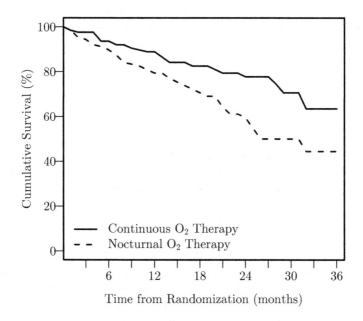

Figure 2.5 *Cumulative all-cause mortality in NOTT. (Figure adapted from Noctur-nal Oxygen Therapy Trial Group (1980))*

Heart failure is a disease in which the heart is weakened and unable to ad-equately pump blood. Heart failure symptoms include dyspnea (shortness of breath) and fatigue and sufferers are often unable to carry on normal daily activities. A class of drugs known as *inotropes* are known to increase car-diac contractility and improve cardiac function. The PROMISE trial (Packer et al. 1991) was conducted to determine the long term effect of milrinone, an inotrope, that was known to improve heart function. Over 1,000 subjects were randomized to either milrinone or placebo, each in addition to the best available care. In the end, PROMISE was terminated early with a significant increase in mortality for subjects in the milrinone group compared to placebo.

Finally, AIDS is a disease in which the immune system of those infected with the HIV virus becomes increasingly compromised until the infected individual becomes vulnerable to opportunistic infections and other fatal insults to the immune system. With the AIDS epidemic raging in the late 1980s, there was a great deal of pressure to find effective treatments as quickly as possible. The use of CD4 cell counts as a measure of immune system function appeared to be an effective alternative to trials assessing long term mortality or other clinical outcomes. Eventually, additional studies demonstrated that drugs improving immune function do not necessarily improve mortality or increase the time to progression of AIDS in subjects with HIV. In addition, treatments were found that did not improve the immune system's CD4 cell count but did improve time to progression of AIDS or survival. CD4 cell count seems not to be a valid surrogate measure for clinical status (Fleming 1994).

2.4.3 Statistical Surrogate Validation

Statistical validation of potential surrogate outcomes has been an area of great interest and research. Burzykowski et al. (2005) discuss many proposed approaches and we will follow their notation. In order to statistically check Prentice's criteria directly, in the case of a continuous (normal) clinical outcome, a common approach is to use the linear models

$$T_j = \mu + \gamma S_j + \varepsilon_j \qquad\qquad (2.16)$$

and

$$T_j = \tilde{\mu}_T + \beta_S Z_j + \gamma_Z S_j + \tilde{\varepsilon}_{Tj}, \qquad\qquad (2.17)$$

where j indexes subjects and ε_j and $\tilde{\varepsilon}_{Tj}$ are normal with mean 0. The failure of condition (2.14) implies the null hypothesis that $\gamma = 0$ in (2.16). The criterion is confirmed if the hypothesis is rejected at, say, the 0.05 level. The second criterion (2.15) is equivalent to the null hypothesis that $\beta_S = 0$ in (2.17). In this case, however, rejecting this hypothesis would result in rejection of the candidate as a valid surrogate. Validation of a surrogate requires that we *accept* the null hypothesis. This situation, for which traditional hypothesis testing does not provide resolution, presents researchers with a difficult and controversial decision.

An alternative approach to formal hypothesis testing is to quantify the extent to which a candidate outcome captures the effect of treatment on a particular clinical outcome. One of the first measures developed for this purpose, the *proportion of treatment effect explained by the surrogate*, or simply *proportion explained* (*PE*), was first introduced in the context of a logistic regression model (Freedman et al. 1992). For continuous outcomes, we use equation (2.17), as well as the following:

$$T_j = \mu_T + \beta Z_j + \varepsilon_{Tj}, \qquad\qquad (2.18)$$

where ε_{Tj} is normally distributed with mean 0 and variance σ_{TT}. *PE* is defined as

$$PE = \frac{\beta - \beta_S}{\beta}.$$

If a certain outcome is a "perfect" surrogate, one would expect $PE = 1$. In contrast, a poor surrogate should give a value for *PE* at or near 0. Thus, the idea does have some intuitive appeal. Confidence intervals for *PE* can be calculated using Fieller's Theorem or the δ-method (see Appendix A.1). It has been suggested that a surrogate outcome may perform well if the lower limit of the 95% confidence interval for PE is greater than 0.5 or 0.75 (Freedman et al. 1992; Lin et al. 1997).

One of the difficulties with this measure is that it is not truly a proportion at all. In theory, PE can take any real value and in many practical situations the estimate is outside the interval $[0,1]$. Examples can also be constructed in which only the beneficial effect of the treatment is captured by the surrogate (Hughes 2002). In this case, PE can be greater than 1, which one might incorrectly interpret as evidence for an effective surrogate. Thus, interpretation of values taken by PE can be difficult. This difficulty is even greater if a treatment by surrogate interaction term is required in model (2.17). In addition, the confidence intervals for PE tend to be wide in practice (Lin et al. 1997; Burzykowski et al. 2005). Even when the point estimate for PE lies in the interval $[0,1]$, the corresponding confidence interval may contain all of $[0,1]$. These and other unreliable statistical properties make PE a measure that is not recommended (DeGruttola et al. 2001).

Burzykowski et al. (2005) suggest the use of two alternatives to PE. The first, called the *relative effect* (RE), is based on (2.18) and an additional relation

$$S_j = \mu_S + \alpha Z_j + \varepsilon_{Sj}$$

where ε_{Sj} is normally distributed with mean 0, variance σ_{SS}, and the covariance between ε_{Sj} and ε_{Tj} is $\mathrm{Cov}(\varepsilon_{Sj}, \varepsilon_{Tj}) = \sigma_{ST}$. RE is defined by

$$RE = \frac{\beta}{\alpha}$$

and compares the aggregate effect of treatment on the true clinical outcome to its effect on the surrogate. A value of 1 indicates that the magnitude of the treatment effect is the same for both the surrogate and the true outcome. Note, however, that the relative magnitude of the values of the two outcomes and the scale on which they are measured must be considered when interpreting the observed value of RE. The second alternative measure, called *adjusted association*, is

$$\rho_Z = \frac{\sigma_{ST}}{\sqrt{\sigma_{SS}\sigma_{TT}}}.$$

Note that ρ_Z is the correlation between the clinical outcome and the surrogate, after adjusting for the treatment. PE, RE, and ρ_Z are related by

$$PE = \frac{\lambda \rho_Z}{RE},$$

where $\lambda = \sqrt{\sigma_{TT}/\sigma_{SS}}$, the ratio of the standard deviations of the two outcomes (a nuisance parameter). In contrast to PE, RE can be interpreted outside the interval $[0,1]$. ρ_Z, on the other hand, is restricted to the interval $[0,1]$. Although these two measures are more easily interpreted than PE, confidence intervals for RE still tend to be very wide.

These measures have been derived in the situation where one has normally distributed outcome variables. As mentioned, PE was first developed using a binary outcome and logistic regression coefficients (Freedman et al. 1992) and has also been used for a survival outcome (Lin et al. 1997). The calculation of PE in this case was based on Cox model coefficients. Burzykowski et al. (2005) discuss extensions of RE and ρ_Z, including cases when surrogates and clinical outcomes are of different data types, for example, longitudinal or ordinal surrogates for survival clinical outcomes.

Since one of the shortcomings of both PE and RE is the tendency to have wide confidence intervals, meaningful surrogate validation requires large sample size. Several authors have recommended the use of meta-analyses for surrogate validation (Burzykowski et al. 2005; Lin et al. 1997; DeGruttola et al. 2001; Hughes 2002). By assessing the performance of possible surrogate outcomes from several related trials, future trials can make better use of existing information and the results will have a better foundation for extrapolation to other treatments or populations. The quantities RE and ρ_Z have been generalized to provide, respectively, trial-level and individual-level measures for surrogate evaluation (Molenberghs et al. 2002; Burzykowski et al. 2005) using meta-analyses.

While meta-analysis is the recommended approach for surrogate outcome validation, it also presents challenges (DeGruttola et al. 2001; Hughes 2002). Extensive follow-up data must be collected for all subjects. This gives rise to another difficulty: access to the raw data and combining data from multiple trials may be difficult (see Chapter 6). The trials included must also be sufficiently similar. It would be unusual to find a large number of trials with the same clinical outcome, the same surrogate outcome, and the same treatment. While it may be possible to combine trials that differ in one or more of the features, more sophisticated statistical methods are required.

While the methods for surrogate validation that we have discussed can be useful, one must keep in mind that no statistical analysis can definitively establish the validity of a potential surrogate outcome. Statistical analyses should be combined with informed medical judgment regarding the underlying diseases processes and the treatments involved. In addition, an outcome that is accepted as a valid surrogate for one drug in a class may not be valid for other drugs in the same class. Far less certain is the validity across drug classes. When definitive evidence of efficacy and safety is required, one should rely on surrogates only when the obstacles to the use of clinical outcomes make their use impractical.

2.5 Composite Outcomes

We use the term *composite outcome* to refer to any outcome that is obtained by combining two or more distinct responses into a single outcome. Composite outcomes serve several purposes.

- Often, the full effect of treatment cannot be captured meaningfully by a single outcome and a hierarchy of responses is required. For example, for subjects with a respiratory disorder such as emphysema, both survival and pulmonary function are of interest and a composite outcome could be constructed using 6 month survival and 6 month pulmonary function among the survivors. As described previously (page 54), an outcome score can be constructed in which subjects who die are assigned a low value, otherwise the pulmonary function score is used. The effect of treatment would be assessed using the Wilcoxon rank-sum test.

- If treatment is expected to provide benefit for several different responses, it may be possible to increase power by combining them into a single outcome. For example, Zhang et al. (1997) describe a trial in subjects with asthma with 4 outcomes: forced expiratory volume in 1 second (FEV_1), peak expiratory flow rate (PEFR), symptoms score (SS) on 0-6 scale, and additional (rescue) medication use. Each of these measures a different manifestation of the disease and collectively measure the overall burden on a subject.

- Failure time outcomes frequently involve multiple event types. For example, a composite failure time outcome might be the first of all-cause death or nonfatal myocardial infarction.

Outcomes of the first type were discussed in Section 2.3.1, and we will not discuss them further. In the following sections, we discuss combining multiple response variables into a single outcome and composite failure time outcomes.

2.5.1 Combining Multiple Outcomes

When there is an expectation that the effect of treatment on each of several equally important outcomes is roughly the same, study power may be increased by combining them into a single outcome. O'Brien (1984) discussed two procedures; a nonparametric rank-sum procedure and a procedure based on multivariate normality assumptions. We take each in turn.

O'Brien's Rank-sum Procedure

Suppose that for subject i in treatment group j we observe response y_{ijk} for outcome k. For each k, assign rank r_{ijk} to observation y_{ijk} according to equation (2.10). For subject i, in group j, the overall score is $s_{ij} = \sum_k r_{ijk}$. The rank sum from equation (2.11) becomes

$$S = \sum_i s_{i1} - K \frac{n_1(n_1 + n_2 + 1)}{2}.$$

The variance of S is more complicated than in the ordinary Wilcoxon rank sum case, and the recommended analysis is simply a two-sample t-test using the s_{ij}. See O'Brien (1984) or Zhang et al. (1997) for examples.

O'Brien Test Based on Multivariate Normal Distribution

Another approach discussed by O'Brien (1984) and Pocock et al. (1987) is based on the assumption of multivariate normality. Let $t = (t_1, \cdots, t_k)'$ denote a vector of k two-sample t-test statistics, R the estimated common correlation matrix of k outcomes in each treatment group, and J a k-dimensional vector of ones. The test statistic

$$Z = \frac{J'R^{-1}t}{\sqrt{J'R^{-1}J}} \tag{2.19}$$

has an asymptotic standard normal distribution.

2.5.2 Composite Failure Time Outcomes

It is common practice, especially in cardiology and cancer, for clinical trials to use composite outcomes in either primary or secondary analyses. A composite outcome is an event that is considered to have occurred if at least one of its component events has occurred. Composite outcomes are usually analyzed using survival analysis techniques that are discussed in detail in Chapter 7. Generally, mortality is one of the component events so that one can consider the time to the first composite event as "event-free survival" time. In cancer trials, the nonfatal component may be recurrence of a tumor. In cardiology, there may be multiple nonfatal components including nonfatal myocardial infarction, nonfatal stroke, or an urgent revascularization procedure (surgical procedure to remove or bypass blockages in critical arteries). Similar combinations of fatal and nonfatal events are used in other disease areas.

Rationale for the use of Composite Failure Time Outcomes

The rationale for the use of composite failure time outcomes is both clinical and statistical and has been discussed by a number of authors (Moyé 2003; Neaton et al. 2005; DeMets and Califf 2002; Montori et al. 2005). We briefly outline some of them here. Clinically, a treatment for a serious, life-threatening disease should target the processes that lead to intermediate outcomes such as irreversible injury (for example, myocardial infarction or stroke) or disease recurrence (new tumors). An effective treatment should be expected to reduce not only the incidence of death, but also the incidence of certain of these intermediate events. Hence, a composite outcome can be used to capture a broader effect of treatment, beyond mortality alone. In addition, the effect of treatment on intermediate events is often expected to be greater than the effect on mortality—especially since new treatments for patients with many acute conditions continue to reduce mortality rates. The target of a therapy may be solely the nonfatal component and mortality is included as a part of the composite outcome for statistical reasons to be discussed below.

Other reasons for the use of composite outcomes are statistical. A frequent motivation is increased study power, or a corresponding decrease in sample size. Power and sample size will be discussed in detail in Chapter 4, so for the purpose of this discussion, we note only that when the primary outcome is a failure time outcome, the sample size is generally a function of the relative effect size ("relative risk") and the incidence rate of the event. As additional components are added to the primary composite outcome, the overall incidence rate increases. Provided that the relative effect of treatment on the expanded composite outcome is sufficiently large, adding an event type to the primary outcome can reduce the required sample size for the trial.

A second, more important, statistical reason for using a composite outcome arises when the target of the therapy is a nonfatal event for diseases in which mortality is a significant *competing risk*. By *competing risk* we mean an event that, when it occurs, precludes observation of the event of interest. Specifically, subjects who die during follow-up are obviously no longer at risk for nonfatal events, and therefore the rate at which we observe nonfatal events is intrinsically linked to mortality. If we restrict our attention to nonfatal events in the presence of mortality, the interpretation of the analysis becomes murky.

To illustrate, consider the simple example shown in Table 2.4, in which, for simplicity, we ignore the timing of the events. In this example, the first row

Table 2.4 *Simple example of interaction between treatment, mortality, and a nonfatal outcome. Nonfatal events are not observed for subjects who die. Observable quantities are shown in bold. Treatment has an effect on the nonfatal outcome but not on mortality.*

| | | Treatment A | | | Treatment B | | |
		Dead	Alive	Total	Dead	Alive	Total
Nonfatal outcome	Y	10	**25**	35	10	**20**	30
	N	10	**55**	65	10	**60**	70
		20	**80**	**100**	**20**	**80**	**100**

corresponds to subjects who, in the absence of mortality, would experience a nonfatal outcome event, while the first column of each table corresponds to subjects who die. We assume that subjects die prior to experiencing the nonfatal event and so we cannot observe the nonfatal event. The numbers in bold are observable quantities.

Treatment has no effect on mortality, but treatment B reduces the number or subjects who, in the absence of mortality, would experience the nonfatal event from 35 to 30. Because mortality precludes observation of the nonfatal outcome, however, the *observed* number of nonfatal outcome events in each group changes as a results of subject deaths. The *observed* number of nonfatal events in group A is 25 versus 20 in group B. In this example, the inference that the nonfatal event rate is lower in group B is correct (although it is interesting to further note that the observed relative reduction overstates the true relative reduction—20% versus 15%.)

A second example is shown in Table 2.5. First note that the observable quantities are the same as those in Table 2.4 and that the only differences appear in the unobservable quantities. Here treatment has no direct effect on the nonfatal outcome so the number of subjects in the first row is the same, 30, in each treatment group. On the other hand, even though the total number of deaths is the same in the two treatment groups, the allocation of

Table 2.5 *Simple example of interaction between treatment, mortality, and a nonfatal outcome. Nonfatal events are not observed for subjects who die. Observable quantities are shown in bold. Treatment has a subject level effect on mortality, but no net effect on mortality or the nonfatal outcome.*

		Treatment A			Treatment B		
		Dead	Alive	Total	Dead	Alive	Total
Nonfatal outcome	Y	5	**25**	30	10	**20**	30
	N	15	**55**	70	10	**60**	70
		20	**80**	**100**	**20**	**80**	**100**

treatments between subjects potentially experiencing the nonfatal event differs by treatment. Because more deaths occur in the first row for treatment B than for treatment A, the *observed* number of subjects with nonfatal events is smaller in treatment B than in treatment A. The effect of treatment B relative to treatment A is to shift mortality from subjects not at risk for the nonfatal event to subjects who are at risk for the nonfatal event. Thus, if we consider the nonfatal outcome in isolation we might conclude, erroneously, that treatment B has a beneficial effect on the nonfatal outcome. The critical feature of this example is that the true underlying model is *unidentifiable*, that is there are at least two distinct underlying relationships between treatment, mortality, and the nonfatal outcome that generate precisely the same observed data.

In each case we can consider the composite of fatal and nonfatal events; there are 45 in group A and 40 in group B. A best (statistical) interpretation of these data is that at the *population level*,

- there is no net treatment difference in mortality, and

- there is a beneficial effect of treatment B relative to treatment B with respect to the composite outcome of fatal and nonfatal events.

As we note, the inference is restricted to the population level—inference at the subject level is difficult. In Table 2.4, 5 individual subjects who would have experienced a nonfatal event on treatment A no longer do if given treatment B. In 2.5, however, 5 subjects who would have died instead experience a nonfatal event while 5 subjects, who would have survived event free, die. It is not possible from the data to distinguish these two scenarios.

One might argue that the scenario in Table 2.5 is biologically unrealistic. This scenario could arise if, for example, treatment A actually has benefit with respect to disease progression so that subjects at risk for the nonfatal event survive; however, there is offsetting toxicity independent of disease that results in increased mortality for subjects not at risk for the nonfatal event. The lack of identifiability implies that it is not possible to statistically rule out this possibility. Any such inference must be conducted based on other external information or scientific insight.

Multiple Nonfatal Event Types

Thus far we have considered only the case in which we have a single nonfatal event in addition to all-cause mortality. When there are several nonfatal events under consideration, for example, myocardial infarction and unstable angina, there is another operating principle at work. Specifically, that when possible, the hierarchical structure of the set of events be respected. That is, if a particular event type is to be included, all related events of greater severity should also be included. To illustrate, consider myocardial infarction and unstable angina. *Unstable angina* (UA) is a condition in which people experience chest pain when at rest or under minimal physical exertion. UA results from blockages in coronary arteries that significantly reduce blood flow, and hence oxygen, to portions of the heart. If a coronary artery becomes completely blocked, a portion of heart muscle may be completely deprived of oxygen and either die or become permanently damaged. This condition is known as a *myocardial infarction* (MI). Thus, an MI can be thought of as a more severe instance of UA.

Now suppose that a proposed treatment, rather than decreasing the underlying arterial blockages, actually made them worse in some subjects, causing them to experience MI rather than simply UA (see Fleiss et al. (1990) for a similar example). The observed rate of UA could in fact decrease, not because the treatment made the underlying condition better, but because it made it worse. If the composite outcome includes UA but not MI, one can be completely misled about the true benefit of treatment.

Recommendations Regarding the use of Composite Failure Time Outcomes

Here we present recommendations regarding the use of composite outcomes. The principle underlying these recommendations is that the conclusions resulting from the analysis of a randomized clinical trial should be based on sound statistical practice combined with informed clinical judgment. Many authors (Montori et al. 2005; Moyé 2003; Yusuf and Negassa 2002) have made statistical recommendations based on the clinical questions of greatest interest, but have not always given adequate attention to the statistical complexities of the data that we can observe. Many clinical questions cannot be answered statistically and analyses are often performed that answer different questions than those that have been posed.

In the simplistic examples of Tables 2.4 and 2.5, we recommended two analyses:

- a comparison of rates of all-cause mortality in the two treatment groups, and

- a comparison of the composite outcome of all-cause mortality and the nonfatal outcome (disease-free survival).

From these analyses, sound statistical reasoning would first conclude that there is no difference in overall mortality between the treatment groups. Second, it would conclude that there is a difference in the occurrence of the *composite* outcome between the treatment groups. Informed clinical judgment would then be brought to bear to interpret these results. One issue to be considered is the plausibility of an interaction between mortality and the nonfatal outcome of the type that appears in Table 2.5. If informed clinical judgment suggests that such a scenario is unlikely, the alternative conclusion is that the underlying structure may be like that of Table 2.4, and that the most likely explanation for the observed data is that treatment B in fact has a beneficial effect on the nonfatal outcome. Caution must be advised, however, since one can never be certain that a scenario such as that shown in Table 2.5 does not hold.

Thus, when there are compelling reasons—both clinical and statistical—for including a particular nonfatal event procedure we propose that a composite outcome be used and constructed according to the following principles.

- All-cause mortality should always be a component of a composite outcome.
- If a particular nonfatal event is to be included in the composite outcome, all related events of greater severity should also be included.
- Subject to the previous principle, if a particular nonfatal event is to be included in the composite outcome, there should be an expectation of a sufficient treatment benefit with respect to this event. The only exception to this principle is the case where an event is included because a related event of lesser severity is also included.

Contrary to the recommendation of some authors, these principles do not require that there is an expectation that the size of the treatment effect be comparable across the outcome components. Statistically, the composite outcome should be treated as a single outcome that satisfies the assumptions that are discussed for failure time outcomes in Chapter 7. The problem of the apparent inhomogeneous treatment effects across outcome components is not solved by considering each outcome separately as some authors suggest, since as indicated previously, these hypothesis tests either test hypotheses regarding conditional parameters (conditional on the subject being alive) or are subject to the phenomenon described above—that rates at which less severe events occur are decreased by increasing the severity of the event. Rather, the problem of apparent inhomogeneous treatment effect is best addressed using a series of analyses that respect the hierarchy of event types and bringing informed clinical judgment to the results. For example, we would consider separate analyses of all-cause mortality, the composite of all-cause mortality and nonfatal MI, and finally the composite of all-cause mortality, nonfatal MI, and unstable angina.

2.5.3 Use of Baseline Measurement

Many trials enroll subjects with a history of abnormal values of a physiological measurement such as blood pressure or cholesterol and the goal of the trial is to alter this parameter and thereby reduce the risk of serious adverse consequences such as heart attacks or strokes. It seems natural in this setting to use the subject's change from baseline (the value recorded immediately before treatment start) as the outcome measure. This strategy is particularly appealing if there is substantial variability in baseline measures and the expected changes within subjects are relatively small. In this case using change from baseline eliminates between-subject variability from the estimate of the treatment effect and potentially increasing power. If, however, the population is relatively homogeneous, so that the variability in individual measurements is greater than the between-subject variability, using change from baseline may actually increase the variability in the observed treatment difference because the baseline value is not closely related to the follow-up value, and subtracting the baseline value merely contributes additional noise.

To make this idea concrete, consider the following simple model. Suppose that subject i has two values, Z_{i0} and Z_{i1}, for the true parameter at baseline and follow-up respectively. Suppose further that we do not observe Z_{ij} exactly, but instead we observe $Y_{ij} = Z_{ij} + \epsilon_{ij}$ where the ϵ_{ij} are i.i.d. Gaussian with mean zero and variance σ^2. Assume further that $Z_{i1} - Z_{i0} = \mu + \gamma z$, where z is an indicator of treatment group, and Z_{i0} is Gaussian with mean ν and variance τ^2 (note that we are assuming that the baseline and follow-up values have the same variance). Then the variance of the observed Y_{i1} is $\mathrm{Var}[\epsilon_{i1}] + \mathrm{Var}[Z_{i1}] = \tau^2 + \sigma^2$. On the other hand, the variance of $Y_{i1} - Y_{i0} = \mu + \gamma z + \epsilon_{i1} - \epsilon_{i0}$ is $\mathrm{Var}[\epsilon_{i1}] + \mathrm{Var}[\epsilon_{i0}] = 2\sigma^2$. Thus, we would prefer Y_{i1} over $Y_{i1} - Y_{i0}$ as the outcome measure if $\sigma^2 > \tau^2$.

It may not be known in advance which of these is preferred unless sufficient knowledge of the values of σ^2 and τ^2 is available at the design stage. An alternative to either of these choices is to use the baseline value as a covariate in a linear regression model. First, note that the covariance matrix of the vector $(Y_{i0}, Y_{i1})^T$ is

$$\begin{bmatrix} \tau^2 + \epsilon^2 & \tau^2 \\ \tau^2 & \tau^2 + \epsilon^2 \end{bmatrix}.$$

By the properties of bi-variate normal distributions, we have that the conditional mean of Y_{1i} given Y_{i0} is $E[Y_{i1}|Y_{i0}] = \mu + \gamma z + \rho(Y_{i0} - \nu)$ and the conditional variance is $\mathrm{Var}(Y_{i1}|Y_{i0}) = \sigma^2(1 + \rho)$ where $\rho = \tau^2/(\tau^2 + \sigma^2)$ is the correlation between Y_{1i} and Y_{i0}. Therefore, the observations at follow-up satisfy the linear model of the form

$$Y_{i1} = \beta_0 + \rho Y_{i0} + \gamma z + \epsilon_i', \qquad (2.20)$$

where ϵ_i' is Gaussian with mean zero and variance $\sigma^2(1+\rho)$. When $\rho = 0$, the baseline and follow-up observations are independent, and the baseline value provides no useful information, so it is ignored. If ρ is near one, then σ^2 is small relative to τ^2, and we gain efficiency by subtracting the baseline value. Thus, the linear model given in (2.20) is a compromise between the analysis of change from baseline and the analysis using only the follow-up observation. When the sample size is sufficient to provide a reliable estimate of $\beta_1 = \rho$, this analysis will be more efficient than either of the other two analyses. The asymptotic variances of $\hat{\gamma}$ using the three approaches is given in Table 2.6

when there are two equal sized treatment groups of size m. Note that the

Table 2.6 *Asymptotic variances for three approaches to the use of baseline values in the estimation of the treatment difference. We assume that there are m subjects per treatment group and ρ is the correlation between baseline and follow-up measurements.*

Method	Variance
Ignore baseline	$2\sigma^2/m(1-\rho)$
Change from baseline	$4\sigma^2/m$
Model (2.20)	$2\sigma^2(1+\rho)/m$

estimate of γ using model (2.20) always has smaller asymptotic variance than both of the other estimates. Frison and Pocock (1992) extend this model to situations with multiple baseline and follow-up measures. Thisted (2006) also investigates the use of baseline in the context of more general longitudinal models.

One drawback to the analysis using equation (2.20) is that it assumes that the observations, $(Y_{i0}, Y_{i1})^T$, are approximately bivariate normal. A nonparametric version of this approach can be implemented by first replacing the observed Y_{ij} by their rank scores (separately for baseline and follow-up) and performing the analysis based on equation (2.20).

Table 2.7 *Power for treatment difference in 3-month LDL for TNT data using samples of 15 per group and 6 different analyses based on 100,000 samples.*

		Significance Level		
		.05	.01	.005
Observed Data	Ignore baseline	88.9	74.0	66.4
	Change from Baseline	94.0	85.5	81.1
	Linear model (2.20)	94.4	86.6	82.8
Ranked Data	Ignore baseline	91.3	76.1	68.1
	Change from Baseline	98.3	93.0	89.0
	Linear model (2.20)	96.5	88.9	83.8

Example 2.3. Returning to the TNT example, we drew samples of both baseline and 3-month LDL size 15 per group and performed six analysis: t-test using only 3-month LDL, t-test using change in LDL at month 3, the linear model in equation (2.20), these three analyses repeated using the ranks of the respective responses. Table 2.7 shows power for each of these analysis and 3 different significance levels. For the analysis using the observed responses, the analysis using change from baseline yields higher power than does the analysis

ignoring baseline, and the analysis based on model (2.20) has slightly higher power than the analysis using change from baseline. Each of the analyses using ranked data has greater power than the corresponding unranked analyses. Unlike the unranked analysis, the analyses using the ranks of the change from baseline appears to have greater power than does the analysis using model (2.20) applied to the ranks.

$\square$

2.6 Summary

At all stages of design, conduct of analysis of a clinical trial, one must keep in mind the overall question of interest. In most cases, the question has a form such as "do subjects treated with agent A have better outcomes than those treated with agent B?" All design elements from the definition of the primary outcome and the associated statistical test, to the sample size and interim monitoring plan, are created with this question in mind. Secondary and supplemental analyses will prove to be important aids to the interpretation of the final result, but cannot be a valid substitute when the primary question does not provide a satisfactory result. The foundational principles of causal inference require that we adhere as much as possible to the intent-to-treat principle.

2.7 Problems

2.1 Find a clinical trial article in a medical journal. Determine how the investigators/authors have defined the question. Identify the study population. Identify the primary, secondary, and other questions. What kind of outcome measure(s) was(were) used? What was the approach used to analyze the data? Is there any part of defining the question you would have done differently? Explain why or why not.

2.2 Find an example of a clinical trial in which a surrogate outcome was used but results were later questioned because the surrogate perhaps did not satisfy the criteria.

CHAPTER 3

Study Design

Once the hypothesis has been formulated, including what outcome variables will be used to evaluate the effect of the intervention, the next major challenge that must be addressed is the specification of the experimental design. Getting the correct design for the question being posed is critical since no amount of statistical analysis can adjust for an inadequate or inappropriate design. While the typical clinical trial design is usually simpler than many of the classical experimental designs available (Cochran and Cox 1957; Cox 1958; Fisher 1925; Fisher 1935), there are still many choices that are being used (Friedman et al. 1998).

While the concept of a randomized control is relatively new to clinical research, starting in the 1950's with first trials sponsored by the Medical Research Council, there are, of course, examples in history where a control group was not necessary. Examples include studies of the effectiveness of penicillin in treating pneumococcal pneumonia and a vaccine for preventing rabies in dogs. These examples, however, are rare and in clinical practice we must rely on controlled trials to obtain the best evidence of safety and efficacy for new diagnostic tests, drugs, biologics, devices, procedures, and behavioral modifications.

In this chapter, we first describe the early phase trial designs that are used to obtain critical data with which to properly design the ultimate definitive trial. As discussed, once a new intervention has been developed, it may have to go through several stages before the ultimate test for efficacy. For example, for a drug or biologic one of the first challenges is to determine the maximum dose that can be given without unacceptable toxicity. This is evaluated in a *phase I* trial. A next step is to determine if the new intervention modifies a risk factor or symptom as desired, and to further assess safety. This may be accomplished through a *phase II* trial or a series of phase II studies. Once sufficient information is obtained about the new intervention, it must be compared to a control or standard intervention to assess efficacy and safety. This is often referred to as a *phase III* trial. Trials of an approved treatment with long-term follow-up of safety and efficacy are often called *phase IV* trials. (See Fisher (1999) and Fisher and Moyé (1999) for an example of the U.S. Food and Drug Administration (FDA) approval process.) While these phase designations are somewhat arbitrary, they are still useful in thinking about the progression of trials needed to proceed to the final definitive trial. Once the classical phase I and II designs have been described, we discuss choices of control groups, including the randomized control. The rest of the chapter will focus on randomized control designs, beginning with a discussion of trials designed to show superiority of the new experimental intervention over a standard intervention. Other trials are designed to show that, at worst, the new intervention is not inferior to the standard to within a predetermined margin of indifference. These trials can be extremely difficult to conduct and interpret, and we discuss some of the associated challenges. Finally, we address *adaptive designs* which are intended to allow for design changes in response to intermediate results of the trial.

3.1 Early Phase Trials

Medical treatments are subjected to a rigorous evaluation process between the time of their conception, preclinical testing, and confirmation with a definitive phase III trial. Most, in fact, do not complete the process. "Every year the pharmaceutical industry develops thousands of new compounds in the hope that some of them will ultimately prove useful in the treatment of human disease" (Ryan and Soper 2005). In the case of potential cancer treatments, for example, only one in ten succeeds (Goldberg 2006). There are a number of possible development pathways that a particular treatment can take. Generally, new compounds are initially subjected to extensive biochemical and pharmacological analysis, progressing to experiments using animal and *in vitro* models and, increasingly, *in silico*, or computer, models. Once these non-clinical studies are completed, the compound may make the transition from "mouse to man" (Schneiderman 1967; Gart et al. 1986). Investigators will then have to rely completely on prospective studies in humans for preliminary clinical information. On the other hand, a new application may be proposed for a treatment about which much is already known. For example, when aspirin was proposed as an anticlotting agent for those at risk of heart attack, it had already been in use as a pain reliever for more than eighty years with attendant information on side-effects, overdoses, and other risks.

The first clinical problem (that is, one that is directly related to human treatment) is to determine an acceptable dose and form of administration for an agent. Although "dose" usually refers to the quantity of a drug, it may also apply to other regimens and procedures such as amount or duration of therapeutic radiation. Initial dose-setting studies, often with 20 to 50 subjects, are called phase I trials (Storer 1989). They may be undertaken using healthy voluntary or paid subjects when the expected toxicities are minor or, alternatively, extremely ill patients administered fairly toxic therapies for diseases such as cancer, having failed all standard options. Phase II trials (Thall and Simon 1995) are typically small prospective studies that evaluate a therapy's potential and may be randomized or not.

Although the distinctions between study phases are useful, they are continually evolving and new intermediate or combination designs are introduced, so the lines aren't always clear. Proposed phase I/II trials (Hardwick et al. (2003) and Gooley et al. (1994), for example) investigate both toxicity and short-term efficacy on the same subjects. Phase II/III designs (Gallo et al. 2006; Storer 1990), also termed *adaptive designs*, begin with an exploratory study of efficacy and, if successful, proceed to a larger confirmatory trial incorporating the same subjects. The FDA has even suggested "phase 0" exploratory studies of cancer drugs (Goldberg 2006). Microdoses much smaller than those to be used for therapy would be given to willing cancer patients and healthy volunteers. Metabolic properties and effects on biomarkers would be assessed and imaging studies performed. Despite these hybridizations, we will associate the term "phase I" with dose-finding trials and "phase II" with efficacy screening trials.

3.1.1 Phase I trials

A phase I trial as defined by Meinert (1996) is "[b]roadly, a trial involving the first applications of a new treatment to human beings and conducted to generate preliminary information on safety." Phase I trials of therapies in cancer and other severe diseases usually have the specific goal of finding the *maximum tolerated dose* (MTD) to use in further testing of efficacy. This dose is quantitatively defined as the largest dose of a drug or other therapeutic agent that induces at most a set proportion, usually 1/3, of subjects with predefined toxicities. Ethical considerations require that the MTD is found by giving the first subjects a very low dose and then sequentially escalating the dose in subsequent patients or subjects until toxicities are observed. The sequential nature of traditional phase I trials requires these toxicities to be short-term, usually occurring within four to eight weeks of initial treatment. See Figure 3.1 for an illustration of the phase I approach in which the goal is to estimate the MTD as the 33rd percentile of the dose-toxicity curve, while minimizing the number of subjects receiving toxic doses.

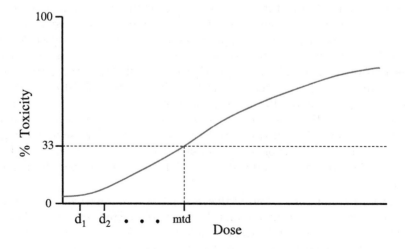

Figure 3.1 *Schematic of phase I trial.*

Typically, investigators pick a set of three to ten doses for evaluation in a phase I trial based on earlier experience in humans, if prior data exists, or, lacking such data, a fraction of the weight-adjusted dose found to be toxic or fatal to laboratory animals. The intervals between doses are commonly large for low doses and then, for safety's sake, progressively shorten. That is, the second dose might double the first, the third add 50% to the second, and subsequent doses increase by smaller amounts. The details vary between trials but the general pattern of diminishing intervals is known inscrutably as the "Fibonacci method" (it does not necessarily correspond to the mathematical sequence). It is also sensible to specify an even lower level than the starting dose in the trial protocol in the event that the latter unexpectedly proves toxic. In addition to the dose levels, investigators must formulate definitions for adverse events severe enough so that their presence would curtail the use of the treatment. These are called *dose-limiting toxicities* (DLTs).

The so-called *traditional design*, used for cancer drugs and still common despite generally preferable alternatives, uses a simple algorithm applied to cohorts of size three. The first three subjects are assigned to the starting dose; if none experience DLTs, three additional subjects are given the next higher dose. If one subject has a DLT then three more subjects are given the same dose and if none of these has another (so that one of six subjects experiences a DLT at that dose) the next cohort is given the next higher dose; otherwise (that is, if at least two out of three or at least two out of six subjects have DLTs) the trial stops. The algorithm is repeated until either the DLT criterion is met or the maximum dose is reached. The dose below the one at which excessive toxicity is observed is called the MTD.

The traditional design has no fixed sample size—the maximum is six times the number of doses. Its most serious drawback is that because there are multiple opportunities for stopping, on average the MTD can have a DLT rate substantially less than $1/3$. Storer (1989) shows that this underestimation varies with the unknown dose-response curve and can be substantial. He presents a similar but more appropriate algorithm, the *modified design*, in which, again, cohorts of three subjects are used: if none have a DLT then the next cohort receives a higher dose; if one has a DLT then the current dose is maintained; and if more than one DLT is observed then the dose is *decreased*. The trial proceeds until a preset sample size is achieved. The recommended MTD could be the most recent dose at which excessive toxicity was not observed or, more efficiently, estimated from a logistic regression or perhaps a Bayesian model. Also, cohort sizes of one or two can be used until an DLT is observed in order to facilitate rapid initial dose escalation when this is deemed safe.

There are many variations of this design that can implemented to suit particular circumstances. At the first de-escalation, increments can be halved in order to refine the MTD estimate; information from sub-dose-limiting toxicities can be used not to de-escalate the dose but to slow its increase, for example, to enlarge the cohort size after a sub-DLT is observed; similarly, toxicity scores can be created that equate a sub-DLT with a fraction of a DLT and exceptionally severe toxicities with more than a unit DLT.

In some circumstances it may be possible to speed up dose escalation by assigning some subjects more than one dose. Simon et al. (1997), in what they called accelerated titration, proposed intra-subject dose escalation. They suggested that if a subject in the first portion of a study does not experience a DLT then he or she could be given a second higher dose. Once an initial estimate of an MTD is made then another group of subjects is assigned to it as their sole dose for confirmation. Obviously, this design is limited to situations where multiple dose assignment to the same subject is feasible.

A fundamentally different approach to dose-escalation can be implemented by using parametric models to dynamically estimate DLT probabilities as a function of dose. This requires prior assumptions regarding likely values of the model parameters and so is essentially a Bayesian model, the earliest and most thoroughly investigated form of which is known as the *continual reassessment method* (CRM) (see O'Quigley et al. (1990), and Garrett (2006) for a tutorial and summary of further developments). Other Bayesian designs such as *Escalation with Overdose Control* (EWOC Babb et al. (1998)) focus on minimizing toxicities to subjects. See Babb and Rogatko (2004) for an overview of Bayesian methods in phase I trials.

The CRM for binary toxicities can be briefly described as follows. Denote the probability of a toxicity at dose $d_{[i]}$ as $F(d_{[i]}, \beta)$, where β is a vector of low (one or two) dimension. (Even though a single scalar parameter is an unrealistic way to characterize a typical dose response curve, it is useful here because of the small sample size and limited goal of estimating the MTD rather than the entire curve.) Let $p(\beta)$ be a prior distribution for the dose-response parameter, whose choice is discussed below. Then, if y_i toxicities are observed at dose $d_{[i]}$, the likelihood for β after n dose cohorts is

$$L_n(\beta) = \prod_{i=1}^{n} F(d_{[i]}, \beta)^{y_i} [1 - F(d_{[i]}, \beta)]^{n_i - y_i}$$

where n_i is the number of subjects receiving dose $d_{[i]}$. The posterior distribution of β is proportional to $p(\beta) L_n(\beta)$ and its mean or mode can be used to estimate the MTD. The next subject, or subjects, is then simply assigned the MTD. That is, each subject receives what is currently estimated to be the best dose. CRM sample sizes are generally fixed in advance. The final MTD estimate would merely be the dose that would be given the next subject were there to be one. Use of a vague prior distribution for β reduces to maximum likelihood estimation, requiring algorithmic dose modification rules for use in early subjects, where little information is available.

The CRM shares several advantages with many other model-based designs. It unifies the design and analysis process—as described above, subjects are assigned to current best estimates. It is very flexible, allowing predictors, sub-dose limiting toxicities, and incomplete information to be incorporated. McGinn et al. (2001) illustrated the latter feature in a trial of radiation dose escalation in pancreatic cancer. Instead of waiting for full follow-up on a cohort of subjects treated at the current dose, they used the time-to-event CRM (TITE-CRM) method of Cheung and Chappell (2000) to utilize interim outcomes from subjects with incomplete follow-up to estimate the dose to assign the next subject. Full follow-up is used at the trial's end to generate a final estimate of the MTD. They note that trial length is shortened without sacrificing estimation accuracy, though at the cost of logistical complexity.

Bayesian methods can build on the results of previous human exposure, if any, and in turn provide prior distributions for future studies. A disadvantage of model-based designs compared to algorithmic ones is their lack of transparency, leading clinicians to think of them as "black box" mechanisms, yielding unpredictable dose assignments.

A phase I trial's operating characteristics have ethical and scientific implications, so the prior distribution must be sufficiently diffuse to allow data-driven dose changes but strong enough to disallow overly aggressive escalation. The latter can be restricted by forbidding escalation by more than one dose level per cohort and by conservatively setting the initial dose at less than the prior MTD. Therefore, since prior distributions used for the CRM and similar methods are often chosen based on the operating characteristics of the designs they produce in addition to, or instead of, scientific grounds, one might use a different prior distribution for the analysis.

3.1.2 Phase II Trials

A phase II trial is a small study of efficacy intended to provide experience with a treatment and its administration in order to inform the decision to conduct a larger trial and, if this is favorable, to inform its planning. "Small" is a flexible term here, depending on event frequency among other factors, but sample sizes in most phase II trials are sixty or less. The outcome is an indicator of treatment effectiveness. Because most phase II studies are performed in one or two stages, their outcomes usually require short to moderate follow-up, often a year or less, but these are intended as guidelines rather than absolute rules. Phase II studies in neurology may look for improvement in clinical symptoms by, say, six months; in cancer, tumor shrinkage (yes/no) and time to tumor progression (as a failure time variable, with maximum follow-ups of 6 to 24 months) are common. Only in the most severe illnesses is overall survival feasible as a primary outcome.

In their simplest form as small one-arm studies with short term outcomes, phase II trials have a long history. Gehan (1961) was one of the first to describe such trials and to formalize them into two subtypes, preliminary and follow-up. A preliminary trial is intended to screen a treatment for initial evidence of efficacy. Its minimum sample size is sometimes given as fourteen using the following argument. Suppose we have the following pair of hypotheses,

$$H_0: \quad \pi_T = 0.20$$
$$H_1: \quad \pi_T > 0.20,$$

where π_T is the probability of tumor response or other measure of treatment efficacy, and let y denote the number of observed successes in our initial sample. One approach is to use a procedure that controls the type II error rate, i.e., the probability that we fail to reject H_1 when it is true. This approach is proper if we want to ensure that we do not prematurely discard promising therapies.

Thus if we wish to use the decision rule that dictates that we pursue further study of a compound unless $y = 0$, a type II error is made if $y = 0$, yet $\pi_T > 0.20$. With a sample of n subjects, the type II error rate is $\Pr\{y = 0|\pi_T\} = (1 - \pi_T)^n$. We note that for $n=13$, this probability is $0.8^{13} = 0.055$, and for $n = 14$, it is $0.8^{14} = 0.044$. Therefore, the design that ensures a type II error rate less than 0.05 requires $n \geq 14$. Using the Gehan design, if $y > 0$, an additional cohort of subjects is treated and a different decision rule is employed at the second stage.

Trials of this nature in diseases for which no treatment exists (or advanced stages of diseases, at which patients have exhausted available treatments) are sometimes known as phase IIA trials. Trials comparing outcomes to existing treatments having known efficacy can be classified as phase IIB trials, although this distinction is not necessarily sharp.

Often, several phase II trials using the same or similar treatments are carried out at different institutions. This compensates for their small sizes and provides a more varied experience with a particular approach, allowing for a more informed choice of the optimal mode of treatment to be used in a subsequent phase III trial. Simon et al. (1985) point out possible inter-institutional variations in patient selection, definition of or ability to detect outcomes, drug dose and schedule and other aspects of the treatment, and sample size. They therefore advocate randomized phase II trials. They also point out that in such studies it may be practical to investigate several schedules (different doses, timings, and/or modes of administration), and proposed designs with several arms, assuming that one has effectiveness probability equal to $\pi + \delta$ and the rest have effectiveness probability π. They give a table of sample sizes yielding a 90% chance of selecting the best treatment. For example, for $\pi = 0.2$, $\delta = 0.15$, and three schedules, a total sample size of 132 (44 per schedule) gives a 90% chance that the schedule observed to have the best efficacy proportion is truly the best one. One can show that randomization increases the sample size required to detect a given difference between two groups, at the same power and type I error, by a factor of four over that for a trial using a historical control; however, this inflation is in part artifactual because it assumes the historical control rate to be known exactly. Nonetheless, many researchers believe that the elimination of bias using randomization justifies its extra costs: randomized phase II trials are becoming increasingly common in many disciplines.

Fleming (1982) formalized the process of deciding whether to conduct further research on a treatment by proposing three hypotheses for binary measures of efficacy:

$$H_0: \quad \pi_T \leq \pi_1$$
$$H_1: \quad \pi_1 < \pi_T < \pi_2$$
$$H_2: \quad \pi_T \geq \pi_2,$$

where for a phase IIA study we might take $\pi_1 = 0.05$ $\pi_2 = 0.2$ (among other possibilities). The sample proportion is compared to two critical values, determined by prespecifying bounds on the type I error probabilities. Two values, α_1 and α_2, are chosen so that $P(H_0 \text{ rejected}|H_0 \text{ true}) \leq \alpha_1$ and $P(H_2 \text{ rejected}|H_2 \text{ true}) \leq \alpha_2$. Rejection of H_2 is evidence of the treatment's lack of efficacy. Rejecting H_0 indicates promise and consideration of a phase III or another phase II trial. Failure to reject one of these two hypotheses suggests that further investigation may be required.

Preliminary and follow-up stages of phase II studies are increasingly integrated into a single trial with an interim analysis. At a mild cost in complexity, this has the administrative advantage of generating a single protocol needing approval only once by each regulatory committee. It also allows continual subject accrual and obviates the logistical problems of shutting down one study and starting another. Finally, a formal two-stage design allows the joint statistical properties of the entire process to be evaluated. These last will be illustrated by a simple one arm study with a binary outcome and an analysis halfway through.

Example 3.1. Researchers at the University of Wisconsin Cancer Center, in a protocol called RO 9471, examined the effects of concurrent hyperthermia using microwaves during radiation treatment of eye tumors. Although the primary outcome was toxicity to eye tissues, it was a single-dose study and, therefore, the desired design features were similar to those of a phase II trial for efficacy and the goal was to show that the probability of toxicity, π_T, is small. The hypotheses were

$$H_0: \quad \pi_T = 0.3$$
$$H_1: \quad \pi_T < 0.3$$

with type I error, the probability of erroneously rejecting H_0, at most 0.05. This can be achieved in a one-stage design with a sample of 29 subjects, rejecting H_0 if there are four or fewer experiencing toxicity. The type I error rate, given $\pi_T = 0.3$, is $0.0260 + 0.0093 + 0.0024 + 0.0004 + 0.0000 = 0.038$ via the binomial formula. By a similar calculation, the power to detect H_1 at $\pi_T = 0.1$ is 0.84.

Now consider the properties under H_0 of a trial with 28 subjects equally divided into two stages as shown in Figure 3.2. Using this design, if no events are observed among the 14 subjects in the first stage, we can stop and reject H_0 (region A). Similarly, if we observe at least 5 events in stage one we can stop but not reject H_0. If between one and four events are observed, we continue to stage two (region B). If the total number of events after the second stage is no more than four, we reject H_0 (region C), otherwise we cannot reject H_0 (region D). Table 3.1 gives the probabilities of rejecting and failing to reject H_0

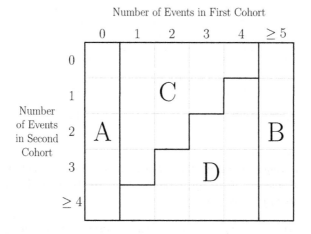

<table>
<tr><td colspan="2">Region</td><td>Action</td></tr>
</table>

Region	Action
A	Reject H_0, stop at stage 1
B	Fail to reject H_0, stop at stage 1
C	Reject H_0 after stage 2
D	Fail to reject H_0 after stage 2

Figure 3.2 *Example schematic of a phase II trial.*

at the end of each stage, under the null and the alternative hypotheses. The probability of erroneously rejecting H_0 is $0.043 + 0.007 = 0.05$. (The calculations are more complex using a failure time outcome in which subjects who are accrued in the first stage can continue to be followed during the second.) Under the alternative hypothesis, there is a 23% probability of stopping and rejecting H_0 after the first stage and a 63% probability of rejecting H_0 after the second stage, yielding 86% power.

Note that the investigators also utilized deterministic curtailment (discussed in Chapter 10), stopping the trial at a point in which its eventual outcome was certain. Regions B and D in Figure 3.2 indicate situations in which, during or after the first stage, they knew that the trial's outcome would be to fail to reject the null hypothesis. There is a 41.7% chance under H_0 of ending the trial after fourteen or fewer subjects. The chances of stopping for the same reason at particular points during the second stage or of stopping near the end of the second stage because five or more events are unobtainable (so rejecting H_0 is certain) are easily calculated.

This example shows a situation in which the power, type I error rate, and maximum sample size for a two-stage design are all about the same as those for

Table 3.1 *Probabilities corresponding to the regions in Figure 3.2.*

Region	Probability Under H_0 ($\pi = 0.3$)	Probability Under H_1 ($\pi = 0.1$)
A	0.007	0.23
B	0.417	0.009
C	0.043	0.63
D	0.533	0.13

the corresponding single stage trial. The former, however, offers the substantial possibility of greatly shortening study duration by stopping early, offering ethical and logistical advantages.   □

Although the two-stage phase II designs discussed here are simple, many refinements are possible such as the use of three or more stages. Failure time outcomes can be used in which case the length of follow-up at each stage will influence total trial duration (Case and Morgan 2001). Thall and Simon (1995) discuss Bayesian phase II designs. As was the case with phase I trials, Bayesian considerations may inform the analysis of a study even when they did not motivate its design.

As a further refinement on two- (and, in principle, three- or more) stage trials Simon (1989) describes designs in which the numbers of subjects in each stage may be unequal. Subject to fixed type I rates (denoted by α, usually specified to be 5% or 10%) and type II error rates (β, usually between 5% and 20%), many designs satisfy the criteria

$$\text{Pr(Reject } H_0 | \pi_T = \pi_1) \le \alpha$$

and

$$\text{Pr(Reject } H_0 | \pi_T = \pi_2) \ge 1 - \beta$$

where π_1 is the value of π_T under H_0 and π_2 is a possible value under H_1. Two strategies for choosing subject allocation between two stages are so-called *optimality* and the *minimax* criterion. Both have been widely applied. Optimality minimizes the expected sample size under the null hypothesis, while minimax refers to a minimization of the maximum sample size in the worst case. Because these goals conflict, optimal designs tend to have large expected sample sizes. Jung et al. (2001) present a graphical method for balancing the two goals. In practice, equal patient allocation to the two stages often serves as a simple compromise. Also, the actual sample size achieved at each stage may deviate slightly from the design. This is particularly true for multi-institutional phase II trials, in which there may be a delay in ascertaining the total accrual and in closing a stage after the accrual goal is met.

3.2 Phase III/IV Trials

The typical phase III trial is the first to definitively establish that the new intervention has a positive risk to benefit ratio. Trials intended to provide additional efficacy or safety data after the new intervention has been approved by regulatory agencies are often referred to as phase IV trials. The distinction is not always clear, however, and we shall focus our discussion on phase III trials since most of the design issues are similar for phase IV trials.

3.2.1 Types of Control Groups

As described earlier, there are a number of potential control groups that could be used in a phase III trial. We shall discuss three: the historical control, the concurrent control, and the randomized control.

Historical Controls

One of the earliest trial designs is the historical control study, comparing the benefits and safety of a new intervention with the experience of subjects treated earlier using the control. A major motivation for this design is that all new subjects can receive the new intervention. Cancer researchers once used this design to evaluate new chemotherapy strategies (Gehan 1984). This is a natural design for clinicians since they routinely guide their daily practice based on their experience with the treatment of previous patients. If either physicians or patients have a strong belief that the new intervention may be beneficial, they may not want to enroll patients in a trial in which they may be randomized to an inferior treatment. Thus, the historical control trial can thereby alleviate these ethical concerns. In addition, since all eligible patients receive the new intervention, recruitment can be easier and faster, and the required sample size roughly half that of a randomized control trial, thereby reducing costs as well. One of the key assumptions, however, is that the patient population and the standard of care remain constant during the period in which such comparisons are being made.

Despite these benefits, there are also many challenges. First, historical control trials are vulnerable to bias. There are many cases in which interventions appeared to be effective based on historical controls but later were shown not to be (Moertel 1984). Byar describes the Veterans Administration Urological Research Group trial of prostrate cancer, comparing survival of estrogen treated patients with placebo treated patients.[1] During this trial, there was a shift in the patient population so that earlier patients were at higher risk. Estrogen appeared to be effective in the earlier high risk patients but not so in the patients recruited later who were at lower risk. A historical control study would have been misleading due to a shift in patient referral patterns. Pocock (1977b) describes a series of 19 studies that were conducted immediately after

---

[1] Veterans Administration Cooperative Urological Research Group (1967), Byar et al. (1976)

an earlier study of the same patient population and with the same intervention. In comparing the effects of the intervention from the consecutive trials in these 19 cases, 4 of the 19 comparisons were "nominally" significant, suggesting that the treatment in one trial was more effective in one study than the other, even though the patients were similar and the interventions were identical.

A recent trial of chronic heart failure also demonstrates the bias in historical comparisons (Packer et al. 1996; Carson et al. 2000). The initial PRAISE trial evaluated a drug, amlodipine, to reduce mortality and morbidity in a chronic heart failure population. The first trial, referred to as PRAISE I, was stratified by etiology of the heart failure: ischemic and non-ischemic. Earlier research suggested that amlodipine should be more effective in the ischemic population or subgroup. The overall survival comparison between amlodipine and placebo treated patients, using the log-rank test, resulted in a p-value of 0.07, almost statistically significant. There was a significant interaction between the ischemic and non-ischemic subgroups, however, with a hazard ratio of 1.0 for the ischemic subgroup and 0.5 for the non-ischemic subgroup. While the result in the non-ischemic group alone might have led to its use in clinical practice, the fact that the result was opposite to that expected persuaded the investigators to repeat the trial in the non-ischemic subgroup alone. In the second trial, referred to as PRAISE II, the comparison of the amlodipine and placebo treated arms resulted in a hazard ratio of essentially 1.0. Of interest here, as shown in Figure 3.3, is that the placebo treated patients in the second trial were significantly superior in survival to the placebo treated patients in PRAISE I. No adjustment for baseline characteristics could explain this phenomenon.

In addition, to conduct an historical control trial, historical data must be available. There are usually two main sources of historical data; a literature resource or a data bank resource. The literature resource may be subject to publication bias where only selected trials, usually those with a positive significant benefit, are published and this bias may be introduced into the historical comparison. In addition, to conduct a rigorous analysis of the new intervention, access to the raw data would be necessary and this may not be available from the literature resources. Thus, researchers often turn to existing data banks to retrieve data from earlier studies. Quality of data collection may change over time as well as the definitions used for inclusion criteria and outcome variables.

Even if data of sufficient quality from earlier studies are available, caution is still required. Background therapy may have changed over time and diagnostic criteria may also have changed. For example, international classification of disease changes periodically and thus there can be increases or decreases in disease prevalence. For example, the seventh, eighth, and ninth revisions of the international classification system resulted in a 15% shift in deaths due to ischemic heart disease. Besides changes in diagnostic criteria and classification codes, disease prevalence can also change over time as shown in Figure 3.4.

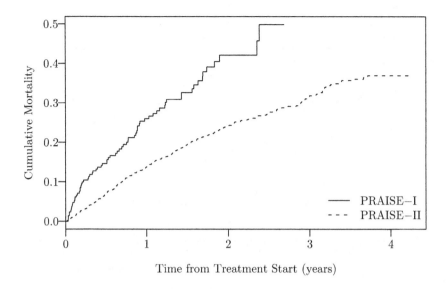

Figure 3.3 *PRAISE I vs. PRAISE II: all-cause mortality for placebo groups by study.*

In this case, historical comparisons of two periods for cardiovascular disease might indicate that more recent interventions were successful. The difference in rates may, however, be due solely to a change in prevalence.

Historical comparisons can be useful to a limited extent but may have bias. Thus, such comparisons may be used early in the assessment of a new intervention to suggest further research and may be used to help design definitive trials.

Concurrent Controls

The concurrent control trial compares the effect of the new intervention with the effect of an alternative intervention applied at some other site or clinic. This design has many of the advantages of the historical control trial but eliminates some of the sources of bias. The primary advantage is that the investigator can apply the new intervention to all participants and only half as many new participants are needed, compared to the randomized control trial. Thus, recruitment is easier and faster. The biases that affect historical controls due to changes in definitions or diagnostic criteria, background therapy, and changing time trends in disease prevalence are minimized if not eliminated. These types of comparisons are somewhat common in medical care as success rates of various institutions in treating patients are often compared and evaluated.

The key problem with the concurrent control trial is selection bias, both from patients or participants and the health care provider. Referral patterns

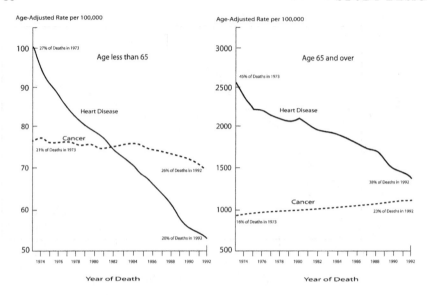

Figure 3.4 *Cancer and heart disease deaths. Cancer and heart disease are the leading causes of death in the United States. For people less than 65, heart disease death rates declined greatly from 1973 to 1992, while cancer death rates declined slightly. For people age 65 and older, heart disease remains the leading killer despite a reduction in deaths from this disease. Because cancer is a disease of aging, longer life expectancies and fewer deaths from competing causes, such as heart disease, are contributing to the increase in cancer incidence and mortality for those age 65 and older. Reprinted with permission from McIntosh (1995).*

are not random but based on many factors. These may include whether the institution is a primary care facility or a tertiary referral center. Patient mix would be quite different in those two settings. Patients may choose to get their care from an institution because of its reputation or accessibility. With the development of large multidisciplinary health care systems, this source of bias may not be as great as it otherwise might be. Even within such systems, however, different clinics may have different expertise or interest and select patients accordingly.

The key to any evaluation of two interventions is that the populations are comparable at the start of the study. For a concurrent control trial, one would have to examine the profile of risk factors and demographic factors. There are many other important factors, however, that may not be available. Even with a large amount of baseline data, establishing comparability is a challenging task. In the previous section, the PRAISE I & II example indicated it was not possible to explain the difference in survival between the same placebo subgroups in the two back to back studies by examining baseline risk factors. Thus, covariate adjustment cannot be guaranteed to produce valid treatment comparisons in trials using concurrent controls.

Randomized Control Trials

As indicated earlier, the randomized control trial is viewed as the "gold standard" for evaluating new interventions. The reason for this, as summarized in Table 3.2, is that many of the sources of bias present in both the historical and concurrent control trials are minimized or eliminated (Friedman et al. 1985).

Table 3.2 *Sources of bias as a function of the control group.*

Design	Sources of Bias
Randomized	Chance
Concurrent (Non-randomized)	Chance & Selection Bias
Historical (Non-randomized)	Chance, Selection Bias, & Time Bias

In a randomized control trial, all intervention arms are assessed at the same time under the same conditions. Since a randomized control trial assigns participants to either the standard control or the new intervention at random, selection bias is eliminated. Neither participant nor health care provider can influence which of the two or more interventions are received. This influence may be conscious or subconscious but in either case, the selection bias can be substantial. A randomized control trial minimizes this possibility. In addition, the process of randomization tends to produce, on average, comparable groups of patients in each of the intervention arms. This is true both for measured and unmeasured risk factors. Investigators typically present a baseline covariate table in their trial results publication, demonstrating comparability for those risk factors that were measured.

Another benefit of randomization is that the process of randomization justifies the common statistical tests used to evaluate the interventions (Byar et al. 1976; Kempthorne 1977). Through randomization, the validity of the statistical tests can be made without invoking assumptions about the distribution of baseline variables. Often these assumptions are not strictly true or, at least, are difficult to establish.

Table 3.3 provides an example of the degree of bias that can occur with different designs (Chalmers et al. 1977; Peto et al. 1976). A series of randomized and non-randomized trials for the evaluation of anticoagulant therapy in patients with a myocardial infarction (heart attack) were summarized, noting the estimate of the intervention effect in each class of designs. In this series, there were 18 historical control trials, 8 non-randomized concurrent trials, and 6 randomized control trials. Each class of designs involves several hundred or more participants. As shown, the historical control series and the concurrent control series estimate a 50% intervention effect while the randomized control trials give a smaller estimate of 20%. This example demonstrates the consid-

erable bias that non-randomized designs can produce, bias likely due to time
trends and patient selection.

Table 3.3 *Possible bias in the estimation of treatment effects for published trials
involving anticoagulation for patients with myocardial infarction as a function of the
control group. The randomized control is the most reliable.*

Design	Patients	P<0.05	Observed Effect
18 Historical	900	15/18	50%
8 Concurrent	3000	5/8	50%
6 Randomized	3000	1/6	20%

Despite the advantages of randomization for minimizing bias, some investigators or participants may object to the randomization process. They may
believe that half of the participants are being deprived of access to the new
intervention that may be beneficial, regardless of the strength of the evidence
or lack thereof. There is an ethical imperative for the physician to do what
they believe is best for their patient and what might be considered ethical behavior by one investigator might not be for another. Byar et al. (1993) argue
that the most ethical behavior, when evidence for the safety and benefit of a
new intervention is not well established, is to find out as quickly as possible
with the best, most unbiased methods available. The randomized control trial
satisfies this requirement according to Chalmers et al. (1983) who, among others, pioneered the use of this design. Of course, if a physician or a participant
strongly believes that the new intervention is better or less toxic than the
standard being used for comparison, they should not participate in the trial.

3.2.2 Common Randomized Control Designs

The designs for randomized control trials that we will describe are, in general,
basic and straightforward. More complicated designs are available but have not
seen widespread use. Basic designs are also simpler to analyze, requiring fewer
assumptions. Other authors have also summarized these designs (Friedman
et al. 1985).

Parallel Group Design

The most common design used in clinical research is the randomized *parallel
group* (or *parallel control*) design depicted in Figure 3.5. Using this design,
participants are screened for eligibility, provide informed consent, have baseline information collected, and are then randomized to one of the intervention
arms. After a period of follow-up, participants are evaluated for compliance to
the interventions, side effects and toxicities, and the primary and secondary

outcome variables. The intervention arms are compared with respect to the outcome variables specified in the protocol.

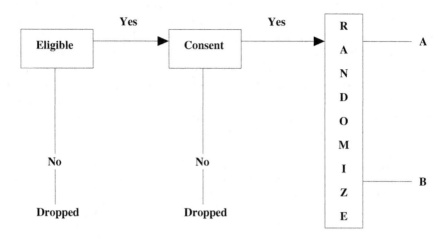

Figure 3.5 *Parallel group design.*

There are many clinical trials in various fields that have successfully used this trial design.[2] The parallel control design has the advantage of simplicity and can give valid answers to one or two primary questions. For example, the Coronary Drug Project (CDP), one of the early randomized control multi-center clinical trials, compared several intervention strategies with a placebo control arm using a parallel design in a population of men who had recently suffered a heart attack. The primary outcome was mortality with cardiovascular mortality as a secondary outcome. The intervention strategies used various drugs that were known to lower serum cholesterol levels but it was not known whether any could safely lower mortality. The Diabetic Retinopathy Study (DRS) was a trial to evaluate a new laser treatment in a diabetic population to reduce the progression of retinopathy, an eye disease that reduces visual acuity. The primary outcome was visual acuity and a retinopathy score which measures disease progression and is based on photographs of the eye fundus (i.e., back of the eye). The Beta-blocker Heart Attack Trial (BHAT) was a randomized double-blind parallel design trial in a group of individuals having just survived a heart attack, comparing a beta-blocker drug with a placebo control. Again, mortality was the primary outcome variable. The Breast Cancer Prevention Trial (P-1) was a cancer prevention trial evaluating the drug tamoxifen to prevent the occurrence of breast cancer in a population at risk (Fisher et al. 1998). Here, the primary outcome was disease free sur-

---

[2] The International Steering Committee on Behalf of the MERIT-HF Study Group (1997), Domanski et al. (2002), HDFP Cooperative Group (1982), The Coronary Drug Project Research Group (1975), The DCCT Research Group: Diabetes Control and Complications Trial (DCCT) (1986), Diabetic Retinopathy Study Research Group (1976)

vival; that is, alive without the occurrence of breast cancer. Most phase III trials use this basic design because of its simplicity and utility.

A variation of the parallel design utilizes a *run-in* period. A schema for this design is shown in Figure 3.6. The primary departure from the basic parallel design is that participants are screened into a prerandomization phase to evaluate their ability to adhere to the protocol or to one of the interventions under evaluation. If they cannot adhere to the intervention schedule such as taking a high percentage of the medication prescribed, then their lack of compliance will affect the sensitivity or power of the trial. If a potential participant cannot comply with some of the required procedures or evaluations, then that individual would not be a good candidate for the main trial.

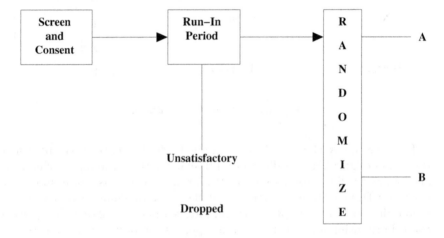

Figure 3.6 *Run-in design.*

There are many trials that have used a "run-in" period. For example, the Cardiac Arrhythmia Suppression Trial (CAST) used a run-in phase to determine if a patient's cardiac arrhythmia could be suppressed using one of the three drugs being tested.[3] CAST was a trial involving patients with a serious cardiac arrhythmia, or irregular heartbeat. Individuals with these irregular heartbeats are known to be a high risk for death, usually suddenly and without warning. Researchers developed a class of drugs that would suppress or control these irregular heartbeats, on the theory that this would reduce the risk of sudden death. Not all patients could tolerate these drugs, however, and in some patients the treatment failed to control the arrhythmia. Therefore, to improve the efficiency and power of the main CAST trial, patients were screened to determine both their ability to tolerate these drugs and the susceptibility of the arrhythmia to pharmacological control. If they met the screening criteria, they were randomized into the main trial, either to one of the 3 drugs or to a matching placebo control. Ironically, these drugs were

[3] The Cardiac Arrhythmia Suppression Trial (CAST) Investigators (1989)

shown to be harmful in a patient population who had passed the screening run-in phase with a successful suppression of their arrhythmias.

Another trial, the Nocturnal Oxygen Therapy Trial (NOTT), evaluated the benefit of giving 24 hours of continuous oxygen supplementation, relative to giving 12 hours of nocturnal use, in patients suffering from advance chronic obstructive pulmonary disease (COPD). Potential participants were entered into a run-in phase to establish that their disease was sufficiently stable to ensure that the outcome variables, pulmonary function, could better reflect the treatment effect. A similar strategy was used in the Intermittent Positive Pressure Breathing (IPPB) Trial.[4]

Randomized Withdrawal Design

A variation in the parallel design is the randomized withdrawal study. Many treatments are shown to be beneficial for a specified period of time, but the required duration of treatment is often not well known. Longer exposure to a drug, for example, may increase the risk of toxicity. If there are no long term benefits, then this risk may not be justified. A randomized withdrawal trial allows design researchers to evaluate the optimal duration of treatment. All participants are given the intervention for a prespecified period of time during which the intervention has been shown to be beneficial. After a predetermined period of exposure, participants are randomly withdrawn from the intervention, as shown in Figure 3.7. The analysis will focus on outcomes starting from the point of randomization. The randomized withdrawal design should be used

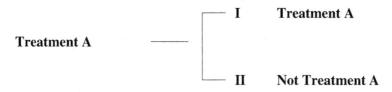

Figure 3.7 *Withdrawal design.*

more often to give better evidence that can help maximize benefit and minimize long term risk. There are few examples of the randomized withdrawal design.

Crossover Design

The crossover design has often been used in the early stages of the development of new therapies to evaluate their effects compared to a standard control. Crossover designs are commonly used for studies of analgesic and psychotropic drugs. One of the unique features of this design is that each patient receives both treatments and, hence, serves as his or her own control. In the simple two-period crossover design, as depicted in Figure 3.8, the participants are

[4] The Intermittent Positive Pressure Breathing Trial Group (1983)

randomly divided into two groups and each participant is exposed to the new treatment (A) and to the control (B), each for a prespecified period of time. In Figure 3.8 these time periods are labeled as period I and period II. Group 1 is exposed to treatment A in period I and treatment B in period II, while group 2 is exposed to treatment B in period I and treatment A in period II.

H_0: A vs. B Scheme

Group	Period	
	I	II
1	TRT A	TRT B
2	TRT B	TRT A

Figure 3.8 *Two-period crossover design.*

The model, according to Brown (1980) and Grizzle (1965), can be written as

$$Y_{ijk} = \mu + \pi_k + \phi_u + \lambda_v + \xi_{ij} + \varepsilon_{ijk},$$

where $i = 1, 2$, $j = 1, \ldots, n_i$ (n_i is the number of subjects in group i), $k =$I,II, $u =$A,B, and $v =$A,B. The terms in the model are defined as follows:

$$
\begin{aligned}
Y_{ijk} &= \text{the measurement for subject } j \text{ in group } i \\
&\quad \text{during period } k, \\
\mu &= \text{the overall mean,} \\
\pi_k &= \text{the effect of period } k, \\
\phi_u &= \text{the effect of treatment } u, \\
\lambda_v &= \text{the carryover effect of treatment } v \text{ from} \\
&\quad \text{period I on the response in period II,} \\
\xi_{ij} &= \text{the subject effect,} \\
\varepsilon_{ijk} &= \text{random error.}
\end{aligned}
$$

In addition, $\mathrm{E}[\xi_{ij}] = \mathrm{E}[\varepsilon_{ijk}] = 0$, $\mathrm{Var}(\xi_{ij}) = \sigma_\xi^2$, $\mathrm{Var}(\varepsilon_{ijk}) = \sigma_\varepsilon^2$, and the ξ_{ij} and ε_{ijk} are assumed to be mutually independent. The carryover effect, λ_v, has a value of 0 for all measurements in period I. Its value in period II is of particular interest and may not be 0. For example, if treatment A cures the disease in period I, then there is no possibility of a response to treatment B in period II. The validity and efficiency of the crossover design depends strongly on whether or not there is any carryover effect. The presentation here follows Brown (1980).

First, we consider at the case in which we assume that $\lambda_v = 0$.[5] In this case, we impose the additional constraint that $\phi_A + \phi_B = 0$, and the difference between the two treatment effects, $\delta = \phi_B - \phi_A$, can be estimated by

$$\hat{\delta}_{co} = \frac{1}{2} \left[(\bar{Y}_{1\cdot 2} - \bar{Y}_{1\cdot 1}) + (\bar{Y}_{2\cdot 1} - \bar{Y}_{2\cdot 2}) \right],$$

---

[5] Actually we need only assume that $\lambda_A = \lambda_B$; however, if carryover effects are present, it is unlikely that they will be the same for both treatments.

where $\bar{Y}_{i \cdot k}$ is the average measurement of all subjects in group i during period k. It is easy to check that

$$\mathrm{E}\left[\hat{\delta}_{co}\right] = \delta \quad \text{and} \quad \mathrm{Var}\left(\hat{\delta}_{co}\right) = \frac{\sigma_\varepsilon^2}{2}\left(\frac{1}{n_1} + \frac{1}{n_2}\right),$$

where σ_ε^2 can be estimated by the subject differences between periods with $n_1 + n_2 - 2$ degrees of freedom. As pointed out by Chassan (1970), the efficiency of the crossover design can be compared to that of the randomized parallel control design using simple calculations. Let the number of subjects in each group in the crossover design be n and the number of subjects in each arm in the parallel design be m. The variance of the estimator in the crossover trial becomes $\mathrm{Var}(\hat{\delta}_{co}) = \sigma_\varepsilon^2/n$ and the variance of the estimator in the parallel design experiment will be

$$\mathrm{Var}(\hat{\delta}_p) = \frac{2}{m}\left(\sigma_\xi^2 + \sigma_\varepsilon^2\right) = \frac{2\sigma_\varepsilon^2}{m(1-\rho)}$$

where ρ is the correlation between measurements in period I and period II for a randomly selected subject. The ratio of the variances for the two experiments will be

$$\frac{\mathrm{Var}(\hat{\delta}_{co})}{\mathrm{Var}(\hat{\delta}_p)} = \frac{m}{2n}(1-\rho).$$

Thus, to achieve the same precision, we require that $m = 2n/(1-\rho)$ which, depending on ρ, is at least twice the sample size, and likely much more. Another observation made by Chassan (1970) is that if the analysis of the parallel design experiment was based on change from baseline, then the appropriate estimator, say $\hat{\delta}_{p(bl)}$, would have variance

$$\mathrm{Var}(\hat{\delta}_{p(bl)}) = \frac{4}{m}\sigma_\varepsilon^2.$$

This is four times the variance of the estimator for the crossover experiment when the two have the same sample sizes. Similarly if the estimate is based on equation (2.20) from Chapter 2, the variance is $2(1+\rho)\sigma_\varepsilon^2/m$, which is between two and four times greater than $\mathrm{Var}(\hat{\delta}_p)$.

The efficiency results are valid only when $\lambda_v = 0$, however. When this assumption is not reasonable, adjustments need to be made that ultimately defeat the purpose of the crossover design. Grizzle (1965) noticed that the hypothesis of no carryover effect can be tested in the simple two-period crossover design. Letting $\gamma = \lambda_B - \lambda_A$ (i.e., the difference in carryover effect between the two treatments), an unbiased estimator of γ is

$$\hat{\gamma} = \left(\bar{Y}_{2 \cdot 1} + \bar{Y}_{2 \cdot 2}\right) - \left(\bar{Y}_{1 \cdot 1} + \bar{Y}_{1 \cdot 2}\right),$$

with variance

$$\mathrm{Var}\left(\hat{\gamma}\right) = \left(4\sigma_\xi^2 + 2\sigma_\varepsilon^2\right)\left(\frac{1}{n_1} + \frac{1}{n_2}\right).$$

We can estimate $4\sigma_\xi^2 + 2\sigma_\varepsilon^2$ by estimating the variance of the sum of the two observations for each individual with $n_1 + n_2 - 2$ degrees of freedom. Once these estimates are available, we can test the hypothesis of no carryover effect. If it is determined that carryover effect is present, then $E[\hat{\delta}_{co}] \neq \delta$. A valid (unbiased) estimate of the treatment effect is $\bar{Y}_{1\cdot2} - \bar{Y}_{1\cdot1}$—the estimate from a parallel group trial and which does not make use of the period II data, subverting the entire benefit of the crossover design.

When in doubt about the carryover effect, Grizzle (1965) recommends testing $\gamma = 0$ at a significance level of 0.1. If this hypothesis is not rejected, $\hat{\delta}_{co}$ can be used. If it is rejected, only information from the first period should be used. On the other hand, in order to have sufficient power for both this test *and* the test for treatment effect, one would need a larger sample size and a simple parallel design would be a more efficient choice. Thus, when there is a very strong belief that $\gamma = 0$, a crossover design may be used. If there is a possibility of carryover effect, however, one should avoid the crossover design.

These results are a summary of those presented by Brown (1980). Another discussion, arriving at many of the same conclusions, is given by Hills and Armitage (1979). Many other possible designs for crossover trials have been explored. These involve a larger number of treatments or periods and may involve various patterns of treatment assignment. Some of these have been discussed in Koch et al. (1989) and Carriere (1994).

Factorial Designs

The factorial design is the most complex of the designs typically used in clinical trials. Using this design, two or more classes of interventions are evaluated in the same study compared to the appropriate standard or control for each. As shown in Figure 3.9 for a two-by-two factorial design, evaluating two interventions A and B compared to a control, there are four cells, each reflecting an intervention strategy. Approximately 25% of the participants are in each cell; that is, 25% receive both interventions AB, 25% receive A and control, 25% receive B and control, and 25% receive both controls. The factorial design allows researchers to evaluate more than one intervention in the same participant population, thus reducing costs and increasing efficiency. Furthermore, as in the Physicians Health Study (PHS) example described later in this section, each treatment comparison may be associated with a different outcome.

	Control	Trt B	Tot
Control	$N/4$	$N/4$	$N/2$
Trt A	$N/4$	$N/4$	$N/2$
Tot	$N/2$	$N/2$	N

Figure 3.9 *Balanced 2×2 factorial design.*

There are several possible effects of interest including,
1. the overall effect of treatment A on its primary outcome,

2. the overall effect of treatment B on its primary outcome,

3. the interaction effect, or equivalently, the modification of the effect of treatment A by treatment B or vice versa,

4. the effect of treatment A on its primary outcome, in the presence of treatment B, or

5. the effect of treatment B on its primary outcome, in the presence of treatment A.

In trials using factorial designs solely for efficiency (PHS, for example), interest is likely to be in (1) and (2), the overall effects of each treatment, ignoring the other. Other studies may be conducted to determine if the effect of the two treatments together is different than the effects of the two separately. In this case interest will be in (3), and probably one or both of (4) and (5). If interest were solely in (4) or (5), there would be no reason to use the factorial design.

The typical model used in the analysis of the two-by-two factorial design is given by

$$Y_{ijk} = \mu + \alpha_i + \beta_j + (\alpha\beta)_{ij} + \varepsilon_{ijk}, \qquad (3.1)$$

where $i = 1, \ldots, I$, $j = 1, \ldots, J$, and $k = 1, \ldots, K$. Y_{ijk} is the outcome of interest for the kth subject receiving level i of intervention A and level j of intervention B. In the design depicted in Figure 3.9, $I = J = 2$ and $K = N/4$. The errors ε_{ijk} are assumed to be independent and normally distributed with mean zero and variance σ^2. μ is interpreted as the overall mean, α_i is the (additional) effect due to level i of intervention A, β_j is the (additional) effect due to level j of intervention B, and $(\alpha\beta)_{ij}$ is the effect due to the combination of level i of intervention A with level j of intervention B. The constraints assumed here are $\alpha_1 + \alpha_2 = 0$, $\beta_1 + \beta_2 = 0$, and $\sum_{i,j}(\alpha\beta)_{ij} = 0$. If each treatment comparison involved a different outcome, there would be two such models. Note that unless one can a priori rule out an effect of, say, treatment B on the outcome associated with treatment A, each model should involve effects for both treatments.

Now consider the marginal effect of treatment A. One school of thought suggests that if the interaction, $(\alpha\beta)_{ij}$, is non-zero, then treatment B is an effect modifier for treatment A and analyses of the effect of treatment A must be performed separately for each level of treatment B. This would be technically true if the primary question solely involved point estimation of treatment effects. On the other hand, recall from Chapter 2 that the primary goal of randomized trials is to test hypotheses regarding the effects of the treatments. From this point of view, the tests of the overall effect of treatment A are still valid, regardless of the presence of the interaction. Furthermore, unless the interaction is quite large, so that, for example, there is little or no effect of treatment A in the presence of treatment B, the test for the overall effect of treatment A should still have good power. In fact, there is, in principle, no reason why treatment B should be considered any differently than baseline variables such as age, comorbidities, or concomitant medications, all of which are potential effect modifiers.

In addition, unless the interaction is such that the effect of treatment A is reversed by treatment B, the interaction is likely to be *removable*, in the sense that a transformation can be applied that will make the interaction zero. For example, if the outcome is dichotomous (success or failure), there may be an interaction using the probability scale (the difference in failure rates is a function of the level of treatment B), but the interaction disappears if the log-odds scale is used (example 4.2 in Section 4.6). Thus, the choice of scale may be more important when factorial designs are used than in other trials.

Under the assumption of no interaction, the test of H_0: $\alpha_1 = 0$ is based on the statistic $D = (\bar{Y}_{21.} - \bar{Y}_{11.} + \bar{Y}_{22.} - \bar{Y}_{12.})/2$, where $\bar{Y}_{ij.}$ is the mean of the observations in cell i, j. For robustness against the actual presence of interaction, the best estimate of $\text{Var}(D)$ is $16\,\hat{\sigma}^2/N$, where $\hat{\sigma}^2$ is the pooled estimate of σ^2 derived from the within-cell variances of the Y_{ijk} (hence with $N - 4$ degrees of freedom) rather than the residual mean square error from the additive model. Alternatively, if outcomes are not assumed to be normal, other analyses, stratified by levels of treatment B, can be performed as given in Section 2.3.1. For example, if Y_{ijk} is dichotomous, a Cochran-Mantel-Haenszel test can be used, or if Y_{ijk} is ordinal, the Van Elteren test may be appropriate.

If interactions are of interest, for normal data, the t-test or F-test corresponding to the interaction term in (3.1) can be performed. Alternatively, for dichotomous data, the Breslow and Day test for interaction (Breslow and Day 1980) may be used, or a logistic regression model may be used, although both of these tests consider only interactions on the log-odds scale. Interaction tests for other types of responses such as failure time outcomes are also available. Note, however, because interactions are intrinsically linked to a particular parameterization, they are necessarily model-based and nonparametric tests are not available. Also note that failure to reject the null hypothesis that there is no interaction does not imply that none exists. In fact, unless the trial is sufficiently large, interaction tests are not likely to be adequately powered (see Section 4.6). Since the sample size required to detect all but the most extreme interactions is many-fold larger than that required for the main effects, doing so will likely more than offset the efficiency gained by using a factorial design.

Next, after the tests of hypotheses have been completed, point estimates will generally be required. Unless the interactions are quite large, in most cases one should report both overall differences by treatment (either adjusted or unadjusted for the potential effect of the other factor—although the primary difference may be solely in the estimates of standard errors). If desired, the interactions and within-stratum effects may also be reported.

Finally, with multiple factors come multiple tests and multiple testing issues. Adjustments for multiple comparisons should be built into the design of the trial (see Section 11.5). Maintaining power while accounting for multiple tests typically requires increased sample sizes, but in the case of factorial designs, not enough to offset the gain in efficiency.

An example of a factorial design is the Physicians' Health Study (PHS), a trial evaluating two potential prevention agents, aspirin and beta-carotene.[6] The PHS was a randomized double-blind placebo controlled trial in a population of U.S. male physicians. These participants were randomized to either aspirin, beta-carotene, both, or neither, as shown in Figure 3.9. The primary questions involved only the main effects and each treatment comparison used a different outcome. The primary outcome for the aspirin versus placebo comparison was cardiovascular mortality and for beta-carotene versus placebo it was cancer incidence. Mortality was a leading secondary outcome in both comparisons. There was no interest in the interactions of the two treatments. The aspirin component of the trial was terminated early with a highly significant reduction in fatal and nonfatal myocardial infarction with a trend in cardiovascular mortality. The overall mortality rate was much lower than anticipated in the design so that the PHS was not adequately powered to detect a mortality effect (see Chapter 4) within the planned follow-up time. The beta-carotene arm continued to the scheduled termination and no difference was observed in either cancer incidence or mortality (Hennekens et al. 1996).

Another example of a factorial design was the Alpha-Tocopheral Beta-Carotene (ATBC) trial, conducted in over 29,000 Finnish male smokers.[7] In this trial, two potential prevention agents, alpha-tocopheral and beta-carotene, were evaluated, compared to a matching placebo control. ATBC was also randomized and double-blind. The primary outcome for both beta-carotene versus placebo and alpha-tocopheral versus placebo was lung cancer incidence. Total cancer incidence was a leading secondary outcome. In ATBC, neither prevention agent reduced the incidence of lung cancer. In fact, the beta-carotene significantly increased the incidence of lung cancer, an observation repeated by another trial conducted in the U.S. (Omenn et al. 1996).

The Women's Health Initiative (WHI) was a 2×3 partial factorial design, evaluating hormone replacement therapy (HRT), a low fat diet, and calcium supplementation in a very large cohort of high risk women.[8] The HRT intervention was compared to placebo in post menopausal women to test for the reduction in coronary heart disease (nonfatal myocardial infarction and death due to coronary heart disease) and to assess the possible increased risk in breast cancer. The low fat diet was to test for reduction in total cancer incidence and the calcium arm was to evaluate for effect on osteoporosis. The HRT arm had two subcomponents, one that compared estrogen plus progestin with placebo in women with an intact uterus and another component that compared estrogen alone with placebo in women without a uterus. While the primary outcome was coronary heart disease, secondary outcomes included mortality and hip fracture. WHI was a partial factorial because women did not have to participate in all of the three interventions. For the HRT compo-

---

[6] Steering Committee of the Physicians' Health Study Research Group (1989), Hennekens et al. (1996)

[7] The Alpha-Tocopherol, Beta-Carotene Cancer Prevention Study Group (1994)

[8] Writing Group for the Women's Health Initiative Randomized Controlled Trial (2002), The Women's Health Initiative Steering Committee (2004)

nent comparing estrogen plus progestin, the trial was terminated early with
an adverse effect due to blood clotting and an adverse effect on breast cancer.[9] Osteoporosis was reduced as measured by the hip fracture rate. There
was no observed reduction in mortality. The estrogen alone arm was also terminated early due to a significant adverse effect due to blood clotting, with no
significant reduction in mortality but with a significant improvement in hip
fracture.[10]

Group-randomization Designs

There are situations in which the intervention of interest cannot be easily administered at the individual level. For example, new sanitation practices in a
hospital may prevent certain kinds of infections. It would be difficult to create
a large trial to test this hypothesis if practitioners were required to follow
different procedures for each patient within a hospital. Instead, it would be
easier to treat all patients in a given hospital equally while assigning entire
hospitals to different practices. This is the idea behind group-randomized designs. These designs differ from designs randomizing individuals because the
groups themselves are not created through the experiment, but rather they
arise from relationships among the group members (Murray et al. 2004). This
usually induces a correlation among observations from members of each group.

One example of a group-randomized trial was the Seattle 5 a Day study
(Beresford et al. 2001). In this study, the intervention consisted of a number
of strategies for individual-level and work environment changes. A total of 28
worksites in the Seattle area were randomized, half with intervention and half
without. The primary outcome was the consumption of fruits and vegetables,
as measured by a modified food frequency questionnaire. Other self-reported
measures were used as secondary outcomes. These measures were assessed
at baseline and at 2 years, using independent cross-sectional samples of 125
workers at each worksite. After 2 years, the estimated intervention effect was
0.3 daily servings of fruits and vegetables, which was statistically significant.

A similar trial was known as Teens Eating for Energy and Nutrition at
School (TEENS) (Lytle et al. 2006). The intervention was similar to that in
the 5 a Day study and consisted of classroom-based curricula, newsletters,
and changes in the school food environment in favor of fruits, vegetables, and
other nutritious foods. The group units were 16 schools in Minnesota that were
randomized to either the intervention or the control arm. Outcome measures
included assessments of both the home food environment and the school food
environment. The home food environment was assessed with a one time parent survey sent to random subsamples of parents at the end of the study. The
results showed that parents of children enrolled in schools receiving the intervention made significantly healthier choices when grocery shopping. Other
measures derived from the parent survey did not show significant differences.

[9] Writing Group for the Women's Health Initiative Randomized Controlled Trial (2002)
[10] The Women's Health Initiative Steering Committee (2004)

The Trial of Activity in Adolescent Girls (TAAG) (Stevens et al. 2005) also used group randomization. The design called for 36 middle schools to be randomized to control or an intervention with special provisions for opportunities for physical activity. The primary goal was to increase the intensity-weighted minutes of moderate to vigorous physical activity engaged in by girls.

Most group-randomized studies are analyzed using linear mixed-effects models or related approaches. Models of this type are described in Chapter 8 in the context of longitudinal data analysis. The group randomization setting is similar to that of repeated measures data because of the correlation between measurements within randomized units (i.e., schools, worksites, etc.). When entire groups are randomized, the notion of "sample size" becomes more complex. Both the number of groups and the number of individuals to be sampled from within those groups must be determined. The necessary calculations are described in Chapter 4.

3.3 Non-inferiority Designs

Historically, most trials have been designed to show that a new intervention is better than or superior to a standard intervention, or that a new intervention added to standard of care is superior to standard of care alone. There are also many situations, however, where a new intervention need not be superior to a standard to be of interest. For example, compared to the standard the new intervention may be less toxic, less expensive, or less invasive and thus have an advantage over the standard, as long as it is not worse than the standard in clinical effect. Many industry sponsors may also want to show that their drug, biological agent, or device is not inferior to a leading competitor product. In cancer or AIDS treatment, a new intervention might have less toxicity and would be of great interest to physicians and patients as long as the effect on recurrence and mortality was almost as good as the standard drug regimen. Trials designed to show that the new intervention is "at least as good as" the control are known as *non-inferiority* trials.

Trials involving diseases that have life-threatening or other severe complications, and for which known effective treatments are available, cannot ethically be placebo controlled if the placebo would be used in place of a treatment known to be effective. (Placebo controls can be used if the new treatment is being used *in addition to* the existing standard.) Thus, unless the new treatment is expected to be superior the current standard, non-inferiority trials must be conducted. On the other hand, the design and conduct of non-inferiority trials can be extremely challenging. For example, in superiority trials, deficiencies in either design or conduct tend to make it more difficult to demonstrate that the new intervention is superior to control, providing incentives that help ensure proper study conduct. For non-inferiority trials, deficiencies can often serve to attenuate treatment differences. In the extreme case, if no subjects in either treatment arm comply with the protocol, the two groups will be indistinguishable and non-inferiority based solely on the formal statistical test will be confirmed (although the result will have no scientific credibility). Based on this logic, it is commonly believed that sloppy conduct increases the likelihood of showing non-inferiority (in Chapter 11, however, we show that this is not necessarily the case). Thus, a non-inferiority trial must strive to achieve quality as good as or better than the corresponding superiority trials.

There are also other challenges in non-inferiority trials. One is the choice of the control group. This issue is directly addressed by the ICH-E10 guidance document *Choice of Control Group and Related Issues in Clinical Trials*.[11] In order to demonstrate convincingly that the new intervention is not inferior, the new intervention needs to compete with the best standard available, not the least effective alternative. The selection of the control is not always straightforward. Different alternatives may have different risks and benefits, leading to different levels of compliance. Members of the medical community may not all agree on the treatment to be considered the best standard. One concern that regulatory agencies have is that if the least effective alternative is chosen, then a new intervention might be found to be non-inferior to a less than optimal alternative or control. A series of such non-inferiority trials could lead to acceptance of a very ineffective new intervention. This specific concern leads to an often used requirement that will be discussed later.

Another challenge results from the fact that it is impossible to show statistically that two groups are *not* different. Specifically, any statistic summarizing the difference between groups has an associated variance or confidence interval. To show absolute equivalence requires that the confidence interval have width zero and this would require an infinite sample size. Similarly, to show that one group is strictly non-inferior requires that the confidence interval is strictly to one side of zero (but possibly including zero) in which case we have essentially shown superiority. To overcome this technical difficulty, researchers construct a *zone of non-inferiority* within which the groups are considered *practically* equivalent (see Figure 3.10). The challenge, therefore, is to determine the maximum difference that can be allowed, yet for which the new treatment would still be considered non-inferior. This maximum value is referred to as the *margin of indifference*. The margin of indifference may be expressed as an absolute difference or a relative difference such as relative risk, hazard ratio, or odds ratio. (Mathematically, this distinction is artificial in the sense that relative differences can be expressed as absolute differences on a log scale.) As shown in Figure 3.10, researchers typically use the confidence interval for an intervention effect to draw inferences and conclusions. Figure 3.10 illustrates that if the confidence interval for the treatment difference excludes zero, the new intervention is concluded to be either better (case A) or worse (case D and E). For the non-inferiority trial, researchers want the confidence interval not to exclude zero difference, but rather want the upper limit to be below the margin of indifference (cases B and C). In case B, the estimate of the intervention effect indicates improvement with the upper limit being less

---

[11] http://www.fda.gov/cber/ich/ichguid.htm

than the margin of indifference. For case C, the intervention effect estimate indicates a slightly worse outcome but the upper limit is still less than the margin of indifference.

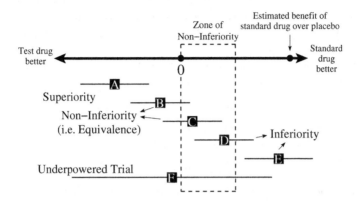

Figure 3.10 *Non-inferiority design (absolute difference) (modified from Antman (2001)).*

Choosing the value of the margin of indifference is difficult (Gao and Ware *to appear*). The choice must be based on a combination of clinical, ethical, and statistical factors. The size of the margin of indifference depends on the disease and the severity of toxicity or magnitude of the cost or invasiveness relative to the degree of benefit from the standard intervention. For example, researchers may decide that an increase in mortality by 20% may be tolerated if the new intervention had little to no toxicity, or did not require an invasive procedure. Thus, the design would be based on a margin of indifference corresponding to a relative risk of 1.2.

Regulatory agencies often take an approach that imposes two requirements on non-inferiority trials. First, a non-inferiority trial must meet the prespecified margin of indifference, δ, when comparing, say, a relative risk of RR_{TC} for the new treatment (T) to the standard (C). Second, the researchers must have relevant data that provides an estimate of the relative risk, RR_{CP}, of the standard to a placebo (P). This estimate is typically based on previous studies, often used to demonstrate the effectiveness of the standard intervention. Then, regulatory agencies may infer the relative risk (RR_{TP}) of the new intervention to a placebo control by multiplying the two relative risks, $RR_{TP} = RR_{TC}RR_{CP}$. If, for example non-inferiority is demonstrated versus the control, but the control has only minimal efficacy relative to placebo, RR_{TP} may show, for example, that despite strong evidence of non-inferiority, the effect against placebo may still be relatively weak. Of course, this imputation makes a key assumption—that the control relative risk is based on data that is still relevant. This may be difficult to determine as background therapy, patient referral patterns, and diagnostic criteria may change over time.

In fact, these arguments are similar to those that were used in section 3.2.1 to indicate why historical control trials have inherent bias.

To make the inference more precise, following Fleming (2007), we transform the relative risks to the log scale, letting $\beta_{XY} = \log(RR_{XY})$ and $\sigma_{XY}^2 = \mathrm{Var}(\hat{\beta}_{XY})$. Using this notation, we assume that the effect of T relative to C is given by $\beta_{TP} = \beta_{TC} + \beta_{CP}$. Note that since we are assuming that C is effective, $\beta_{CP} < 0$ (i.e., $RR_{CP} < 1$).

Now suppose that we wish to ensure that a fraction, p, of the effect of C relative to placebo is preserved; $\beta_{TP} < p\beta_{CP}$, or equivalently,

$$\beta_{TC} < p\beta_{CP} - \beta_{CP} = -(1-p)\beta_{CP}. \qquad (3.2)$$

Assuming that β_{CP} is known exactly, choose $\delta = -(1-p)\beta_{CP}$. Then, non-inferiority of T relative to C requires that

$$\hat{\beta}_{TC} + Z_{1-\alpha/2}\sigma_{TC} < -(1-p)\beta_{CP},$$

i.e., the upper limit of the $1 - \alpha$ confidence interval is below δ.

The assumption that β_{CP} is known exactly is unrealistic, so we will need to use an estimate, $\hat{\beta}_{CP}$, and also consider its variance σ_{CP}^2, both based on the results of previous trials. Rewriting (3.2), we require $\beta_{TC} + (1-p)\beta_{CP} < 0$ so that the criterion for showing non-inferiority is

$$\hat{\beta}_{TC} + (1-p)\hat{\beta}_{CP} + Z_{1-\alpha/2}(\sigma_{TC}^2 + (1-p)^2\sigma_{CP}^2)^{1/2} < 0 \qquad (3.3)$$

or

$$\hat{\beta}_{TC} + Z_{1-\alpha/2}\sigma_{TC}$$
$$< -(1-p)\hat{\beta}_{CP} + Z_{1-\alpha/2}[(\sigma_{TC}^2 + (1-p)^2\sigma_{CP}^2)^{1/2} - \sigma_{TC}], \qquad (3.4)$$

so the choice of δ is the right-hand side of (3.4). We note, however, that in this case δ depends on σ_{TC}^2 which may not be known until the trial is completed. When this might be of concern, one may simply prespecify the other parameters, p, $\hat{\beta}_{CP}$, and σ_{CP}^2, and apply (3.3) once $\hat{\beta}_{TC}$ and σ_{TC}^2 are known.

Certainly, following this approach requires assumptions. One is that the historical estimate of the control effect relative to placebo (e.g., RR_{PC}) is still relevant to the present population and standards of practice. For example, background therapy may have been developed and the patient mix may have changed in important but possibly unknown ways. In addition, the initial trial or trials were based on a particular set of patients or participants who volunteered and they may be different in important respects from the current population being studied. Whether these differences exist or not is usually difficult to determine. This assumption is sometimes referred to as the *constancy* assumption and it may not hold in all cases. Examples exist where two trials conducted consecutively with the same control intervention had significant differences in the control arms between trials (Packer et al. 1996; Carson et al. 2000). In some cases, the historical data may not even exist if the control was established on the basis of an intermediate marker such as lowering blood pressure, and the next treatment is being evaluated on reducing mortality or morbidity. Second, the percent of the initial control vs placebo effect, p, to maintain (e.g., 50%) is arbitrary but has a major impact on the choice of δ.

Another consideration in setting the value of δ is the magnitude of the difference or relative difference that would change clinical practice or patient preference. While the methods described in this section may be of value in providing guidance, other medical considerations should also be considered and adjustments made before the trial design is finalized. Nonetheless, it may be more important to focus on the trial that is being conducted, making sure that the appropriate or best control intervention is being utilized, that the trial is being conducted in the best possible way, and that the new treatment or intervention is compared with the statistically and medically determined value of δ. The imputation of the new intervention effect compared to placebo, had a placebo arm been present, while relevant, should not necessarily be the main focus of the interpretation. Control intervention "creep", that is, sequentially choosing weaker and less effective controls, can probably be best prevented by discussions between trial investigators and sponsors with the appropriate regulatory agencies when necessary.

An example of a non-inferiority trial is the OPTIMAAL trial, a trial of a new drug losartan and a standard drug captopril for patients with chronic heart failure (Dickstein et al. 2002). The primary outcome was total mortality. The margin of indifference was determined to be a relative risk of 1.2. Cough is a side effect of captopril use and, as a result, many patients are non-adherent. If the new drug losartan could be shown to be not inferior to captopril, it may be a viable alternative treatment. The standard drug captopril had previously been shown to be superior to placebo with a relative risk, RR_{CP}, of 0.805. As shown in Table 3.4, the relative risk for the losartan-captopril comparison, RR_{TC}, was 1.12 indicating an increase in mortality for patients treated with the new drug losartan. The imputed relative risk was obtained by multiplying the two relative risks together to get an estimate of 0.906. While this imputed relative risk of 0.906 is favorable, the upper level of the confidence interval, 1.26 for the losartan-captopril comparison, did not meet the OPTIMAAL prespecified margin of indifference 1.2. As a result, the new drug losartan was rejected as an alternative to captopril. Of course, the prespecified margin of indifference was a decision based on judgment of the investigators.

Another example that illustrates important issues is two simultaneous trials of a new agent, ximelagatran, compared to the standard control of warfarin. Warfarin is the generally accepted standard to prevent clotting of the blood, but requires frequent monitoring to maintain the correct dose levels and avoid either over- or under-clotting. New agents that could provide the same clinical benefit but without the inconvenience of the intensive monitoring are of great interest. Ximelagatran had been shown in earlier studies to effectively prevent clotting and two trials, SPORTIF III, conducted largely in Europe, and SPORTIF V, conducted largely in the U.S., were designed as non-inferiority trials to assess the ability of ximelagatran to reduce mortality and morbid-

Table 3.4 *Results related to the OPTIMAAL trial.*

	Rel. Risk	% change
catopril vs. placebo[*]	0.805	-19.5
losartan vs. captopril[†]	1.126	12.6
losartan vs. putative placebo	0.906	-9.4 ($RR = 0.805 \times 1.126$)

[*]Derived from previous trials
[†]Derived from OPTIMAAL

ity.[12] The subjects in both trials suffered from atrial fibrillation, increasing the risk of stroke and thereby the risk of mortality or morbidity. Clearly, warfarin was the appropriate control and the trials were conducted extremely well, achieving excellent clotting control.

Two issues arose, however, that are instructive for non-inferiority trials. The first issue is that the margin of indifference was based on an absolute difference in event rates, assuming an annual event rate of approximately 3%. In fact, the annual event rate observed in the trial was half the assumed rate, raising doubts regarding whether δ was in fact too large. The second issue is that there is little reliable data comparing warfarin to placebo, making the imputation of the effect of ximelagatran to placebo problematic. In retrospect, it would have been better to design these trials using a relative scale that would have automatically accounted for the lower than expected event rate. Nevertheless, the lack of historical data regarding the clinical effect of warfarin precludes meaningful imputation of effectiveness relative to placebo. These issues, combined with an observed increase in serious adverse effects related to abnormal liver function, led to the decision by the FDA to not approve ximelagatran based on these trials.

The design and conduct of non-inferiority trials is especially challenging. Many authors have discussed advantages and challenges of non-inferiority trials.[13] While such trials are necessary, the precise design and methods of analysis are still not completely determined and more experience is necessary before such methods will be established.

3.4 Screening, Prevention, and Therapeutic Designs

Phase III clinical trials may serve a variety of purposes. Screening or diagnostic trials may evaluate two methods or devices that are designed to detect disease or identify individuals at high risk for disease or an event. Examples of diagnostic procedures include mammography for detecting breast cancer or

---

[12] Halperin and Executive Steering Committee, SPORTIF III and V Study Investigators (2003), Albers, G. W. on behalf of the SPORTIF Investigators (2004)

[13] Fleming (2000, 1990), Temple and Ellenberg (2000), Ellenberg and Temple (2000), Hung et al. (2003), Hung et al. (2005)

ultrasound for measuring the degree of atherosclerosis in the carotid artery. Prevention trials are designed to intervene in a population at risk for disease but not yet diagnosed, comparing the proposed intervention to standard health care. An example would be giving a cholesterol lowering drug, such as a statin, to individuals identified to have high serum cholesterol, or giving a blood pressure lowering drug to a population with high blood pressure. Therapeutic trials evaluate a new intervention intended to reduce morbidity or risk of death due to diagnosed disease. Using a clot busting drug such as streptokinase in a patient with a heart attack, placing a stent in the coronary arteries for patients with blockage in those arteries, or surgical removal of a tumor in a cancer patient are examples of treatments that could be evaluated in a therapeutic trial to determine if morbidity or mortality would be reduced compared to a patient population not receiving those therapies.

These trials present different design challenges, even if a basic randomized parallel design is utilized. Screening trials such as mammography screening for breast cancer often are very large since, fortunately, the prevalence of breast cancer is low in the general population (Miller et al. 1992). The goal is to identify those individuals in the general population who have early stage breast cancer so that early intervention can be employed. Thus the design must include a strategy for efficiently evaluating a large number of individuals who may have no symptoms or reason to be seeking medical assistance. The false positive rate and false negative rates of the diagnostic procedure are critical in the design of screening trials (Prorok et al. 2000).

Prevention trials typically assess whether a new intervention can reduce the risk of disease developing in disease-free individuals, defined as *primary prevention*,[14] or preventing the recurrence of the disease, defined as *secondary prevention*.[15] In primary prevention trials, individuals at high risk for the incidence of a disease are treated with a drug, device, or procedure to prevent the disease occurrence. For example, in individuals with high cholesterol or high blood pressure, a primary prevention trial using cholesterol or blood pressure lowering drugs assess whether these interventions reduce the incidence of heart attacks or death from the heart attack. Here the individuals entered into the trial may be at higher risk but generally are disease-free and not seeking medical assistance. Thus, recruitment strategies must target otherwise healthy individuals, and convince them to enter the trial. Experience suggests that the yield of patients potentially eligible will likely be no more

---

[14] Steering Committee of the Physicians' Health Study Research Group (1989), Multiple Risk Factor Intervention Trial Research Group (1982), Writing Group for the Women's Health Initiative Randomized Controlled Trial (2002), Diabetes Control and Complications Trial Research Group (1993), The Alpha-Tocopherol, Beta-Carotene Cancer Prevention Study Group (1994), Hypertension Detection and Follow-up Program Cooperative Group (1979), Lipid Research Clinics Program (1984)

[15] Beta-Blocker Heart Attack Trial Research Group (1982), MERIT-HF Study Group (1999), Packer (2000), Bristow et al. (2004), ALLHAT Collaborative Research Group (2000), Aspirin Myocardial Infarction Study (AMIS) Research Group (1980), The Coronary Drug Project Research Group (1975), Hulley et al. (1998)

than about 20%, perhaps as low as 5–10%. Therefore, large numbers of individuals must be screened for eligibility and willingness to participate in order to get the desired number of randomized participants.

Since these individuals are not ill, the trial design must account for the likelihood that not all of them will comply with the intervention. That is, the individuals are less likely to take all of their medication, especially if there are undesirable side effects and the sensitivity of the trial to detect a benefit of the intervention will be reduced. In Chapter 4 we discuss sample size calculations that attempt to take into account the anticipated level of compliance. Failure to account for non-compliance can be problematic.

Secondary prevention trials are designed to evaluate whether an intervention can prevent the recurrence of the disease in a population who have had a defining event. For example, we may assess whether drugs such as beta-blockers reduce the occurrence of a second heart attack in a patient surviving a heart attack or whether longer term use of tamoxifen following standard treatment reduces the risk of the breast cancer recurrence. Secondary prevention trials require a different recruitment strategy since these individuals are now identified through an event or occurrence of a disease. Secondary prevention trials, like primary prevention trials, are often large because the recurrence rates may be low. On the other hand, there may be a large number of eligible individuals. While these individuals have been diagnosed with a disease, they may still not fully comply with the intervention being tested. Thus, compliance must be considered in the design of the trial.

For both primary and secondary prevention trials, designing the trial to address the compliance to intervention is critical. As shown in Chapter 4, the sample size increases nonlinearly with the degree of non-compliance. Thus, every attempt must be made in the design to maximize compliance. Characteristics of the participant population may be used to identify individuals likely to have a high degree of compliance. For example, individuals with other competing risks or diseases may have difficulty with compliance. If individuals are not able to come to the clinic for evaluation and intervention support, they may not be able to comply optimally. Once every consideration in the entry criteria and logistical aspects has been covered, then the sample size must be adjusted to account for the remaining degree of non-compliance.

As we will discuss further in Chapter 11, the "intent to treat" principle requires that all participants randomized into the trial must be accounted for in the analysis. Failure to comply with this principle can lead to serious bias in the analysis and interpretation of the results. It is not appropriate to remove participants who do not comply fully with the intervention. Thus, potential non-compliance must be addressed in the design.

Therapeutic trials evaluate new treatments or interventions for patients who are in the acute phase of their disease for the effectiveness in reducing mortality and morbidity.[16] For example, treatments such as clot busting drugs for a

---

[16] The TIMI Research Group (1988), Volberding et al. (1990), The Global Use of Strategies

patient with an evolving heart attack has proven to be effective in reducing death due to the heart attack. Recruitment strategies for therapeutic trials depend on access to patients and their willingness to participate in the trial. The recruitment pool is generally much smaller than for a primary prevention trial and the yield also much less than 100%, probably also in the neighborhood of 20%.

3.5 Adaptive Designs

There are many uses of adaptive methods in the design and conduct of clinical trials. As described earlier, phase I and phase II trials are by their very nature adaptive. In a phase I trial, dose depends on the patient response to the most recent dose. The next stage in a phase II trial does not proceed unless the results from the first stage are favorable. For phase III trials, trial design can be modified as well during the conduct of a trial.

3.5.1 Sequential Designs

A large class of adaptive designs will be described in Chapter 10. Briefly, sequential methods are used to determine when the accumulating results on safety measures and efficacy assessment are so convincing, either favorable or unfavorable to the new intervention, that the trial should be terminated or that the protocol should be modified. The statistical methods are described that also identify when a trial is not going to meet its objectives and continuation is futile.

3.5.2 Outcome Based Adaptive Design

In contrast to the previous section where no data analyses comparing interventions are used for sample size adjustment, *outcome adaptive* trials use the evolving estimate of the intervention effect to make design modifications. Historically, designs such as "play-the-winner" use the success or failure of the last participant to determine the next treatment assignment (see Chapter 5). These designs, however, have not been widely used in clinical trials, despite their superficial appeal.

Other methods have been proposed to modify study design based on the interim estimate of the intervention (Lan and Trost 1997; Fisher 1998; Cui et al. 1999; Shen and Fisher 1999; Chen et al. 2000). One of these is referred to as the weighted Z-statistic method. This method is based on the idea that the type I error rate of the trial is maintained, even if the sample size is changed in response to the observed treatment difference, provided that the

to Open Occluded Coronary Arteries (GUSTO III) Investigators (1997), Moss et al. (1996), Cardiac Arrhythmia Suppression Trial II Investigators (1992), The Diabetic Retinopathy Study Research Group (1978), Fisher et al. (1995), Gruppo Italiano per lo Studio Della Sopravvivenze Nell'Infarcto Miocardico (GISSI) (1986) total information content is unchanged. This is achieved at the conclusion of the trial by decomposing the Z usual statistic into two components—the Z-statistic at the time of the design modification and a Z-statistic derived from the post modification observations.

For simplicity, assume that $X_i \sim N(\theta, 1)$, $i = 1, \ldots, N_0$, where N_0 is the initial total sample size. Let n be the sample size at the time the adjustment is made and t the information fraction, $t = n/N_0$. The observed treatment difference is

$$\hat{\theta} = \sum_1^n X_i/n,$$

and the interim Z statistic for testing $H_0 : \theta = 0$ is

$$Z^{(n)} = \sum_1^n X_i/\sqrt{n}.$$

With no modification the trial would complete with sample size N_0, and a final test statistic

$$
\begin{aligned}
Z^{(N_0)} &= \sum_1^{N_0} X_i/\sqrt{N_0} \\
&= \sqrt{\frac{n}{N_0}} \sum_1^n X_i/\sqrt{n} + \sqrt{\frac{N_0 - n}{N_0}} \sum_{n+1}^{N_0} X_i/\sqrt{N_0 - n} \\
&= \sqrt{t}\, Z^{(n)} + \sqrt{1-t}\, \overline{Z}^{(N_0-n)}
\end{aligned}
\tag{3.5}
$$

where $\overline{Z}^{(N_0-n)}$ is the Z statistic using only the final $N_0 - n$ subjects. Note that this a weighted sum of the Z statistics involving the first n and final $N_0 - n$ subjects where the weights are the square roots of the corresponding information fractions.

It can be shown that, provided that the weights remain fixed, we can adjust the final sample size any way that we like, in particular based on $\hat{\theta}$, and use the corresponding Z statistic in place of $\overline{Z}^{(N_0-n)}$ in (3.5) and still preserve the overall type I error rate.

Suppose that, based on $\tilde{\theta}$, we propose a revised total sample size N and the end of the trial we use the test statistic

$$Z^{(N)} = \sqrt{t}\, Z^{(n)} + \sqrt{1-t}\, \overline{Z}^{(N-n)}.$$

Then, under an alternative hypothesis $H_1 : \theta = \theta_A$, unconditionally,

$$EZ^{(N)} = \frac{n + \sqrt{(N_0 - n)(N - n)}}{\sqrt{N_0}} \theta_A.$$

Thus, if $N > N_0$, we have $EZ^{(N)} > EZ^{(N_0)}$, and the power for H_1 will be increased, although the increase will be smaller than if we had used N as the planned sample size at the start of the trial. Using this approach, the outcomes for the final $N - n$ subjects are down-weighted (provided $N > N_0$) so that the effective information contributed is the fixed.

The choice of N can be subjective, possibly using both prior expectations regarding the likely effect size and the interim estimate, $\hat{\theta}$, and its associated variability. Note that since $Z^{(n)}$ is known, one likely would base the decision on the conditional expectation of $\overline{Z}^{(N)}$ given $Z^{(n)}$.

Tsiatis and Mehta (2003) have criticized this method, suggesting that it is not efficient. Others have worried that these trials are prone to bias since speculations about the size of the treatment effect in a blinded trial might arise, based on the size of the sample size adjustment. These more recent response adaptive designs have been used (Franciosa et al. 2002; Taylor et al. 2004) but as yet not widely due to concerns. Jennison and Turnbull (2006) suggest that efficient trials can be designed using common group sequential methods by considering *a priori* a number of possible effect sizes.

Lan and Trost (1997) proposed using conditional power to make an assessment of whether the interim results are sufficiently encouraging to justify an increase in sample size. This concept was further developed by Chen, DeMets, and Lan (2000). Conditional power is the probability of obtaining a statistically significant result at the end of the trial, given the current observed trend in the intervention effect compared to control and given an assumption about the true but unknown treatment effect for the remainder of the trial. Conditional power will be described in more detail in the data monitoring chapter (Chapter 10). Let $Z(t)$ be the normalized statistic observed at information fraction t in the trial. The conditional power is $\Pr(Z(1) \geq C | Z(t), \theta)$, where C is the critical value at the conclusion of the trial, and θ is the standardized treatment difference. The computational details can be found in Section 10.6.3.

Chen, DeMets, and Lan showed that if the conditional power for the observed trend is greater than 0.50 but less than desired, the sample size can be increased up to 75% with little practical effect on the overall type I error rate and with no serious loss of power.

The methods described above have many attractive features and many control the type I error, as desired. The primary concern with adaptive designs that adjust sample size based on emerging trends is not technical but rather logistical. Trials are designed and conducted to minimize as many sources of bias as possible. If the sample size is adjusted based on emerging trends according to one of the methods described, it is straightforward for those with knowledge of both the size of the adjustment and the adjustment procedure to obtain an estimate of the emerging treatment difference. Of course, following any interim analysis, investigators may have been given clues regarding the current trend—if the recommendation is to continue, investigators might assume that the current results have exceeded neither the boundary for benefit nor the boundary for harm. If there is a formal futility boundary, then additional clues may be given about where the current trend might be. Of course, the difficulty is that data monitoring committees may have reasons to recommend that a trial continue even if a boundary for the primary outcome has been crossed. (Related issues are discussed further in Chapter 10.) Investigators, therefore, may be able to glean knowledge regarding the range for current trends whether or not the trial is using any adaptive design. For adaptive designs modifying sample size based on current trends, however, the clues may be stronger. The concern is whether this information biases the conduct of the trial in any way. For example, would investigators alter their recruitment or the way participants are cared for? If the trial is double-blind, biases may be less than for non-blinded trials. As of today, there is inadequate experience with these types of adaptive designs to be confident that bias might not be introduced. These designs are still somewhat controversial.

3.6 Conclusions

An engineer or architect must finalize the design of a large project before construction of a project begins, for it is difficult, if not impossible, to correct a design flaw once construction has been begun. The same is true for the design of a clinical trial. No amount of statistical analysis can correct for a poor or flawed design. In this chapter, we have discussed a variety of designs, all of which have an appropriate application. Each design may need to be modified somewhat to meet the needs of the particular research question. For the phase III clinical trial, the randomized control trial is the most widely used design. While simple, it can be used to address many research questions and is very robust, not relying on many additional assumptions beyond the use of randomization.

A clinical trial should not use a research design that is more complicated than necessary. In general, the practice should be to keep the design as simple as possible to achieve the objectives. In recent years, clinical trials have increasingly utilized the factorial design with success, getting two or more questions answered with only a modest increase in cost and complexity. Greater use of the factorial design has the potential to improve efficiency in cases for which they are appropriate. Statistical methods for adaptive designs that allow for modification of sample size during the course of the trial based on interim trends are available, but there remain concerns regarding their practical implementation. Use of this kind of adaptive design should be considered with caution.

3.7 Problems

3.1 Suppose we conduct a phase I trial to find the MTD. We use the daily doses $1g$, $1.9g$, $2.7g$, $3.4g$, $4.0g$, and $4.6g$ which correspond to true (unknown) toxicity levels of $0\%, 10\%, \ldots, 40\%$, and 50%, respectively. For this exercise, you may need to use a computer for simulation or, where possible, direct calculation.

(a) First, consider using the traditional design. The trial begins with the $1g$ dose and proceeds according to the algorithm described in Section 3.1.1; the last dose without excessive toxicity is the MTD estimate.

      i. What is the expected value of the MTD estimate in this case?

      ii. What is the expected value of the sample size?

      iii. What is the expected number of subjects that would be treated at or over the 40% toxicity level (i.e., $4g$) in this case?

      iv. What modifications could you make in the design so that the expected value of the toxicity of the MTD estimate will be approximately 1/3?

(b) Next, consider the modified design (allowing steps down in dose), starting at the third level ($2.7g$), stopping after 15 patients.

      i. What is the expected value of the MTD estimate (use the stopping dose to estimate the MTD)?

      ii. What is the expected number of patients who would be treated at or over the 40% toxicity level?

(c) Finally, consider using another design with single-patient cohorts. Start at the first dose level, increasing the dose for the next subject when a non-toxic response is observed. When a toxic response is observed, a second stage begins at the previous (lower) dose level. If two subsequent non-toxic responses are observed, the dose increases. If a toxic response is observed, the dose is reduced. Stop after a total of 15 patients.

      i. What is the expected value of the MTD estimate (again, use the stopping dose to estimate the MTD)?

      ii. What is the expected number of patients who would be treated at or over the 40% toxicity level?

(d) How would you derive confidence intervals for the MTD using data from the three designs above? Demonstrate your confidence intervals' coverage properties via simulation.

3.2 Consider Fleming's three-hypothesis formulation for phase II trials with binary outcomes. Suppose you have a single arm trial where $\pi_1 = 0.05$, $\pi_2 = 0.25$, and the total sample size is 30. Set the level for H_0 and H_2 each to 0.05, i.e.,

$$P(\text{reject } H_0 | \pi_T = 0.05) \leq 0.05 \quad \text{and}$$
$$P(\text{reject } H_2 | \pi_T = 0.25) \leq 0.05$$

(a) Give the three critical regions that would be used at the trial's conclusion. State the probabilities of observing an outcome in each of the three regions, given that H_2 is true ($\pi_T = 0.3$).

(b) Suppose that, after fifteen patients, only one success is observed. What is the probability, conditional on the interim results, of rejecting H_0, given that H_2 is true ($\pi_T = 0.3$)? What is the probability, conditional on the interim results, of rejecting H_0, given that H_0 is true ($\pi_T = 0.05$)?

(c) Before the trial starts, suppose it is determined that another identical trial, using the same critical regions, will be performed following this one in the event that no hypothesis is rejected. What is the probability, given H_0 is true ($\pi_T = 0.05$), that H_0 will be rejected? What is the probability, given H_2 is true ($\pi_T = 0.25$), that H_2 will be rejected? Should the critical regions be adjusted to conserve the overall error rates? Explain.

3.3 Consider a non-inferiority study in which we are interested in the probabilities of failure π_C and π_E in the control and experimental arms, respectively. In particular, we are interested in the following two pairs of hypotheses: absolute (additive) non-inferiority,

$$
\begin{aligned}
H_0 &\quad : \quad \pi_E - \pi_C \geq 0.1 \\
H_1 &\quad : \quad \pi_E - \pi_C < 0.1;
\end{aligned}
$$

and relative (multiplicative) non-inferiority,

$$
\begin{aligned}
H_0 &\quad : \quad \frac{\pi_E}{\pi_C} \geq 2 \\
H_1 &\quad : \quad \frac{\pi_E}{\pi_C} < 2.
\end{aligned}
$$

There are 80 subjects in each arm. Assume the sample is large enough to use the normal approximation.

(a) What test statistic do you suggest for the hypotheses of absolute non-inferiority?

(b) For a one-sided test at the 0.05 level, show the rejection region on a plot with axes corresponding to the observed failure proportions in the two arms.

(c) What test statistic do you suggest for the hypotheses of relative non-inferiority?

(d) For a one-sided test at the 0.05 level, show the rejection region on a plot as in the previous case.

(e) Which test do you think will be more likely to reject H_0 when $\pi_E = \pi_C = 0.1$?

(f) In general, supposing that $\pi_E = \pi_C = 0.1$, for what values (approximate) of these probabilities, if any, do you think that your absolute non-inferiority test will be more likely to reject H_0? For what values, if any, do you think that your relative non-inferiority test will be more likely to reject H_0?

CHAPTER 4

Sample Size

One of the most important design features of an experimental study is the sample size. A clinical study that is too small to yield meaningful results wastes resources and puts patients at risk with minimal potential for benefit. A study that is too large may be able to identify effects that are too small to be of clinical interest while potentially exposing more subjects than necessary to inferior treatments.

The dilemma faced at the design stage is that typically the information required to compute the sample size is not known prior to the initiation of the study. Often sample sizes are based on available resources, and the detectable effect sizes are determined from the sample size, rather than reverse.

Most trials are designed with a fixed (maximum) sample size determined prior to study start, possibly with provisions for early stopping for either benefit, safety, or futility. In addition to the traditional fixed size trial based on tests of significance, there is increasing interest in the literature in adaptive trials that make use of information acquired early in the trial to adjust the sample size and may use either Bayesian or frequentist criteria. A brief discussion of procedures of this type appears in Section 3.5.2.

Because most studies are currently conducted using the frequentist significance testing approach, the material in this chapter will be presented from a frequentist point of view, the key principle of which is illustrated by Figure 4.1. Suppose that $X_1, X_2, \ldots, X_N$ are a sample of normally distributed random variables with mean μ and known variance, σ^2. Suppose that we want to test the hypothesis $H_0: \mu = 0$ with low type I error and reject H_0 with high probability when a particular alternative hypothesis, $H_1: \mu = \mu_1$, is true (low type II error). To ensure low type I error, we will reject H_0 if $\overline{X}_N > C_N$ where $\overline{X}_N$ is the mean of N observations and C_N is a constant defined by $\Pr\{\overline{X}_N > C_N | \mu = 0\} = \alpha$ for a small value of α. Because the variance of $\overline{X}_N$, σ^2/N, is a decreasing function of N, the distribution of $\overline{X}_N$ becomes more concentrated about its mean as N increases. For small samples, $N = 10$, the distribution is diffuse and C_{10} is large. In particular, $C_{10} > \mu_1$, and most samples of size 10 from the alternative distribution ($\mu = \mu_1$) will have mean less than C_{10}. That is, when $H_1: \mu = \mu_1$ is true, we will reject H_0 less than half the time. When $N = 30$, the distribution of $\overline{X}_{30}$ is a bit more peaked about its mean, and C_{30} is below μ_1, and under H_1 we will reject H_0 a bit more than half the time. Finally, when $N = 120$, both distributions are quite concentrated about their respective means, and $\overline{X}_{120}$ will almost certainly be larger than C_{120}, and thus power under H_1 will be quite high. The methods

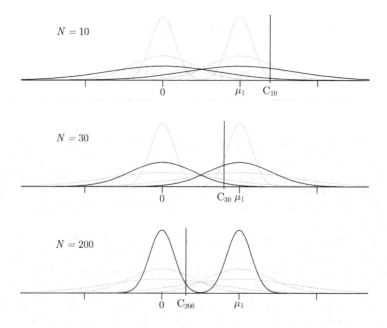

Figure 4.1 *Illustration of the fundamental principle underlying sample size calculations. Curves represent the densities for the mean of N observations from normal distributions with mean either 0 or μ_1 for $N = 10, 30, 120$. The black curves represent the densities for the sample sizes indicated for each panel. The vertical lines indicate the location of the critical value for a (one-sided) test of $H_0: \mu = 0$.*

described in this chapter are focused on finding the sample size that ensures that the trial will have the desired type I and type II errors. Intuitively, this is equivalent to selecting N so that C_N is properly situated between the true means under H_0 and H_1—if C_N is too close to μ_1 we will have high type II error, and if C_N is too close to 0, we will enroll more subjects than necessary.

4.1 Sample Size versus Information

Before describing the methods for sample size calculation we need to understand what is meant by the term "sample size." While in many trials it is clear, in others it is less so. For example, in a longitudinal study, we may have multiple baseline/pre-treatment and/or follow-up observations. In this case, the "effective sample size", closely related to *information*,[1] is a function of both the number of subjects and the number of observations per subject. Similarly,

---

[1] See Appendix A.5 for a discussion of *statistical information*. Informally, one can think of information as the reciprocal of the variance of a parameter estimate. When the variance of each observation is known and fixed, information is directly proportional to sample size.

in a study of long-term survival, "effective sample size" may be a function of a combination of the number of subjects and the length of follow-up per subject (for example, the total person-years of exposure). Hence, in some settings it may be more useful to define the study size by the total information required rather than by the number of subjects, the number of subjects being only one component of a strategy to achieve the desired total information. Ideally a study would be designed so that it would end not when a predetermined number of subjects had been followed to their prescribed end of follow-up, but rather when the desired level of information had been obtained (Lachin 2005).

To illustrate, suppose that we have n subjects, whose data are i.i.d. (independent and identically distributed) within treatment group, and let Δ denote the effect of treatment. Suppose further that the score function[2] is $U_n(\Delta) = \sum_{i=1}^{n} u(y_i, \Delta, z_i)$ where z_i is the indicator of treatment group, so that an efficient (two-sided, level α) test of the null hypothesis $H_0 : \Delta = 0$ is obtained by rejecting H_0 if $-U(0)^2/U'(0) > \chi^2_{1,1-\alpha}$, where $\chi^2_{1,1-\alpha}$ is the $100 \times (1 - \alpha)$-percentage point of the χ^2 distribution with 1 degree of freedom. Under H_0, the Fisher information is $\mathcal{I}(0) = -E[U'(0)|\Delta = 0] = -\sum_{i=1}^{n} Eu'(y_i, 0, z_i)$. The Fisher information will be larger if the information per subject, $-Eu'(y_i, 0, z_i)$, is larger, or, alternatively, for fixed $-Eu'(y_i, 0, z_i)$, if the number of subjects is increased. Consider the following examples.

- Let $y_i \sim N(\Delta, 1)$, i.e., y_i has a Gaussian distribution with mean Δ and variance one. The score function is $U(\Delta) = \sum_{i=1}^{n} y_i - \Delta$ so $\mathcal{I}(0) = n$ and the Fisher information and the sample sizes coincide.

- Suppose x_i is an exponential random variable (e.g., time to death) with rate $\lambda = \exp(\mu)$ and that we follow all subjects until a fixed time τ. Let $T_i = \min(x_i, \tau)$, and $y_i = 1$ if $x_i \leq \tau$ and $y_i = 0$ otherwise. In other words, y_i indicates whether the failure occurs during the follow-up time so that it can be observed. The score function is $U(\mu) = \sum_{i=1}^{n}(y_i - \exp(\mu)T_i)$ (see Example A.6 in Appendix A.5). The Fisher information is $\mathcal{I}(\mu) = n(1 - \exp(-\lambda\tau))$. Thus, we can increase information either by increasing n, or increasing the follow-up time τ, although if $\lambda\tau$ is already large, so that $\exp(-\lambda\tau)$ is near zero, the information gain achieved by further increasing τ is minimal. If we take $\tau = \infty$, then, again, $\mathcal{I}(\mu) = n$, the sample size.

- In example A.9 (Appendix A.5, page 402), m_j, $j = 1, 2, \ldots, n$, measurements are obtained on n subjects and we wish to conduct inference regarding the overall mean μ. If the correlation between observations within subjects is ρ and the variance is σ^2, the Fisher information is

$$\mathcal{I}(\mu) = \sum_{j} \frac{m_j}{\sigma^2(1 + m_j\rho)}.$$

In this setting, one might consider initiating the study fixing $m_j = m$ in

---

[2] See Appendix A.2 for a discussion of the score function, Fisher information, and likelihood based inference.

advance, but without fixing the sample size, n, estimating ρ and σ^2 from the data and sampling until $mn/\hat{\sigma}^2(1+m\hat{\rho})$ reaches a predetermined value.

The information based approach to study design is commonly used in studies with long-term follow-up and a time-to-failure (i.e., disease-free survival) outcome. In survival studies, information is usually proportional to the number of subjects experiencing the failure of interest. Typically a fixed number of subjects are enrolled, but the total length follow-up is not fixed in advance. The study ends when a predetermined number of subjects fail. Total information is also an essential component of studies with sequential monitoring procedures based on the triangular test promoted by Whitehead (1983) (see Section 10.5). Studies using designs of this type end either when sufficient evidence either for or against the efficacy of treatment is obtained, or when a maximum, prespecified amount of information, equivalent to $\mathcal{I}(0)$, has accrued. A more complete discussion of information based designs can be found in Lachin (2005).

In this chapter we will only formally consider information based designs in the context of time-to-failure outcomes (Section 4.4).

4.2 A General Setup for Frequentist Designs

We begin by describing a very general setup involving two treatment groups. Typically studies with more than two treatment groups are designed with particular pairwise comparisons of primary interest, so there is usually little lost by considering only two groups at a time. Let X_{jN}, $j = 1, 2$ represent the observed data with total sample size N for each of treatment groups 1 and 2. In this section we do not make any assumptions regarding the structure of X_{jN}, so the contribution from each subject to X_{jN} might be a single observation (e.g., blood pressure), a dichotomous outcome (e.g., vital status), a vector of follow-up observations, or any of a variety of other possible structures. We will assume that the X_{jN} comes from a family of distributions parameterized by γ_j, $j = 1, 2$, possibly vector valued. The distribution of X_{jN} may depend on additional nuisance parameters, but for simplicity we will suppress this dependence.

Using a typical frequentist significance testing procedure, we wish to test the null hypothesis $H_0 : \gamma_1 = \gamma_2$. At the conclusion of the study we will either reject or accept[3] H_0. A *type I* error occurs if we conclude that H_0 is false when it is true, while a *type II* error occurs if we conclude that H_0 is true when it is false. The goal is to find the smallest sample size, N, so that the type I error rate is at most α and the type II error rate is at most β for a given alternative hypothesis H_1. The *power* of the study is the rejection probability, $1 - \beta$, under H_1. We will assume that

---

[3] It may be more appropriate to say that we *fail to reject* since in many, if not most, settings we take failure to reject H_0 to mean that the true effect size, $\gamma_2 - \gamma_1$, may be non-zero, but not large enough to ensure rejection of H_0. If the trial is adequately powered, it may suggest that the effect size is too small to be of clinical interest.

1. the test of H_0 is based on a univariate test statistic, U, that under H_0 is asymptotically normal (AN) with mean zero and variance V_0 for which we have a consistent estimate, $\hat{V}_0$, and

2. under a fixed, known alternative hypothesis H_1, U is asymptotically normal with mean Δ (independent of N) and variance V_1.

We begin with a one-sided test. The generalization to a two-sided test is straightforward. We let

$$T = U/\sqrt{\hat{V}_0}.$$

Since $T \sim AN(0,1)$, we will reject H_0 if $T > Z_{1-\alpha}$ where $Z_{1-\alpha} = \Phi^{-1}(1-\alpha)$. We will also assume that under H_1,

$$T \sim AN(\Delta/\sqrt{E[\hat{V}_0|H_1]}, V_1/E[\hat{V}_0|H_1]).$$

Then the power is

$$
\begin{aligned}
1 - \beta &= \Pr\{T > Z_{1-\alpha}|H_1\} \\
&= \Pr\left\{ \frac{U - E[U|H_1]}{\sqrt{V_1}} > \frac{Z_{1-\alpha}\sqrt{E[\hat{V}_0|H_1]} - E[U|H_1]}{\sqrt{V_1}} \middle| H_1 \right\}
\end{aligned}
$$

which is equivalent to

$$Z_{1-\alpha}\sqrt{E[\hat{V}_0|H_1]} + Z_{1-\beta}\sqrt{V_1} = \Delta. \qquad (4.1)$$

Equation (4.1) is the most general equation relating effect size, significance level, and power; however, it does not explicitly involve the sample size. In order to introduce the sample size into equation (4.1), we need a bit more.

First, while many, if not most, studies have equal sized treatment groups, occasionally the randomization is unbalanced and we have unequal sized treatment groups. Let ξ_j be the proportion of subjects in treatment group j, so that $\xi_1 + \xi_2 = 1$ (if there are more than two treatment groups, ξ_j will be the proportion out of those assigned to the two groups under consideration).

Second, among the cases that we consider, we will have $NE[\hat{V}_0|H_1] \approx \phi(\bar{\gamma})/\xi_1\xi_2$ where $\bar{\gamma} = \xi_1\gamma_1 + \xi_2\gamma_2$, and $NV_1 = \phi(\gamma_1)/\xi_1 + \phi(\gamma_2)/\xi_2$ for some function $\phi(\cdot)$. $\phi(\gamma)$ may be regarded as the variance contributed to the test statistic by a single observation given that the true parameter is γ. In this case, equation (4.1) becomes

$$\Delta\sqrt{N} = Z_{1-\alpha}\sqrt{\phi(\bar{\gamma})/\xi_1\xi_2} + Z_{1-\beta}\sqrt{\phi(\gamma_1)/\xi_1 + \phi(\gamma_2)/\xi_2} \qquad (4.2)$$

which can be solved for N to find the sample size required to achieve a given power or for $1 - \beta$ to find the power for a given sample size. In many cases $\phi(\gamma_1)/\xi_1 + \phi(\gamma_2)/\xi_2 \approx \phi(\bar{\gamma})/\xi_1\xi_2$ and this equation can be reasonably approximated by

$$\sqrt{\phi(\bar{\gamma})/\xi_1\xi_2}(Z_{1-\alpha} + Z_{1-\beta}) = \Delta\sqrt{N}. \qquad (4.3)$$

Note that using equation (4.3), $N \propto 1/\xi_1\xi_2$, so that if we have an unbalanced

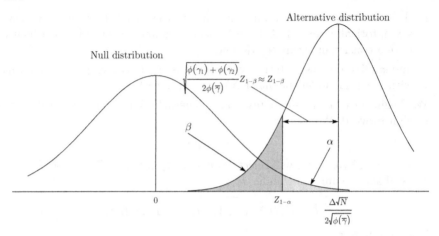

Figure 4.2 *Graphical representation of equation (4.2). For this figure we take $\xi_1 = \xi_2 = 1/2$.*

randomization, a larger sample size will usually be required relative to the balanced case. The increase in sample size is relatively small unless the degree of imbalance is quite large. For example, if we use a 3:2 randomization, so that $\xi_1 = .6$ and $\xi_2 = .4$, then $1/\xi_1\xi_2 = 25/6 = 4.167$ (compared to 4 in the balanced case) and the total sample size will need to be increased only by about 4%. Similarly, a 2:1 randomization requires an increase of 12.5%. An increase of at least 50% is not required unless the degree of imbalance is at least $2 + \sqrt{3} = 3.73$ to 1.

4.2.1 Two Sample Binomial

Suppose we wish to conduct a study of short term mortality (say within one month of treatment) so that the time of death is not of concern. Suppose further that π_1 and π_2 are probabilities of death for experimental and control groups, respectively, and we wish to test $H_0 : \pi_1 = \pi_2 = \pi$ versus $H_1 : \pi_1 \neq \pi_2$. Let a be the number of deaths in the experimental group and b be the number of deaths in the control group so that $a \sim \text{Bin}(n_1, \pi_1)$ and $b \sim \text{Bin}(n_2, \pi_2)$, where n_1 and n_2 are known and fixed, so that $\xi_j = n_j/N, j = 1, 2$.

If we have the table

	Experimental	Control	Total
Dead	a	b	m_1
Alive	c	d	m_2
	n_1	n_2	N

the (uncorrected) Pearson χ^2 statistic is

$$\frac{(a - n_1 m_1/N)^2 N^3}{n_1 n_2 m_1 m_2} = Z^2,$$

where

$$Z = \frac{a/n_1 - b/n_2}{\sqrt{m_1 m_2/n_1 n_2 N}}.$$

So let $U(a,b) = \dfrac{a}{n_1} - \dfrac{b}{n_2}$ and, since $V_0 = \pi(1-\pi)(1/n_1 + 1/n_2)$, $\hat{V}(a,b) = \dfrac{m_1 m_2}{n_1 n_2 N}$. Under H_1, $E[U(a,b)|H_1] = \pi_1 - \pi_2 = \Delta$.

$$\begin{aligned}
V_1 &= \mathrm{Var}[U(a,b)|H_1] \\
&= \frac{\pi_1(1-\pi_1)}{n_1} + \frac{\pi_2(1-\pi_2)}{n_2} \\
&= \frac{1}{N}\left(\frac{\phi(\pi_1)}{\xi_1} + \frac{\phi(\pi_2)}{\xi_2}\right),
\end{aligned}$$

where $\phi(x) = x(1-x)$, and

$$\begin{aligned}
E[\hat{V}(a,b)|H_1] &= E\left[\frac{(a+b)(N-a-b)}{n_1 n_2 N}\right] \\
&= \frac{N\bar{\pi}(1-\bar{\pi})}{n_1 n_2 N} - \frac{n_1\pi_1(1-\pi_1) + n_2\pi_2(1-\pi_2)}{n_1 n_2} \\
&= \frac{\bar{\pi}(1-\bar{\pi})}{\xi_1\xi_2 N} - \frac{\xi_1\pi_1(1-\pi_1) + \xi_2\pi_2(1-\pi_2)}{\xi_1\xi_2 N^2} \qquad (4.4) \\
&\approx \frac{\phi(\bar{\pi})}{\xi_1\xi_2 N}, \qquad (4.5)
\end{aligned}$$

where $\bar{\pi} = \xi_1\pi_1 + \xi_0\pi_0$. The approximation in (4.5) holds for reasonably large N because the second term in equation (4.4) is negligible.

Hence, equation (4.2) becomes

$$\sqrt{N}\Delta = Z_{1-\alpha}\sqrt{\bar{\pi}(1-\bar{\pi})(\frac{1}{\xi_1} + \frac{1}{\xi_0})} + Z_{1-\beta}\sqrt{\frac{\pi_1(1-\pi_1)}{\xi_1} + \frac{\pi_0(1-\pi_0)}{\xi_0}}. \quad (4.6)$$

In the balanced case, $n_1 = n_0$, $\xi_1 = \xi_0 = 1/2$, so $\bar{\pi} = (\pi_0 + \pi_1)/2$, $(\frac{1}{\xi_1} + \frac{1}{\xi_0}) = 4$ and equation (4.2) becomes

$$\sqrt{N}\Delta = 2\left(Z_{1-\alpha}\sqrt{\bar{\pi}(1-\bar{\pi})} + Z_{1-\beta}\sqrt{\pi_1(1-\pi_1) + \pi_0(1-\pi_0)}\right). \quad (4.7)$$

Finally, again in the balanced case, equation (4.3) becomes

$$\sqrt{N}\Delta = 2\left(Z_{1-\alpha} + Z_{1-\beta}\right)\sqrt{\bar{\pi}(1-\bar{\pi})}. \quad (4.8)$$

To evaluate the accuracy of the approximations in equations (4.3) and (4.5), consider a numerical example. Let $\pi_1 = .4$ and $\pi_2 = .3$. Assuming balance, we have $\bar{\pi} = .35$. Equation (4.4) becomes

$$E[\hat{V}(a,b)|H_1] = \frac{4 \times .35 \times .65}{N} - \frac{2 \times .4 \times .6 + 2 \times .3 \times .7}{N^2}$$

$$= \frac{.91}{N} - \frac{.90}{N^2}.$$

Using this value in equation (4.1), taking $\alpha = .05$ and $\beta = .1$, and solving for N (this is now a quadratic equation) we find $N = 952.6$, which we would round up to 953. Using (4.7), we find $N = 952.0$, and using (4.8), we find $N = 956.2$. For comparison, the exact sample size, using the exact binomial distribution, is 950. For practical purposes, there are no meaningful differences between these estimates.

An alternative formulation of this problem is to consider not the difference $\pi_1 - \pi_0$, but the log-odds ratio $\Delta = \log(\pi_1(1 - \pi_0)/(1 - \pi_1)\pi_0)$. Now let $U(a,b) = \log(ad/bc)$, the observed log-odds ratio. By the delta method (Appendix A), we have $\phi(\pi) = 1/\pi(1 - \pi)$. Equation (4.2) becomes

$$\sqrt{N}\Delta = Z_{1-\alpha}\frac{1}{\sqrt{\bar{\pi}(1 - \bar{\pi})\xi_1\xi_2}} + Z_{1-\beta}\sqrt{\frac{1}{\pi_1(1 - \pi_1)\xi_1} + \frac{1}{\pi_2(1 - \pi_2)\xi_2}}.$$

Using the numerical example above, for $\pi_1 = .4$ and $\pi_2 = .3$, $\Delta = \log(.4 \times .7/.6 \times .3) = 0.442$, and $N = 952.2$. The required sample size is virtually unchanged.

4.3 Loss to Follow-up and Non-adherence

For a variety of reasons, it is rare for studies involving humans to proceed entirely according to plan. There are two primary ways in which subjects fail to comply with study procedures that affect the required sample size. First, outcomes for some subjects may not be available because the subjects fail to return for follow-up evaluations. We refer to this as *loss to follow-up*. Second, subjects may fail to receive all or part of the intended therapy. We refer to this as *non-adherence*. Some authors refer to this as *non-compliance* or *drop-out*. Since non-compliance is also used to refer to other deviations from the study protocol, we will not use this term. Drop-out is sometimes also used to refer to loss to follow-up and we will avoid its use.

4.3.1 Loss to Follow-up

In principle, the cases with loss to follow-up are difficult because follow-up status, treatment assignment, and outcome may be associated. That is, observations missing due to loss to follow-up are not missing at random. In most situations it is not possible to properly assess whether or not there are such associations (since, by definition, we cannot observe the responses for missing observations) and, in turn, properly account for them. Issues regarding missing data are further discussed in Chapter 11. For the purpose of this chapter, we will assume that the outcomes for subjects lost to follow-up are *ignorable*, meaning that their omission does not introduce bias into the analysis.

If we assume that the rate at which subjects are lost to follow-up is r, independent of treatment, and we enroll N subjects, then the expected number of subjects on which outcome data is available is $N^* = (1 - r)N$. To achieve the desired power, we first find the value of N^* satisfying equation (4.2), and then the required sample size is

$$N = N^*/(1 - r). \tag{4.9}$$

4.3.2 Non-adherence

As in the previous section, assessing or accounting for non-adherence is difficult because there may be associations between adherence, treatment assignment, and outcome. To avoid these difficulties we will assume that the analysis will be conducted according to the Intent to Treat principle, requiring that all subjects be analyzed using their assigned treatment groups regardless of the treatment actually received (or degree of adherence). The Intent to Treat principle will be discussed in more detail in Chapter 11.

To begin, we will assume that all randomized subjects will receive one or the other of the treatments under study—no other treatments are available and no subjects will receive only partial treatment. We will also assume that both treatments are available to all subjects. That is, a proportion, p, of subjects assigned to the control group, referred to as *drop-ins*, will actually receive the experimental treatment. For cases in which the experimental treatment is unavailable to control subjects, we can take $p = 0$. Similarly, a proportion q of subjects assigned the experimental treatment, referred to as *drop-outs*, will actually receive the control treatment. Since the control treatment will usually be either no-treatment (placebo) or an approved or otherwise accepted treatment, we will generally have $q > 0$.

For simplicity, suppose that Y_{ij} is an observation from subject i in treatment group $j = 1, 2$ and that $EY_{ij} = \mu_j$. If adherence status is independent of outcome and the proportion of subjects in the group assigned the experimental treatment who fail to adhere is q, $EY_{i1} = (1 - q)\mu_1 + q\mu_2$.[4] Similarly, $EY_{i2} = p\mu_1 + (1 - p)\mu_2$. Hence the difference in means is

$$\begin{aligned}
E[Y_{i1} - Y_{i2}] &= ((1 - q)\mu_1 + q\mu_2) - (p\mu_1 + (1 - p)\mu_2) \\
&= (1 - p - q)(\mu_1 - \mu_2), \tag{4.10}
\end{aligned}$$

and the effect of non-adherence of this type is to decrease the expected treatment difference by a factor of $1 - p - q$. Note that under the null hypothesis

---

[4] If adherence status is not independent of outcome, we may have, for example, that there is no effect of treatment on non-adherers. If this were the case, then $E\overline{Y}_1 = \mu_2$ and equation (4.10) would not hold.

$\mu_1 = \mu_2$, so there is no effect on the distribution of the observed treatment difference.

In the case where there is partial adherence—for example, subjects receive a fraction of their assigned treatment—equation (4.10) still holds provided that (1) p and q are the mean proportions of assigned treatment that are received in the respective treatment groups and (2) the dose-response is a linear function of the proportion of treatment actually received. These assumptions are usually adequate for the purpose of sample size estimation and, in the absence of detailed information regarding adherence rates and dose responses, are probably the only reasonable assumptions that can be made. If p and q are small, then equation (4.10) is likely to be a good approximation, and all efforts should be made in the design and conduct of the study to ensure that p and q be made as small as possible. In section 4.4 we will discuss a more general approach in the context of time-to-event analyses.

In the general setting, based on equation (4.10), assumption (2.) becomes $EU = (1 - p - q)\Delta$. Hence, combined with equation (4.9), we can rewrite equation (4.2) to account for both loss to follow-up and non-adherence to yield the general formula

$$N = \frac{\left(Z_{1-\alpha}\sqrt{\phi(\bar{\gamma})/\xi_1\xi_2} + Z_{1-\beta}\sqrt{\phi(\gamma_1)/\xi_1 + \phi(\gamma_2)/\xi_2}\right)^2}{(1 - p - q)^2\Delta^2(1 - r)}.$$

To illustrate the impact of non-adherence and drop-out on sample size, Table 4.1 shows the required sample sizes for non-adherence and loss to follow-up rates between 0 and 50% when the required sample size with complete adherence and follow-up is 1000. Since the adjustment to the sample size depends on the sum $p + q$, the results are shown as a function of $p + q$.

Table 4.1 *Impact of non-adherence and loss to follow-up on required sample size.*

$p+q\backslash r$	0	10%	20%	30%	40%	50%
0	1000	1111	1250	1429	1667	2000
10%	1235	1372	1543	1764	2058	2469
20%	1562	1736	1953	2232	2604	3125
30%	2041	2268	2551	2915	3401	4082
40%	2778	3086	3472	3968	4630	5556
50%	4000	4444	5000	5714	6667	8000

4.4 Survival Data

It is common for large clinical trials to use a time-to-failure outcome, so we will devote a significant portion of this chapter to this topic. We will begin with the simplest case in which the failure time distributions are exponential. Cases with time dependent rates of failure, loss to follow-up, and non-adherence will be discussed in Section 4.4.2.

4.4.1 Exponential Case

We begin with the exponential case (i.e., constant hazard function). Suppose that λ_i, $i = 0, 1$ are the hazards rates for the control and experimental groups so that the failure time, Y_{ij}, for subject i in group j is exponential with mean $1/\lambda_j$. The survivor function is given by $S_j(t) = \exp(-\lambda_j t)$.

Suppose further that subject i in group j is subject to an administrative censoring time (maximum follow-up time) of C_{ij}. Typically, C_{ij} is determined by time of enrollment into the study and will be the time from enrollment to the end of the study. We will assume that the distribution of the C_{ij} are known in advance and independent of treatment group.

Let $T_{ij} = \min(C_{ij}, Y_{ij})$, $\delta_{ij} = 1$ if $T_{ij} = Y_{ij}$ and $\delta_{ij} = 0$ otherwise. If we let $T_j = \sum_{i=1}^{n_j} T_{ij}$ and $D_j = \sum_{i=1}^{n_j} \delta_{ij}$ be the total follow-up time and numbers of failures respectively in group j, then the estimated hazard rate in group j is $\hat{\lambda}_j = D_j/T_j$. Similar to the 2-sample binomial case, the score test for $H_0 : \lambda_1 = \lambda_2$ is equivalent to the comparison of the observed rates, $U(T_1, T_2, D_1, D_2) = \hat{\lambda}_1 - \hat{\lambda}_2 = D_1/T_1 - D_2/T_2$. The variance of $\hat{\lambda}_i$ is asymptotically λ_j/T_j, so $\phi(\lambda) = \lambda/ET_{ij}$. Since T_{ij} depends on both the failure time and the censoring time, we will need to consider the distribution of the censoring times. For simplicity we begin with the case in which there is no censoring.

No Censoring

If there is no censoring, $ET_{ij} = EY_{ij} = 1/\lambda_j$. Hence $\phi(\lambda) = \lambda/ET = \lambda^2$. Thus if $\bar{\lambda} = \xi_1\lambda_1 + \xi_2\lambda_2$, equation (4.2) becomes

$$N = \frac{(Z_{1-\alpha}\bar{\lambda}/\xi_1\xi_2 + Z_{1-\beta}\sqrt{\lambda_1^2/\xi_1 + \lambda_2^2/\xi_2})^2}{(\lambda_1 - \lambda_2)^2}$$

and equation (4.3) becomes

$$N = \frac{(Z_{1-\alpha} + Z_{1-\beta})^2\bar{\lambda}^2}{\xi_1\xi_2(\lambda_1 - \lambda_2)^2}. \tag{4.11}$$

It is worth noting that these formulas are scale invariant. That is, the sample size remains unchanged if both λ_1 and λ_2 are multiplied by a constant. This implies that while the treatment difference is specified in terms of the *difference* in rates, the sample size in fact depends only on the hazard ratio, λ_1/λ_2.

This fact is easier to see if we let $U = \log(\hat{\lambda}_1/\hat{\lambda}_2)$. Then it is easy to show that $\phi(\lambda) = 1$, and we have

$$N = \frac{(Z_{1-\alpha} + Z_{1-\beta})^2}{\xi_1\xi_2\log(\lambda_1/\lambda_2)^2}. \tag{4.12}$$

Common Censoring Time

In the case of a common censoring time, all subjects are followed for a fixed length of time. This may happen in studies involving subjects experiencing an acute episode where, after a period of a few weeks or months, the risk of the event in question will have returned to a background level. In such cases we may choose to terminate follow-up after a relatively short, predetermined time. Here we assume that $C_{ij} = C$, a known common value, and we have

$$ET_{ij} = \int_0^C t\lambda_j e^{-\lambda_j t}dt + Ce^{-\lambda_j C}$$
$$= \frac{1 - e^{-\lambda_j C}}{\lambda_j} \qquad (4.13)$$

so, $\phi(\lambda) = \lambda^2/(1 - e^{-\lambda C})$. Hence, the required sample size will be inflated by approximately $1/(1 - e^{-\bar{\lambda}C})$.

It is useful to note that $1 - e^{-\bar{\lambda}C}$ is approximately the probability that a subject in the trial will be observed to fail by time C, so that $N(1 - e^{-\bar{\lambda}C})$ is approximately the number of expected failures $D. = D_1 + D_2$. Hence, in this case equation (4.11) will apply, not to the total sample size, but to the required number of failures, $D.$. We have now shown that for exponential observations with a common length of follow-up, independent of the underlying rates and the length of follow-up, the number of failures required for given type I and type II error rates depends only on the hazard ratio. Furthermore, since in cases where hazards change with time, if the hazard ratio $\lambda_2(t)/\lambda_1(t)$ is constant, the time scale can always be transformed so that the transformed failure times are exponential and this result will hold. Later we will see that this is true regardless of the pattern of enrollment and the underlying distribution of failure times, provided that the hazard functions are proportional across all follow-up times.

Staggered Entry with Uniform Enrollment

The case of staggered entry with uniform enrollment is one in which the C_{ij} are uniformly distributed on the interval $[F - R, F]$ where R is the length of the enrollment period and F is the total (maximum) length of follow-up. We will assume that all subjects are followed to a common termination date.

If a subject is enrolled at time $s \in [0, R]$, then as in equation (4.13), the expected follow-up time is $(1 - e^{-\lambda_j(F-s)})/\lambda_j$. The overall expected follow-up time will be

$$ET_{ij} = \frac{1}{R}\int_0^R \frac{1 - e^{-\lambda_j(F-s)}}{\lambda_j}ds$$
$$= \frac{R\lambda_j - e^{-\lambda_j(F-R)} + e^{-\lambda_j F}}{R\lambda_j^2}, \qquad (4.14)$$

so $\phi(\lambda) = R\lambda^3/(R\lambda - e^{-\lambda(F-R)} + e^{-\lambda F})$. Equation (4.3) becomes

$$N = \frac{(Z_{1-\alpha} + Z_{1-\beta})^2 R\bar{\lambda}^3}{(R\bar{\lambda} - e^{-\bar{\lambda}(F-R)} + e^{-\bar{\lambda}F})\xi_1\xi_2(\lambda_2 - \lambda_1)^2}.$$

Note that the expected number of events is

$$D. = \left(1 - \frac{e^{-\lambda(F-R)} - e^{-\lambda F}}{R\lambda}\right)N,$$

so that $D.$ satisfies equation (4.11). Again, the total number of events is determined by the hazard ratio, the allocation ratios, ξ_j, and the desired type I and type II error rates, independent of total follow-up time, enrollment rates, and underlying hazard rates.

Loss to Follow-up

In Section 4.3.1, we provided an adjustment to the sample size to account for loss to follow-up when no follow-up information is available for subjects who are lost to follow-up and we can assume that subjects are lost at random. In survival studies, we typically have some amount of follow-up on all subjects and loss to follow-up has the effect of simply reducing the length of follow-up for a subset of subjects. It may be reasonable in many cases to assume that the time of loss to follow-up follows an exponential distribution with rate η. In general, we could assume that the rate is treatment specific, but we will not do that here.

Note that in this setting we still have that $\phi(\lambda, \eta) = \lambda/ET_{ij}$. The follow-up time, T_{ij}, however, will be the minimum of the administrative censoring time, C_{ij}, the failure time, Y_{ij}, and the time that the subject is lost to follow-up, L_{ij}. Assuming that L_{ij} and Y_{ij} are independent, then $\min(L_{ij}, Y_{ij})$ will have an exponential distribution with rate $\lambda + \eta$. Hence, we can use a version of equation (4.14) substituting $\exp(-(\lambda_j + \eta)(F - s))$ for $\exp(-\lambda(F - s))$ in the integral. The result is that we have

$$\phi(\lambda, \eta) = \frac{R\lambda(\lambda + \eta)^2}{R(\lambda + \eta) - e^{-(\lambda+\eta)(F-R)} + e^{-(\lambda+\eta)F}}$$

and the sample size formula is

$$N = \frac{(Z_{1-\alpha} + Z_{1-\beta})^2 R\bar{\lambda}(\bar{\lambda} + \eta)^2}{(R(\bar{\lambda} + \eta) - e^{-(\bar{\lambda}+\eta)(F-R)} + e^{-(\bar{\lambda}+\eta)F})\xi_1\xi_2(\lambda_2 - \lambda_1)^2}.$$

4.4.2 Time-dependent Rates of Failure, Loss to Follow-up, and Non-adherence

The exponential survival models of the previous section are appropriate for chronic disease in which failure rates are approximately constant over time. They may be less than adequate, however, for acute conditions in which the risk of failure is initially high, say in the first few days or weeks following a myocardial infarction. Conversely, risk of cancer recurrence or death may be low immediately after treatment, and increase some months later. Sample size formulas that don't rely on the exponential assumption are essential for these more general settings.

Typically, we approach settings with time-dependent rates of failure, loss to follow-up, and non-adherence in two steps. First, we calculate the number of failures (primary events) necessary to reach the desired power, and second, we consider the number of subjects and length of follow-up required to reach this target. We will assume that the analysis of the failure time outcome is based on the log-rank test which is described in detail in Section 7.3.2. The test is constructed by considering the set of distinct failure times, $t_1, t_2, \ldots$, and for each time, t_j, we have $n_{j\tau}$ subjects at risk in treatment group τ, $\tau = 1, 2$, and d_j failures in the two groups combined. The Fisher information for the log-rank test given in equation (7.8) is a sum over distinct failure times,

$$I(0) = \sum_j \frac{d_j n_{j1} n_{j2}}{(n_{j1} + n_{j2})^2}$$

and under H_0, $E[n_{j1} n_{j2}/(n_{j1} + n_{j2})^2] = \xi_1 \xi_2$. Hence, under H_0, the Fisher information is approximately $D\xi_1\xi_2$ where $D = \sum_j d_j$, and therefore is proportional to the observed number of events. Thus, trials whose size and duration are determined by the target number of events are effectively information-driven trials as described in Section 4.1.

Most long term studies using time-to-failure outcomes are designed to enroll a fixed number of subjects during an initial enrollment period, the length of which may be specified in the protocol. In practice, however, enrollment rates rarely match expectations and actual enrollment periods are occasionally shorter, but more often longer than expected. Subjects are followed until the target number of events is reached. The advantage of this strategy is that study power is maintained regardless of the underlying hazard rates, enrollment rates, duration of enrollment, or number of subjects enrolled, provided that the target number is reached. If hazard rates prove to be higher than expected, this may result in the total duration of the study being shortened, saving time and resources. On the other hand, if hazard rates are lower than expected, or decrease unexpectedly with follow-up time, the total duration of the study may increase beyond what available resources or sponsor time-lines can support.

One example is the CARS study (Coumadin Aspirin Reinfarction Study (CARS) Investigators 1997) that enrolled subjects immediately following an acute myocardial infraction. The study was designed with the assumptions of a constant hazard rate of 0.11 in the placebo group. In fact, hazard rates were initially much higher than the predicted 0.11, but decreased rapidly and after approximately two months, dropped below the expected rate to the extent that when projected to four years, the cumulative rate was approximately half the expected (see the example in Cook (2003)). The result was that enrollment was extended well beyond that specified in the protocol, one of the experimental arms was dropped in order to increase accrual to the remaining two arms, and overall duration extended. While such adjustments may be difficult and expensive, the alternative is that the trial would be under-powered and the results possibly ambiguous.

We begin with a simple formula for computing the target number of events.

Shoenfeld's Formula

Perhaps the most useful formula in this setting is due to Schoenfeld (1983). Shoenfeld's formula provides the number of subjects with events (failure) necessary to achieve the desired power as a function of the hazard ratio, independent of the underlying rates. Shoenfeld derived his formula in the setting with covariate adjustment. For simplicity we will derive his formula without covariate adjustment. We assume that hazard functions depend on time, t, from treatment start and that $\lambda_1(t) = r\lambda_2(t)$, so that r is the hazard ratio. Since the formula provides the required number of failures, we consider only subjects who fail, and will assume that there are no tied failure times. We let x_j be the treatment indicator for the subject failing at time t_j: $x_j = 1$ if the subject is in group 1, and $x_j = 0$ otherwise, $j = 1, 2, \cdots, D$ where D is the total number of failures. Also let n_{j1} and n_{j2} be the numbers of subjects at risk at time t_j in groups 1 and 2, respectively.

In order to fit into the framework from Section 4.2, we will use a rescaled log-rank statistic, equation (7.3), for $H_0 : r = 1$,

$$U = \frac{1}{D\xi_1\xi_2} \sum_{j=1}^{D} \left(x_j - \frac{n_{j1}}{n_{j1} + n_{j2}} \right),$$

where the second term in the sum is the expected value of x_j given n_{j1}, n_{j2}, and H_0. The variance of U under H_0 is

$$\frac{1}{D\xi_1^2\xi_2^2} \sum_{j=1}^{D} \frac{n_{j1}n_{j2}}{(n_{j1} + n_{j2})^2}.$$

Under an alternative hypothesis $H_1 : r = r_1 \neq 1$,

$$E[x_j | n_{j1}, n_{j2}] = \frac{r_1 n_{j1}}{(n_{j1} + n_{j2}r_1)^2}.$$

If we assume that $|r_1 - 1|$ is small, then at each failure time we will have that $n_{jk}/(n_{j1} + n_{j2}r_1) \approx \xi_j$, $\Delta = EU \approx \log(r_1)$, and Var $U = 1/D\xi_1\xi_2$, so that $\phi(r_1) = 1$. Applying equation (4.3), we have Shoenfeld's formula,

$$D = \frac{(Z_{1-\alpha} + Z_{1-\beta})^2}{\xi_1\xi_2(\log r_1)^2}. \tag{4.15}$$

Note that the right hand side is identical to the right hand side of equation (4.12) under the exponential model with no censoring. The difference is that Shoenfeld's formula does not tell us how many subjects and the total follow-up time that are required in order to reach the target number of events.

Note that no adjustment is required for subjects expected to be lost to follow-up. The effect of loss to follow-up (provided that it is not informative) is to decrease the observed number of primary events. Given that we achieve the target number in spite of loss to follow-up, power will be maintained. Non-adherence to assigned treatment will require adjustment, however. For example, if we assume that no control subjects cross over to the experimental arm, a fraction, q, of experimental subjects do not receive any of their assigned treatment, and that the effect of treatment is the same in adherent and non-adherent subjects, the effective hazard rate in the experimental arm will be $\lambda^* = q\lambda_1 + (1 - q)\lambda_2$, and the hazard ratio becomes $r_1^* = qr_1 + 1 - q$. We can now apply Shoenfeld's formula using r_1^* to obtain

$$D = \frac{(Z_{1-\alpha} + Z_{1-\beta})^2}{\xi_1\xi_2(\log(qr_1 + 1 - q))^2}.$$

Since most non-adherence does not result in subjects either receiving all or none of their assigned medication, this calculation is probably unrealistic. It may be more realistic to let q be the proportion of assigned medication actually taken in the experimental group, under the assumption that there is a linear dose response, independent of adherence status. On the other hand, if the effect of non-adherence is to decrease the effectiveness of treatment in a time dependent way—at later follow-up times more subjects are non-adherent increasing the aggregate hazard rate in the experimental group—the assumption of proportional hazards may no longer hold, and Shoenfeld's formula will no longer apply. Methods like those described in the next section are required to deal with this more complex situation.

Shoenfeld also provides techniques for determining the number of subjects required to achieve the target number of events; however, these techniques make simplifying assumptions regarding the failure time distributions and patterns of accrual. A more general method is outlined in the next section.

Markov Chain Model of Lakatos

All the methods for determining sample size discussed prior to this point require restrictive assumptions regarding enrollment patterns and failure distributions. Wu et al. (1980) describe a method in which failure rates and non-adherence rates are allowed to vary on a time-dependent piecewise basis. This idea was generalized by Lakatos (1986, 1988) and Shih (1995) who propose a Markov chain method for accounting simultaneously for time-varying event, non-adherence, loss to follow-up, and enrollment rates. This model allows subjects who cross over from treatment to control or vice versa to cross back over to their assigned treatment groups at arbitrary, prespecified rates. Cook (2003) shows how models fit to existing data sets can be used in the computations.

To motivate the Markov chain model, we imagine that a given subject is followed from the start of treatment until either they withdraw from the study (are lost to follow-up), have a primary event, or the study is terminated. The instantaneous rate at which either of the first two can happen can be both time and treatment dependent. Furthermore, at any time a subject can be non-adherent. That is, a subject assigned the experimental treatment may stop taking the assigned treatment in favor of the control treatment, or a subject assigned the control treatment may begin taking the experimental treatment. Because the times at which subjects crossover, are lost to follow-up, and experience primary events are dependent upon one another in complex ways, finding their exact joint distribution (or more specifically, the marginal distribution of the failure time) is mathematically intractable and we need to resort to numerical methods.

Lakatos and Shih use a Markov chain in which at any given time a subject can be in one of four states: lost to follow-up (L), has had an event (E), and active on either E (experimental treatment) or C (control). As an approximation to the continuous time process, the follow-up time is divided into small equal-length intervals, so that the probability that a subject would experience more than one transition in a given interval is small. Therefore, within each interval we assume that the transition probabilities from state X to state Y do not depend on the transition probabilities from state X to any other states.

In this setting we may specify time dependent rates at which subjects change state, with the constraint that states L and E are absorbing states—subjects who enter these states remain there for the duration of the study. It is assumed that subjects who crossover (drop-ins or drop-outs) immediately acquire the transition rates of the new group, e.g., the hazard rate for a study event for a subject who has dropped out of group E and into group C becomes the hazard rate for subjects assigned C. Lakatos (1988) discusses incorporating lag times, either in initial treatment effectiveness or in changes in effectiveness resulting from crossovers; however, for simplicity we will not discuss this issue here.

It is important to note that because hazard rates are arbitrary, it is no longer necessary to make the proportional hazards assumption. If non-proportional hazards are used, however, it is no longer the case that study power depends only on the observed number of primary events. For example, if the hazard ratio is attenuated (becomes closer to one) with increasing follow-up time, then a given number of events derived from a small number of subjects with long follow-up times will have lower power than if the same number of events accrued in a larger number of subjects with short follow-up times.

At each follow-up time, we assume that subjects are in one of four states:

A_E = Active on treatment E (1)
A_C = Active on treatment C (2)
L = Subject lost to follow-up (3)
E = Subject has had a primary event (4)

where (l) indicates the index used for subscripting the state vector and transition matrix below. We will say that a subject has an event of type l at time t if they enter state l at time t from a different state. The transition probabilities at time t depend on t and are computed using the time-dependent hazard rate specifications.

Let $0 = t_0 < t_1 < t_2 < \ldots$ and $S_{kj} = (q_{kj1}, q_{kj2}, q_{kj3}, q_{kj4})^T$ where q_{kjl} is the probability that a subject assigned to treatment k will be in state l at time t_j. Thus $S_{10} = (1, 0, 0, 0)^T$ and $S_{20} = (0, 1, 0, 0)^T$. Transitions from S_{kj} to S_{kj+1} are determined by time varying transition probabilities and, given S_{kj}, are independent of $S_{kj'}$ for $j' < j$ (that is, the process is Markov).

For subjects assigned treatment k, let $\lambda^*_{klm}(t)$ be the hazard function for the occurrence of an event of type m, $m \neq l$, for a subject assigned to group k who is currently receiving treatment l at time t. Then we let

$$\mu_{klmj} = 1 - \exp\left(-\int_{t_j}^{t_{j+1}} \lambda^*_{klm}(s)ds\right)$$

and

$$\mu_{kllj} = 1 - \mu_{kl(3-l)j} - \mu_{kl3j} - \mu_{kl4j}.$$

In many, if not most, situations one will assume that a subject cannot cross back over to their assigned treatment once they become non-adherent, that is $\lambda^*_{k(3-l)l} = 0$; however, this not required. One may also make other simplifying assumptions, such as that $\lambda^*_{kl3}(t) = \lambda^*_{k'l'3}(t)$ for all k, l, k', l'; that is, loss to follow-up does not depend on assigned treatment or adherence status. The transition probabilities are given in the following matrix, M_k. The columns represent the state at time t_j and the rows the state at time t_{j+1}.

$$M_j = \begin{bmatrix} \mu_{k11j} & \mu_{k21j} & 0 & 0 \\ \mu_{k12j} & \mu_{k22j} & 0 & 0 \\ \mu_{k13j} & \mu_{k23j} & 1 & 0 \\ \mu_{k14j} & \mu_{k24j} & 0 & 1 \end{bmatrix}$$

Beginning with S_{k0} defined above, $S_{k(j+1)} = M S_{kj}$, $j = 1, 2, \ldots$. For example,

$$S_{11} = \begin{bmatrix} \mu_{1110} \\ \mu_{1120} \\ \mu_{1130} \\ \mu_{1140} \end{bmatrix},$$

$$S_{12} = \begin{bmatrix} \mu_{1111}\mu_{1110} + \mu_{1211}\mu_{1120} \\ \mu_{1121}\mu_{1110} + \mu_{1221}\mu_{1120} \\ \mu_{1131}\mu_{1110} + \mu_{1231}\mu_{1120} + \mu_{1130} \\ \mu_{1141}\mu_{1110} + \mu_{1241}\mu_{1120} + \mu_{1140} \end{bmatrix}, etc.$$

This setup allows us to compute the probability that a given subject will be in one of four states given arbitrary time-dependencies for the loss to follow-up, non-adherence. The degree of accuracy will depend on the step size $t_j - t_{j-1}$, and the magnitude of the hazards $\lambda^*_{klm}(t)$.

The calculation of power requires that we find the expected number of subjects at risk and the expected number of events expected to occur in each treatment group at any time during follow-up. This calculation requires assumptions regarding patterns of enrollment and study duration.

To account for staggered entry, we follow Cook (2003), which differs from the approach of Lakatos and Shih. In what follows, where otherwise unclear, we refer to time from study start (enrollment of the first subject) as "study time" and the time from enrollment for individual subjects as "subject time." For each treatment group $k = 1, 2$, we first compute the sequence of state vectors, $S_{kj}, j = 0, 1, \ldots$ out to the maximum potential follow-up time. All intermediate state vectors are saved as a matrix $Q_k = [q_{klj}]$.

Now fix an enrollment strategy, $r_{kj}, j = 1, 2, \ldots$, the number of subjects enrolled to group k between time t_{j-1} and time t_j. The implicit assumption throughout is that the proportion of subjects accrued to each treatment group is constant over time, i.e., r_{2j}/r_{1j} does not depend on j. We let $r_{\cdot j} = r_{1j} + r_{2j}$ and $\rho_j = r_{kj}/r_{\cdot j}$ (the subscript "$\cdot$" represents summation over the corresponding index).

Then if N_{kjp} is the cumulative number enrolled through time t_j, given that we enroll through time τ_p,

$$N_{kjp} = \sum_{x=1}^{j \wedge p} r_{jx}$$

where "$\wedge$" indicates the minimum of the two arguments. Let n_{kljp} be the number of subjects in state l at time t_j (study time) given that we enroll through time τ_p. Then

$$n_{kljp} = \sum_{x=1}^{j \wedge p} r_{kx} q_{kl(j-x+1)}. \tag{4.16}$$

The four dimensional array $D = [n_{kljp}]$ contains the expected number of subjects in treatment group k who are in state l given that the total length of follow-up has been t_j (study time) and enrollment is through time τ_p.

The array D is useful for addressing number of questions regarding the expected results of the trial given various assumptions regarding both length of follow-up and enrollment.

Next, we discuss the algorithm for computing the log-rank statistic. Using the state indices from the table above, let $s_{kj} = \rho_k(q_{11j} + q_{12j})$ be the probability that a subject assigned treatment k will be active at time t_j after enrollment (subject time). Also let $d_{kj} = \rho_k(q_{k4j} - q_{k4(j-1)})$ and e_j be expected number of events accruing between time t_{j-1} and t_j (subject time) for a subject in group E under H_0:

$$e_j = \frac{d_{\cdot j} s_{1j}}{s_{\cdot j}}$$

and the variance of d_{1j} (conditional on $d_{\cdot j}$) at time t_j is

$$v_j = \frac{d_{\cdot j}(s_{\cdot j} - d_{\cdot j}) s_{1j} s_{2j}}{s_{\cdot j}^3}.$$

At study time t_j, with enrollment through τ_p, the expected value of the log-rank statistic is:

$$U_{jp} = \sum_{y=1}^{j \wedge p} r_{\cdot y} \sum_{x=1}^{j-y+1} (d_{1x} - e_x) \qquad (4.17)$$

and the expected value of its variance estimator is:

$$V_{jp} = \sum_{y=1}^{j \wedge p} r_{\cdot y} \sum_{x=1}^{j-y+1} v_x. \qquad (4.18)$$

For given enrollment time and follow-up time let $Z_{jp}^{\text{EXP}} = [U_{jp}/V_{jp}^{1/2}]$ be the expected value of the log-rank Z-score. Since the variance of the observed Z-score under the specified alternative is approximately one, power (for one-sided level α) can be calculated by the formula

$$Z_{1-\alpha} + Z_{1-\beta} = Z_{jp}^{\text{EXP}}.$$

Power for two-sided tests is obtained by replacing α above by $\alpha/2$.

Note that the quantities computed above depend on both the total enrollment and the enrollment pattern. If, prior to the start of enrollment, the pattern of enrollment is held fixed, but rescaled to reflect either a proportionate increase or decrease in the (possibly) time-dependent enrollment rates, these quantities can be simply rescaled. In particular, for fixed enrollment and follow-up times, Z_{jp}^{EXP} will change with the square root of the total sample size. The goal is to find the combination of enrollment pattern, total enrollment, and total length of follow-up that yields the desired value of Z_{jp}^{EXP}. Clearly these computation are complex and require the use of specialized software. This algorithm is implemented in software available from http://www.biostat.wisc.edu/~cook/software.html.

4.5 Clustered Data

Clustered data arise when the observations are naturally grouped according to features that are expected to induce correlations among observations within clusters. Examples include observations repeated over time within subjects and subjects within families, schools, or clinical sites. In some studies, units within the same cluster are assigned different treatments; for example, in an ophthalmology study, subjects may have one treated and one untreated eye, or siblings with a genetic disease may be assigned different treatments. The typical approach in this case is to perform an analysis stratified by cluster, so that subjects are only directly compared to others within the same cluster, effectively eliminating the variability among clusters. In this case the sample size calculations are not significantly affected by the clustering, although in cases where there is a high degree of variability among clusters, one must be careful that the sample size estimate is based on the within-cluster variances and not marginal variances that will include the cluster effects.

There are also situations in which all members of a cluster receive the same treatment. This is certainly the case when we have repeated observations over time within subjects (unless we are using a crossover design), or when group randomization is used (see Section 3.2.2). The sample size calculations will change significantly, however, since, in a sense, the unit of analysis becomes the cluster and not the individual. The approach is effectively the same in all cases; the "effective" sample size is a combination of the number of clusters and the number of observations per cluster.

The typical approach for clustered data is to assume that we have a *within-cluster* variance, ν^2, and a *between-cluster* variance, τ^2. The marginal variance for a single observation is the sum, $\sigma^2 = \nu^2 + \tau^2$. Furthermore, because observations from within the same cluster are conditionally (on cluster) independent, the covariance between them is the cluster variance, τ^2. Thus, the correlation between subjects within a cluster is $\rho = \tau^2/\sigma^2$.

Tests of H_0 can be constructed by first averaging observations with clusters, then comparing the means by treatment. The variance of the mean of cluster i containing m_i observations is $\tau^2 + \nu^2/m_i = \sigma^2(1 + (m_i - 1)\rho)/m_i$.

There are two ways of combining cluster means that we consider. If all clusters are the same size, the methods coincide. First, if the cluster sizes are fixed in advance and under the model assumptions, in the optimal analysis each cluster mean is assigned a weight equal to the reciprocal of the cluster variance, $m_i/\sigma^2(1 + (m_i - 1)\rho)$. The *effective* variance function, ϕ, which in this setting is independent of the mean, is

$$\phi_w = \frac{\sigma^2}{E[m_i/(1 + (m_i - 1)\rho)]},$$

where the expectation is with respect to the cluster sizes. If the cluster sizes are fixed, then this is just the average. If the cluster sizes are all equal, it further reduces to the (common) cluster variance, $\sigma^2(1 + (m - 1)\rho)/m$. Given assumptions regarding σ^2 and ρ, and the cluster sizes m_i, equation (4.3) can be used to determine the required number of clusters. When there is discretion regarding the number of observations per cluster, one can select both the cluster sizes and the number of clusters, weighing the relative costs of each, to optimize efficiency.

Alternatively, if there are concerns regarding the validity of the assumptions, we may prefer to give equal weight to each cluster. If, for example, there is an association between cluster size and outcomes, the weighted estimate will be biased—giving higher weight to clusters with, say, larger values of the outcome variable, and lower weight to lower values. In the unweighted case, ϕ will simply be the mean cluster variance,

$$\phi_u = \sigma^2 E\left[\frac{1 + (m_i - 1)\rho}{m_i}\right].$$

Again, application of equation (4.3) gives the required number of clusters. Note that unless all m_i are equal, $\phi_u > \phi_w$, so when the assumptions hold, the weighted analysis is more efficient.

When outcomes are non-normal—binary, failure time, etc.—more complex models are required and we will not discuss them here.

4.6 Tests for Interaction

Occasionally it may be desirable to be able to identify interactions between either two treatments, or between a treatment and one or more baseline covariates. Sample size requirements can be substantially larger for interaction tests than for main effects. As we will show, this results from both greater variability in test statistics or parameter estimates, and a decrease in the effect size.

Suppose that we have two factors, F_j, $j = 1, 2$, each of which takes two values E_j and C_j. We will assume that for factor 1, assignment to either E_1 or C_1 is random and independent of F_2. Also let ζ_k, $k = 1, 2$, be the proportion of subjects with levels E_2 and C_2 of F_2 and ξ, $k = 1, 2$, be the proportion of subjects with levels E_1 and C_1 of F_1. Because of the random assignment of factor F_1, in what follows it makes no difference whether factor F_2 is a subject baseline characteristic or is randomly assigned.

We illustrate with two examples.

Example 4.1. Suppose that y_{ijk} is the response for subject i with assignments $F_1 = j$ and $F_2 = k$. The responses are assumed independent with $y_{ijk} \sim N(\mu_{jk}, \sigma^2)$. Then the interaction of interest, Δ, can be written as

$$\Delta = (\mu_{11} - \mu_{21}) - (\mu_{12} - \mu_{22}) \qquad (4.19)$$
$$= (\mu_{11} - \mu_{12}) - (\mu_{21} - \mu_{22}). \qquad (4.20)$$

The test statistic is $U = (\bar{y}_{11} - \bar{y}_{12}) - (\bar{y}_{21} - \bar{y}_{22})$ with variance

$$V = \frac{\sigma^2}{N} \left(\frac{1}{\xi_1 \zeta_1} + \frac{1}{\xi_1 \zeta_2} + \frac{1}{\xi_2 \zeta_1} + \frac{1}{\xi_2 \zeta_2} \right)$$
$$= \frac{\sigma^2}{N \zeta_1 \zeta_2} \left(\frac{1}{\xi_1} + \frac{1}{\xi_2} \right).$$

This expression suggests that the sample size formula can be derived from (4.2) by letting $\phi(\mu_{j1}, \mu_{j2}) = \frac{\sigma^2}{\zeta_1 \zeta_2}$. Hence, we find that

$$N = \frac{(Z_{1-\alpha} + Z_{1-\beta})^2 \sigma^2}{\Delta^2 \zeta_1 \zeta_2 \xi_1 \xi_2}.$$

Note that this is the sample size required for main effects using the same σ^2, ξ_j, and Δ, but multiplied by $1/\zeta_1 \zeta_2$. Since $1/\zeta_1 \zeta_2 \geq 4$, at least 4 times as many subjects will be required to detect an interaction of size Δ as will be for a main effect of size Δ. Furthermore, it is likely that interactions that might occur would be smaller than the corresponding main effect of treatment, further increasing the required sample size. □

Unlike main effects, interactions are scale dependent. That is, many interactions can be eliminated by transforming the response variable. We illustrate with another example.

Example 4.2. Suppose that Y_{jk} are binomial with probability π_{jk} and size n_{jk} with n_{jk} as in the previous example. In the example in Section 4.2.1, the score (Pearson χ^2), Wald, and likelihood ratio tests of $H_0 : \pi_1 = \pi_2$ are all asymptotically equivalent, independent of the parameterization, and give quite similar results, even in small samples. On the other hand, the interaction test can be a test of $H_0 : \pi_{11} - \pi_{21} = \pi_{12} - \pi_{22}$ (constant risk difference), $H_0' : \pi_{11}/\pi_{21} = \pi_{12}/\pi_{22}$ (constant risk ratio), or $H_0'' : \pi_{11}(1 - \pi_{21})/(1 - \pi_{11})\pi_{21} = \pi_{12}(1-\pi_{22})/(1-\pi_{12})\pi_{22}$ (constant odds ratio). These are all distinct hypotheses unless $\pi_{11} = \pi_{12}$.

We consider H_0''. We let $U(\mathbf{Y}) = \log(Y_{11}(1-Y_{21})/(1-Y_{11})Y_{21}) - \log(Y_{12}(1-Y_{22})/(1 - Y_{12})Y_{22})$. Note that

$$\text{Var} \log \left(\frac{Y_{1k}(1 - Y_{2k})}{(1 - Y_{1k})Y_{2k}} \right) \approx \frac{1}{n_{1k}\pi_{1k}} + \frac{1}{n_{1k}(1 - \pi_{1k})} + \frac{1}{n_{2k}(1 - \pi_{2k})} + \frac{1}{n_{2k}\pi_{2k}}$$

$$= \frac{1}{N\xi_k} \left(\frac{1}{\zeta_1\pi_{1k}(1 - \pi_{1k})} + \frac{1}{\zeta_2\pi_{2k}(1 - \pi_{2k})} \right).$$

Hence we can apply equation (4.2) with $\phi(\pi_{ik}, \pi_{2k}) = 1/\zeta_1\pi_{1k}(1 - \pi_{1k}) + 1/\zeta_2\pi_{2k}(1-\pi_{2k})$ and $\Delta = \log(\pi_{11}(1-\pi_{21})/(1-\pi_{11})\pi_{21}) - \log(\pi_{12}(1-\pi_{22})/(1-\pi_{12})\pi_{22})$. □

4.7 Equivalence/Non-inferiority Trials

The calculations for sample sizes for equivalence/non-inferiority trials are similar to those for superiority trials. An equivalence trial is one in which the null hypothesis has the form $H_0 : |\gamma_1 - \gamma_2| > \delta$ for some $\delta > 0$ known as the equivalence margin. Typically, H_0 is rejected, and equivalence established, if a confidence interval for the difference $\gamma_1 - \gamma_2$ lies entirely within the interval $(-\delta, \delta)$. For a non-inferiority trial, the null hypothesis generally has the form $H_0 : \gamma_1 - \gamma_2 > \delta$ where larger values of γ correspond to less efficacious treatments. H_0 is typically rejected, and non-inferiority established, if a confidence interval for the difference $\gamma_1 - \gamma_2$ lies entirely below the δ.

The sample size for equivalence/non-inferiority trials will be based on an alternative hypothesis under which either equivalence or non-inferiority holds. For equivalence this will usually be $H_1 : \gamma_1 = \gamma_2$. For non-inferiority, it may be that $H_1 : \gamma_1 = \gamma_2$, or that $H_1 : \gamma_1 - \gamma_2 = \delta_1$ where $\delta_1 < 0$. In the former case it is believed that the two treatments are in fact equivalent, and in the latter that the experimental treatment is in fact superior but that the difference, δ_1, is too small to be demonstrated except by a very large trial. The goal becomes to show that the new treatment is at least as efficacious, and that it may have additional benefits such as easier administration, lower cost, or fewer or less severe adverse reactions.

Equations (4.2) and (4.3) will apply to equivalence/non-inferiority trials with a small modification. The function $\phi(\cdot)$ is unchanged, and the values of γ from H_1 are used in the same way. We replace Δ from these equations by $\Delta + f(\delta)$ for some function $f(\cdot)$.

We illustrate using two examples.

Example 4.3. Suppose y_{ij} are Gaussian with mean μ_j and variance σ^2. We wish to conduct an equivalence trial with equivalence margin δ. The alternative hypothesis is $H_1 : \mu_1 = \mu_2$. Using equation (4.3), we have

$$N = \frac{(Z_{1-\alpha} + Z_{1-\beta})^2 \sigma^2}{\xi_1 \xi_2 (\mu_1 - \mu_2 + \delta)^2} = \frac{(Z_{1-\alpha} + Z_{1-\beta})^2 \sigma^2}{\xi_1 \xi_2 \delta^2}.$$

□

Example 4.4. Suppose y_{ij} are binary with mean π_j and we believe that treatment 1 is superior with odds ratio $\psi = \pi_1(1 - \pi_2)/(1 - \pi_1)\pi_2 = .9$. If we expect that the control rate $\pi_2 = 0.2$, then $\pi_1 = 0.184$. To achieve 90% power with a type I error of 0.01 requires a sample size of nearly 35000. We are willing to accept a result that shows that the odds ratio, ψ, is less than 1.15.

We take $U(\pi_1, \pi_2) = \log(\pi_2/(1 - \pi_2)) - \log(\pi_1/(1 - \pi_1))$. Then $\phi(\pi) = 1/\pi(1 - \pi)$. Under H_1, $\bar{\pi} = (.2 + .184)/2 = .192$, so the required sample size is

$$N = \frac{(2.57 + 1.28)^2/.192(1 - .192)}{(\log(1.15) - \log(.9))^2/4} = 6360.$$

□

4.8 Other Considerations

There may be other considerations that may constrain the desired sample size. For example, one might impose an upper bound based on the smallest treatment effect that is likely to change clinical practice. For example, using equation (4.3), if N is the sample size required to detect an effect of size Δ with power $1 - \beta$ and significance level α, and the observed value of Δ is $\hat{\Delta}$, then $\text{Var}\hat{\Delta} \approx \phi(\hat{\gamma})/\xi_1\xi_2 N \approx (\Delta/(Z_{1-\alpha} + Z_{1-\beta}))^2$. Therefore, the smallest value of $\hat{\Delta}$, Δ', that will reach statistical significance is

$$\Delta' = \frac{Z_{1-\alpha}}{Z_{1-\alpha} + Z_{1-\beta}}\Delta.$$

So, for example, if $\alpha = .025$ and $\beta = .1$, then $\Delta' = 1.96/(1.96 + 1.28)\Delta = .6\Delta$. Therefore, if the observed value of U is 60% of the hypothesized effect size, we will have achieved statistical significance. If this effect size is too small to be of clinical interest, then one can argue that the study is overpowered. With this sample size, any observed difference that is clinically relevant will be guaranteed to be considered statistically significant, provided that the assumed variance is correct. From this point of view, the maximum sample size required is

$$N = \frac{\phi(\bar{\gamma})Z_{1-\alpha}^2}{\xi_1\xi_2\Delta_M^2},$$

where Δ_M is the minimum clinically relevant effect size. Any study larger than this enrolls more subjects than required to find any relevant effect and, from this point of view, may be considered unethical. Note, however, that we may wish to enroll more subjects if we have reason to believe that the assumed variance is unreliable.

4.9 Problems

4.1 Use equation (4.7) to create the following plots.

  (a) Fix $\beta = 0.1$, $\Delta = 0.1$, and $\pi_0 = 0.4$. Plot sample size vs. α for values of α from 0.001 to 0.1.

  (b) Fix $\alpha = 0.05$, $\Delta = 0.1$, and $\pi_0 = 0.4$. Plot sample size vs. β for values of β from 0.05 to 0.3.

  (c) Fix $\alpha = 0.05$, $\beta = 0.1$, and $\pi_0 = 0.4$. Plot sample size vs. Δ for values of Δ from 0.05 to 0.3.

  (d) Fix $\alpha = 0.05$, $\beta = 0.1$, and $\Delta = 0.1$. Plot sample size vs. π_0 for values of π_0 from 0.15 to 0.95.

4.2 Assume that $\phi(\bar{\gamma}) = 1$ and $\xi_1 = \xi_2 = 1/2$.

  (a) Using equation (4.3), calculate the required sample size for a two-sided test (replacing α with $\alpha/2$) having 90% power. Do this for several reasonable values of α and Δ.

  (b) Compare your results with the corresponding sample sizes for a one-sided test.

  (c) Approximate the actual power for the sample sizes you calculated in part 4.2(a) (i.e., you need to include the probability of rejecting H_0 by observing a value below the lower critical value). Discuss.

4.3 Suppose a situation arises in which the number of subjects enrolled in a trial is of no ethical concern. The objective of the trial is to test an experimental drug against standard care. The experimental drug, however, costs 2.5 times as much per subject as the standard care. Assuming normally distributed outcomes with equal variances, what is the optimal sample size for each group if the goal is to minimize the cost of the trial while still controlling type I and type II errors?

4.4 A common variance stabilizing transformation for binomial observations is the arcsine transformation: $T_j = \sin^{-1}(\sqrt{x_j/n_j})$ where $x_j \sim$ Binom(n_j, π_j).

  (a) Show that the variance of T_j is asymptotically independent of π_j.

(b) If $U = T_2 - T_1$, find the function $\phi(\cdot)$ required for equation (4.2).

(c) Derive the sample size formula for the two sample binomial problem using this transformation.

(d) For the case $\pi_1 = .4$, $\pi_2 = .3$, $\xi_1 = \xi_2 = .5$, $\alpha = .05$, and $\beta = .1$, find the required sample size and compare to the numerical example on page 121.

CHAPTER 5

Randomization

Another important feature in clinical trial design is the allocation of subjects to their respective treatments and is typically done through the process of *randomization*, although some allocation schemes make only limited use of randomization. It represents the single most significant difference between clinical trials and other forms of medical investigation (Lachin 1988b). The procedure to be used must be chosen before any treatment is given or any data collected. The particular randomization scheme employed is integral to the trial design and may influence the choice of methods used for the final analysis.

The purpose of this chapter is to give an overview of the important properties of a number of methods used for randomization. The first section outlines the main reasons for randomized allocation. The remaining sections describe many of the methods that have been proposed to carry out the assignment of treatments to subjects. The methods have been divided into two main categories: fixed procedures and adaptive procedures. The latter require information about previous treatment assignments, previous subject outcomes, or subject characteristics in order to generate subsequent treatment assignments. While the overall goals of each method are essentially the same, each possesses distinct properties. Furthermore, optimal statistical analysis depends on the type of randomization employed. Most of these will be discussed for the situation in which two treatments are compared to one another. Multi-treatment versions of many of these procedures are also available and possess essentially the same properties.

5.1 The Role of Randomization

Randomization was proposed by Fisher (1935) as a basis for designed scientific experiments. In particular, he used randomization to assign treatments to plots in agricultural experiments. In clinical research, randomization has become a fundamental part of experiments intended to show effectiveness of drugs or other interventions. The main functions of the randomization process are to protect against sources of bias due to confounding with known and, especially, unknown factors, to eliminate the need for artificial and untestable assumptions, and to provide a sound foundation for statistical inference. As noted in Chapter 2, randomization ensures independence between assigned treatment and outcome, thereby allowing us to attribute observed differences between treatment groups not attributable to chance to the causal effect of the treatment (equation (2.4)). These ideas, presented in this section, have been discussed in detail by Kempthorne (1977) and Lachin (1988b), among others.

5.1.1 Confounding

Suppose we have the following familiar linear regression model:

$$y = \beta_0 + \beta_1 x + \varepsilon,$$

where y is the outcome of interest, x is a predictor (treatment), β_0 and β_1 are model parameters, and ε is the error. Now suppose we observe n pairs (x_i, y_i), $i = 1 \ldots n$, and after an appropriate analysis we find that x and y have significant correlation or that the "effect of x on y" is significant. We cannot automatically assume that x explains or causes y. To see that this is so, let the roles of x and y be reversed in the above model. We might see the same results as before and feel inclined to state that y explains x. A third possibility is that another characteristic, z, referred to as a *confounder* explains or causes both x and y.

Subject characteristics that are associated with both treatment and outcome result in *confounding*, introducing bias into hypothesis tests and the estimates of parameters (i.e., treatment effects) when the nature of the association is not correctly adjusted for. Even when the investigator is aware of the characteristic and it is measurable, adjustment may be problematic. For example, suppose an observational study is conducted and treatment assignment is based on disease diagnosis and patient characteristics, as is the case for observational studies. How could one eliminate the possibility of confounding? Baseline variables can be adjusted for in the analysis using a statistical model, and thus, a model is required. A typical choice is the linear regression model,

$$y = bx + z\boldsymbol{\beta} + \varepsilon,$$

where x is treatment, z is a vector of covariates, b and $\boldsymbol{\beta}$ are the model parameters, and ε is the error, which is assumed to be normal.

The first problem is that it is impossible to include all covariates in z, and we must assume that the form of the model is correct. Some of the relevant (confounding) covariates may not even be known or easily measured. Even a subset of the list of known characteristics may be too large for the model. In other words, we could have more variables than observations, giving no chance of statistical tests. We can select a few covariates to include, however, if we do not include a sufficient number of covariates, we increase the possibility of an incorrect estimate of b due to residual confounding. Conversely, including too many covariates will hurt the precision of estimates. Given that the estimates of the parameters of interest are strongly influenced by the model building process, it will be difficult to assess the validity of results. Of course, when the important characteristics are unknown or not measurable, adjustment is impossible. In short, when confounding is not accounted for in the allocation procedure, it is difficult, if not impossible to adjust for in the analysis. The goal of the allocation procedure becomes to eliminate the possibility of confounding. Since we usually cannot render an outcome independent of a potential confounding characteristic, we require an allocation procedure that can make the characteristic independent of the treatment assignment. The use of randomization ensures this independence.

5.1.2 Selection Bias

A systematic difference between what is observed in a sample of trial participants and what is true for the whole population is sometimes referred to as *bias*. The term is most commonly used to refer to the difference between a parameter estimate and the true parameter value, but it is also used, for example, to refer to differences that can lead to errors in hypothesis tests.

Selection bias results from an association between outcomes and treatment assignments. In observational studies, treatments are assigned based on a patient's diagnosis. Thus those with and without exposure to a particular treatment will usually be quite different—not because of the effect of treatment, but because of differences in underlying disease. Similarly, in a comparative study without randomization, a physician might assign patients to treatments based, at least in part, on medical assessment. While this is a desirable feature of daily medical practice, in a clinical experiment, it may produce selection bias and must be carefully avoided. Neither the clinician nor anyone else with patient contact must know a potential participant's treatment prior to their enrollment.

A classic illustration of the need for randomization to eliminate selection bias is the study of gastric freezing as a treatment for potentially fatal stomach ulcers. Wangensteen et al. (1962) presented a method for treating ulcers in which a patient was anesthetized and a balloon containing a coolant was inserted into the patient's stomach to freeze, and hopefully eliminate, the ulcer. The investigators attempted this procedure in several patients and achieved success in all of them. This study led to the popularization of the technique. The experiment was neither blinded nor randomized.

Ruffin et al. (1969) reported the results of a double-blind clinical trial in which 160 patients were randomized to either gastric freezing (82 patients) or sham freezing (78 patients). The latter was similar to the true procedure except that the coolant was removed before the ulcer could freeze. The outcome of interest was treatment failure measured by the requirement of surgery, recurrent bleeding, or severe pain. The analysis showed no statistical difference between the two groups, with gastric freezing (51% failure) somewhat inferior to the sham procedure (44% failure).

One likely reason for the conflicting conclusions of these two studies was that the first lacked a randomized control. It is likely that in the first study, since these patients had a severe illness and were to undergo total anesthesia—a risky and potentially fatal procedure—that the investigators chose the healthiest subjects for their studies. Bias can arise if the selected subjects' outcomes were compared to historical or other control groups that were not similarly selected. Randomization ensures that patients will not be preferentially chosen for the active treatment and that the eligibility criteria for control participants are identical to those for the treatment participants. This was not the case for the Wangensteen study, in which all patients received treatment. Therefore, the randomized trial should be regarded as more reliable.

Another trial in which randomization was not properly carried out was reported by Hareyama et al. (2002). This was called "a prospective, randomized trial" to compare high-dose-rate vs. low-dose-rate radiation therapy for the treatment of uterine cancer. As stated by the authors, however, "Treatment arm (HDR or LDR) was allocated according to the month of each patients birth. Patients whose birth month was numerically odd were allocated to HDR, and those whose birth month was even to LDR." This was not a randomized trial because the method of assignment was deterministic and known in advance. One problem with this scheme is that patients born in certain months could systematically differ from patients born in other months. A more serious consequence of such an allocation rule is that investigators could know, based on a patient's birth date, the treatment arm to which the patient would be assigned. The physician could use this knowledge and his or her own judgment to recommend that a patient accept or reject participation in the trial. Outside of the clinical trial setting, this would appear to be good medical practice. However, for a valid experiment this must be avoided when possible. From this point of view, randomization serves to protect the scientific process from what would otherwise be good medical practice.

If a trial is double-blind and randomized, there can be no selection bias. On the other hand, when physicians have details in advance about the treatment allocation sequence, selection bias is possible, even when randomization is used, depending on the particular randomization procedure used. For example, if the randomization is designed to enforce equal treatment group sizes and a physician knows how many individuals have been assigned to each group, then the treatment arm with fewer individuals will be the most likely group to which the next participant will be assigned. This type of selection bias will be discussed later in the chapter as each type of randomization scheme is described.

5.1.3 Population vs. Randomization Models

An assumption commonly used to justify comparison of non-randomized groups is that the participants represent a random sample from the whole population. The problem with this approach is that participants in a clinical study never represent a random sample from the whole population. Participants enrolled in clinical trials are very different from those who are not. Furthermore, not all members of the population can be available at the time of the trial. For example, suppose we could take a random sample today from all infants with a certain birth defect. We would not have a random sample from the entire population because infants will be born in the next months or years with the same defect and those infants would not have been available when the sample was taken.

Figure 5.1.3 from Lachin (1988b) illustrates this concept by presenting three models. The first model is the sampling-based population model. In this setting, we begin with two infinitely large populations, each receiving one of the treatments to be compared. We then assume patients' responses are i.i.d. from a probability distribution (e.g., normal) with c.d.f. $G(y|\theta_\tau)$, where τ indexes treatment and θ_τ are parameters (e.g., mean). We then have statistical tools that are valid for testing $H_0: G(y|\theta_1) = G(y|\theta_2)$, once we take a random sample from each population. If we accept that the i.i.d. assumption holds, our subjects become identical units and we can assign treatment by any deterministic method to get valid results.

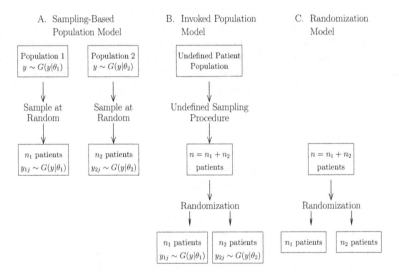

Figure 5.1 *Population sampling models, the patient selection process, and the randomization model for a clinical trial. Modified from Lachin (1988b).*

The second model in Figure 5.1.3 illustrates the case in which one invokes the population model after randomization. This model assumes that, despite having an unspecified population from which patients are drawn using a method that is not random sampling, the distributional assumptions can still be used with the final outcome data. This conclusion has no sound foundation, however, and relies on distributional assumptions that are not verifiable.

The goal of randomization is to avoid having to invoke the population model at all by creating a framework for an assumption-free test. This is the third model shown in Figure 5.1.3. No assumptions are made about the patient population or the underlying probability distribution. Thus, because we cannot truly sample randomly from the entire population of interest or know with certainty the underlying model, randomization is the soundest alternative.

5.1.4 Statistical Inference

Randomization or *permutation* tests are valid, formal tests of equality of treatments that do not rely on the assumptions of the population models mentioned in the previous section (Lachin 1988b; Fisher 1935; Kempthorne 1977). Instead, these tests make use of the distribution induced on the data by the randomization (the *randomization distribution*). To illustrate such a distribution, consider a group of 10 subjects, divided into two groups of 5 (groups A and B) by randomization (this method of randomization will be discussed in greater detail in section 5.2.1). We observe 10 response values and calculate at $\bar{y}_A$, the observed sample mean of the 5 subjects in group A. Figure 5.2 shows the randomization distribution for $\bar{y}_A$, given the observations corresponding to the 10 circles along the axis. We suppose that the filled in circles correspond to those assigned group A in the trial. The vertical line is at $\bar{y}_A$ for the allocation shown. With the given number of subjects and equal group sizes, there are 251 other possible allocation patterns. Th histogram represents the randomization distribution of $\bar{y}_A$ and is quite similar to that of the approximating t-distribution.

When comparing two groups, the basic idea is this: each participant's outcome measure is considered a fixed number for that participant. Under the null hypothesis of no treatment effect, a participant would have the same outcome under any treatment assignment. The observed difference between the two groups, as measured by some predetermined statistic, is compared to the difference that would have been observed under all other possible ways in which randomization could have assigned treatment. Since each subject's outcome is considered fixed, any observed difference must be due either to chance (randomization) or to a treatment effect. The randomization distribution of the statistic gives a probability, under the null hypothesis, of a treatment difference at least as large as the one observed due to chance alone. If this p-value is small enough, the conclusion is that the difference is due to treatment. Formally, as described by Lachin (1988b), let n be the total number of participants, let n_1 be the number assigned to the first treatment, and let $n_2 = n - n_1$ be the number assigned to the second. Given a particular randomization scheme, the *reference set*, S, consists of all possible randomization sequences of n patients to the two groups. Let K be the total number of elements in S, and let T be a test statistic of interest (for example, difference in mean outcome between the two groups). Now, suppose we observe $T = T^*$ and let T_i be the value of T that would have been observed with the same data values and the allocation corresponding to the ith element of S. If all randomization sequences have equal probability, then a one-sided p-value for

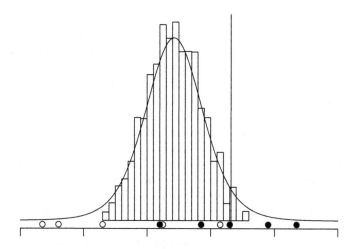

Figure 5.2 *Randomization distribution of the mean in one treatment group of size five randomly drawn from the ten observations shown in circles at the bottom. The vertical line represents the mean of the allocation corresponding to the solid circles.*

the test of no treatment effect is given by

$$p = \frac{1}{K} \sum_{i=1}^{K} I(T_i \geq T^*),$$

where $I(\cdot)$ is the indicator function. We reject the null hypothesis if, for example, $p < \alpha$. There are many possible reference sets. For the *unconditional reference set*, we consider all $K = 2^n$ possible allocations of the participants into two groups. The *conditional reference set* is used when we consider n_1 as fixed. In this case, $K = \binom{n}{n_1}$.

Example 5.1. Suppose we have a trial with $n = 6$ participants and assign $n_1 = 3$ to control and $n_2 = 3$ to intervention by randomly choosing one of the $K = \binom{6}{3} = 20$ possible arrangements. Suppose we observe the arrangement $\{1, 2, 1, 1, 2, 2\}$ where 1 indicates assignment to intervention and 2 indicates assignment to control, and suppose the corresponding observed outcome values at the end of the trial are $\{5, 7.5, 6, 3, 4, 8\}$. Then, the observed difference in means (intervention $-$ control) is $T^* = (7.5 + 4 + 8)/3 - (5 + 6 + 3)/3 \approx 1.83$. Simple calculation will show that there are two other arrangements that give an equal or larger value of T: $\{1, 2, 2, 1, 1, 2\}$ with $T \approx 3.17$ and $\{2, 2, 1, 1, 1, 2\}$

with $T = 2.5$. Thus, the one-sided p-value is $3/20 = 0.15$ and we conclude that there is no significant difference at conventional levels (e.g., $\alpha = 0.05$). □

In the early days of clinical trials, permutation tests were often not computationally feasible. Consider a trial with 50 participants, 25 in each of two treatment arms. In this case there are over 10^{14} possible allocation patterns. Of course, many clinical trials are much larger. Thus, even today, such enumeration is rarely used. A way of performing permutation tests without enumerating every possible randomization sequence uses the fact that the distributions of statistics used for permutation tests are often asymptotically normal under the null hypothesis of no treatment effect. In most cases, especially with moderate sample sizes, tests based on normal theory approximate permutation tests very well, as illustrated even for small samples by Figure 5.2. The mean and variance of these asymptotic distributions depend on the statistic and also the randomization method employed.

Of course, today computation has become much easier and takes much less time. There are many statistical software packages that perform a variety of permutation tests, even with large sample sizes. If possible, one should use a permutation test, or a good approximation, because it uses no assumptions beyond randomization.

5.2 Fixed Randomization Procedures

In this section, three types of randomization are discussed: the random allocation rule, complete randomization, and permuted-block randomization. The first two are sometimes referred to as *simple* randomization schemes because they have fewer restrictions. The methods were compared with respect to certain properties by Lachin (1988a) and Matts and Lachin (1988). These properties are imbalance (i.e., inequality of treatment group sizes), potential for selection bias, accidental bias, and testing issues. Here, we do not discuss accidental bias since, in practice, randomization procedures are most commonly selected based on the other properties. The assessment of these properties is described in greater detail in the context of the first method, the random allocation rule.

5.2.1 Random Allocation Rule

The first simple randomization technique is called the *random allocation rule*. For this rule, the total sample size is a fixed number n and the number in each group is fixed. For two groups, the most commonly desired ratio of patients in each group is 1:1 ($n/2$ in each group), so we will make this assumption. There are two ways in which this method can be implemented. The first is to enroll all participants in the trial at once, randomly allocating half to each treatment. Of course this is feasible only for small trials. The alternative is to generate the random sequence for the entire trial, but assign participants only as they arrive. In the latter case, of interest are the probabilities, conditional and unconditional, that each participant is assigned to a specific treatment. For example, the unconditional probability that any participant is assigned to either treatment is $1/2$. On the other hand, the probability that a participant is assigned to, say, treatment 1, given that all previous assignments are known, may be different. Formally, let n^* and n_1^* be, respectively, the number of participants who have enrolled and the number who have been assigned to treatment 1 at the time a new participant enters the trial. Also, let τ be the new participant's assigned treatment. Then, the probability that this new participant will be assigned to treatment 1 is

$$\Pr(\tau = 1 | n_1^*, n^*) = \frac{n/2 - n_1^*}{n - n^*}.$$

Because total and group sample sizes are predetermined, there can be no imbalance in the number of participants in each arm at the end of enrollment. The exception to this occurs when patients are assigned as they enter the trial and fewer than n subjects are enrolled. For example, let $Q = \max(n_1, n_2)/n$ be used to measure imbalance. If the desired sample size is 6 but the trial only enrolls $n = 4$ participants, the only possible imbalance is $Q = 3/4$ (the other possibility, of course, is balance, $Q = 1/2$). The probability of imbalance is 0.4 and the expected imbalance is 0.6. For arbitrary sample sizes, probabilities of imbalance correspond to probabilities of the hypergeometric distribution. The probability of an imbalance greater than or equal to a specific Q can be calculated using Fisher's exact test or approximated by a χ^2 test (Lachin 1988a).

While imbalance is not usually a problem when using the random allocation rule, selection bias is a concern. Blackwell and Hodges Jr. (1957) give a simple way to assess a randomization procedure's susceptibility to selection bias in an unblinded study in which there is the possibility that the investigator may, consciously or not, select subjects based on guesses regarding next treatment assignment. Under this model, it is assumed that the experimenter always guesses the most probable treatment assignment, conditional on the past assignments. For any particular realization, the *bias factor*, F, is defined as the number of correct guesses minus the number expected by chance alone (i.e., $n/2$). If the random allocation rule is used and all participants enter the trial at once, there can be no selection bias. In the case of staggered entry (i.e., participants enter one at a time), however, each time we have imbalance and the following treatment assignment brings us closer to balance, the result is a correct guess. This will always occur $n/2$ times and the number expected by chance alone is $n/2$. Thus, $E[F]$ is half of the expected number of times during accrual that we have balance. Blackwell and Hodges Jr. (1957) show that this is $2^{n-1}/\binom{n}{n/2} - 1$, so that

$$E[F] = \frac{2^{n-1}}{\binom{n}{n/2}} - \frac{1}{2}.$$

It may be surprising that, as $n \to \infty$,

$$\frac{E[F]}{\sqrt{n}} \to C,$$

where $C = \sqrt{\pi/32}$. This implies that, as the sample size increases, the potential for selection bias increases and can become quite large.

Finally, we consider permutaion tests and their relationship to the randomization scheme. An example of a permutation test for a trial randomized by the random allocation rule was given in Section 5.1.4. A popular general family of permutation tests is the linear rank family. A linear rank statistic with centered scores has the form

$$S = \frac{\sum (a_i - \bar{a}) (T_i - E[T_i])}{\sqrt{\mathrm{Var}\left(\sum (a_i - \bar{a}) (T_i - E[T_i])\right)}}, \qquad (5.1)$$

where a_i is a score that is a function of the participant responses, $\bar{a} = \frac{1}{n} \sum a_i$, T_i is an indicator that the patient received treatment 1, and $E[T_i]$ is the permutational expectation of T_i, based on either the conditional or the unconditional reference set. The statistic S is asymptotically standard normal. For the random allocation rule, $E[T_i] = 1/2$. The variance in (5.1) is

$$V = \sum_i (a_i - \bar{a})^2 \mathrm{Var}(T_i) + \sum_{i \neq j} (a_i - \bar{a})(a_j - \bar{a}) \left(E[T_i T_j] - E[T_i]^2 \right). \quad (5.2)$$

Now, $E[T_i T_j]$ is the probability that participant i and j are both assigned to treatment 1. This is

$$E[T_i T_j] = \frac{\binom{n/2}{2}}{\binom{n}{2}} = \frac{n-2}{4(n-1)}.$$

Using this and the fact that $\mathrm{Var}(T_i) = \frac{1}{2}\left(1 - \frac{1}{2}\right)$ gives

$$V = \frac{n}{4(n-1)} \sum (a_i - \bar{a})^2.$$

5.2.2 Complete Randomization

In contrast to the random allocation rule, *complete* randomization does not assume fixed group sizes. Instead, only a desired total sample size is predetermined. Treatment is assigned to participants as they enter the trial using a method equivalent to flipping a fair coin. Thus, a fixed probability of $1/2$ is given to each treatment and the group sample sizes, n_1 and n_2, conditional on the total sample size, have binomial distributions. Since the probabilities are the same for each participant and the "coin flips" are independent, both the conditional and unconditional probabilities of assignment to either treatment are $1/2$.

Another way in which complete randomization differs from the random allocation rule is the potential for imbalance at the end of the trial. The most important benefit of balance is that increased imbalance results in decreased power for statistical tests. Only a very high amount of imbalance, however, has any substantial effect on power. Lachin (1988b) states that if $Q < 0.7$, loss in power is trivial. To calculate the probability of a particular imbalance from complete randomization, we can either use the binomial distribution directly or invoke the normal approximation. Specifically, n_1 and n_2 are each binomial$(n,1/2)$ or approximately $N(n/2, n/4)$. Using the normal approximation, the probability that the imbalance is greater than a fixed value, say, $R > 1/2$, is

$$\Pr(Q > R) \approx 2\Phi\left((1 - 2R)\sqrt{n}\right),$$

where $\Phi(\cdot)$ is the standard normal c.d.f. Thus, as the sample size increases, the probability of imbalance decreases. Table 5.1 shows the probabilities of imbalance greater than 0.6, 0.7, and 0.75 for a range of sample sizes. For even moderate sample sizes, the probability of a non-trivial power loss due to treatment imbalance is practically zero.

Table 5.1 *Probabilities of imbalance for complete randomization.*

		Sample Size				
		10	30	50	100	150	200
	.60	.344	.200	.119	.035	.011	.004
Imbalance	.70	.109	.016	.003	3×10^{-5}	4×10^{-7}	6×10^{-9}
	.75	.109	.005	.0003	2×10^{-7}	4×10^{-10}	3×10^{-13}

One of the benefits of complete randomization is that there is no possibility of selection bias. The probability of assignment to either treatment is always $1/2$, so the physician has no best guess.

For linear rank tests based on the unconditional reference set, $E[T_i]$ in (5.1) is $1/2$. The variance is

$$V = \sum_i (a_i - \bar{a})^2 \operatorname{Var}(T_i) = \frac{1}{4} \sum_i (a_i - \bar{a})^2.$$

When using the conditional reference set, $E[T_i] = n_1/n$ and

$$E[T_i T_j] = \frac{\binom{n_1}{2}}{\binom{n}{2}} = \frac{n_1(n_1 - 1)}{n(n - 1)}.$$

We can then use (5.2) again and $\operatorname{Var}(T_i) = n_1(1 - n_1)$ to give

$$V = \frac{n_1(n - n_1)}{n(n - 1)} \sum (a_i - \bar{a})^2.$$

Note that, asymptotically, $n_1/n \to 1/2$ and the variance based on the conditional reference set becomes the same as the variance based on the unconditional reference set. These are also asymptotically equivalent to the variance for the random allocation rule. For small or even moderate sample sizes, however, the three variances can be quite different.

5.2.3 Permuted-Block Randomization

One of the most commonly used randomization methods in clinical trials is *permuted-block randomization*. This method periodically ensures treatment balance by repeating the random allocation rule sequentially within blocks, or groups of participants. In the most common configuration, each block has size m (must be even) and within each block $m/2$ subjects are assigned to each treatment. Note that the random allocation rule could be considered a special case of this procedure with one block of size n. Another design, the paired or matched comparison, where participants are randomized as pairs and then the two responses are compared, is a permuted-block design with $m = 2$. The permuted-block method also allows the possibility of using blocks of different sizes, say $m_1, \ldots, m_B$, where B is number of blocks. In addition, one can let these block sizes be random. For example, half of the blocks could be randomly selected to have size 6 and the rest could be given size 4.

In the case where all blocks have size m and a total of n enroll in the trial, treatment balance is achieved if n is a multiple of m. When blocks have different sizes, the last block must be filled to conserve balance. The probability of specific imbalances in each block can be calculated using the same methods as for a random allocation rule with sample size m. The maximum possible imbalance at any given time in the trial is

$$Q_{\max} = \frac{1}{2} + \frac{m_c}{2n^*},$$

where n^* is number enrolled so far and m_c is the current block size.

To evaluate the potential for selection bias, once again we think of each block as a random allocation rule. As with the random allocation rule, there is no possibility of selection bias if, for each block, all participants are randomized at once. This is not difficult in most cases, as block sizes are usually small. If this cannot be done, with equal block sizes we have

$$E[F] = B \left(\frac{2^{m-1}}{\binom{m}{m/2}} - \frac{1}{2} \right).$$

In the general case, with possibly unequal block sizes,

$$E[F] = \sum_{i=1}^{B} \left(\frac{2^{m_i-1}}{\binom{m_i}{m_i/2}} - \frac{1}{2} \right).$$

It is easy to see that $E[F]$ is always greater for permuted-block randomization than for the random allocation rule. Notice that, for fixed m, $E[F]/n$ is constant for any n. For large m, $E[F]/n \approx C/\sqrt{m}$, where C was given in section 5.2.1. Thus, the rate at which the expected bias factor increases is n compared to $\sqrt{n}$ for the random allocation rule. The use of random block sizes does not help to reduce this potential bias. Specifically, $E[F]$ is approximately the same as it is when all blocks have the average block size.

Matts and Lachin (1988) consider another measurement of potential for selection bias. This measurement is denoted F' and it is the number of treatment assignments that can be exactly determined in advance. For example, if a block has size 8, and 4 out of six randomized participants have already been assigned to one treatment, the last two must be assigned to the other treatment. Thus, after $m/2$ assignments have been made to one treatment, the remaining assignments are known. At least 1 assignment (the last) is known in each block and up to $m/2$ could be known. For equal block sizes, we have $E[F'] = 2mB/(m+2)$, and in the general case

$$E[F'] = \sum_{i=1}^{B} \frac{2m_i}{m_i + 2}.$$

This type of selection bias is eliminated if different block sizes are used and the physician does not know the possible block sizes. In the situation where possible block sizes are known, this bias can also be greatly reduced by choosing block sizes randomly. One might expect that selection bias is completely eliminated in this case. Several assignments could be known, however, if the total number assigned to one treatment exceeds the total number assigned to the other by half of the maximum block size.

When permuted-block randomization is used, the permutation test should take the blocking into account. If blocking is ignored, there is no randomization basis for tests. Furthermore, the usual approximate distributions of test statistics that ignore blocking may not be correct. Matts and Lachin (1988) discuss the following three examples:

1. 2×2 Table. When the outcome variable is binary, it is common to summarize the data using a 2×2 table as in Table 5.2. The statistic

$$\chi_P^2 = \frac{4(ad - bc)^2}{n(a+c)(b+d)}$$

may be used. Based on a population model, under the null hypothesis this statistic is asymptotically χ^2 with one degree of freedom. However, when permuted-block randomization is assumed, the asymptotic distribution is not necessarily χ^2. The proper permutation test is performed by creating a 2×2 table for each block. If we use a subscript i to denote the entries in the table for the ith block, the test statistic is

$$\chi_{MH}^2 = \frac{\left(\sum_{i=1}^{B}(a_i - E[a_i])\right)^2}{\sum_{i=1}^{B} \mathrm{Var}(a_i)}, \quad \text{where}$$

$$E[a_i] = \frac{a_i + c_i}{2} \quad \text{and}$$

$$\mathrm{Var}(a_i) = \frac{(a_i + c_i)(b_i + d_i)}{4(m-1)}.$$

This is the Mantel-Haenszel χ^2 statistic, which is based on the hypergeometric distribution. Asymptotically, assuming permuted-block randomization and under H_0, its distribution is χ^2 with one degree of freedom.

Table 5.2 2×2 *table.*

		Disease		Total
		Yes	No	
Treatment	Tmt 1	a	b	$n/2$
	Tmt 2	c	d	$n/2$
	Total	$a + c$	$b + d$	n

2. *t*-test. With a continuous outcome variable, the usual analysis for comparing the two levels of a factor is the familiar ANOVA *t*-test. If a population model is assumed, the *t*-statistic has a *t*-distribution under the null hypothesis. Of course, the observed value of the statistic will depend on whether or not a blocking factor is included in the model. If permuted-block randomization is assumed but blocking is not included for testing, the statistic will not necessarily have the *t*-distribution under the null hypothesis. If the given randomization is assumed and blocking is included, the permutation distribution of the resulting statistic will be well approximated by the *t*-distribution.

3. Linear Rank Test. Linear rank test statistics have been discussed in previous sections. The linear rank test statistic that does not take blocks into account is asymptotically standard normal, assuming either the random allocation rule or complete randomization, as long as the correct variance term is used. This is not the case, however, if permuted-block randomization is assumed. Thus, one must use a version of the statistic that takes the blocks into account:

$$S = \frac{\sum_{i=1}^{m} \sum_{j=1}^{B} w_j \left(a_{ij} - \bar{a}_{.j}\right) \left(T_{ij} - 1/2\right)}{\sqrt{\frac{m}{4(m-1)} \sum_{i=1}^{m} \sum_{j=1}^{B} w_j^2 \left(a_{ij} - \bar{a}_{.j}\right)^2}},$$

where w_j is a weight for block j, $\bar{a}_{.j} = \sum_{i=1}^{m} a_{ij}/m$, and all other terms are as in (5.1), with an added j subscript denoting the jth block. In this case, the scores a_{ij} depend solely on the responses in the jth block. This statistic is asymptotically standard normal under the null hypothesis and permuted-block randomization.

In each of these situations, if the number of blocks is relatively large, it can be shown (Matts and Lachin 1988) that the statistic that does not take blocking into account is approximately equal to $1 - R$ times the statistic that does, where R is the intrablock correlation. R can take values in the interval $[-1/(m-1), 1]$. It is probably reasonable to assume that if there is an intrablock correlation, then it is positive. Furthermore, the lower bound for the interval in which R takes values approaches 0 as m gets larger. So, in the more likely situation that R is positive, the incorrect (without taking blocking into account) test statistic would be smaller in magnitude than the correct statistic, resulting in a conservative test. Many argue that its conservativeness makes using the incorrect test acceptable, but conservativeness reduces efficiency and power. In addition, for small block sizes, the test may be anticonservative, inflating the type I error.

5.3 Treatment- and Response-Adaptive Randomization Procedures

Up to this point, the randomization methods presented have the property that treatment allocation is based only on the randomization scheme and the order in which participants enter. The methods presented in this section have the property that probabilities of treatment assignment may change throughout the allocation process, depending on previous patient assignments or outcomes. In this section, three main randomization procedures are discussed: biased coin randomization, the urn design, and the play-the-winner rule. With the first two, assignment probabilities are adapted based on treatment imbalance. The last is referred to as a *response-adaptive* procedure, because the probabilities change due to observed responses or outcomes. The same criteria addressed in the previous section are discussed here.

5.3.1 Biased Coin Randomization

Recall that one may think of complete randomization as flipping a fair coin. Efron (1971) proposed a modified version of this concept known as a *biased coin design*. A biased coin design with parameter p, denoted $\text{BCD}(p)$, begins with a fair coin flip (i.e., equal probability of assignment to either group). Subsequently, a probability $p > 1/2$ is assigned to the treatment that has fewer participants. For example, if τ is the assigned treatment and $n_1 < n_2$ then $\Pr(\tau = 1) = p > 1/2$. If, at any point, the two groups are equal in size, the next assignment is again based on a fair coin flip. The unconditional probability that a participant is assigned to either treatment is $1/2$. Note that, if $p = 1$, the result is paired randomization, or a permuted-block design with $m = 2$.

In order to evaluate balancing properties of the biased coin design, we let D_n be the absolute value of the difference in group sizes when n participants have been assigned treatment. This forms a Markov chain defined by the probabilities

$$\Pr(D_{n+1} = j - 1 | D_n = j) = p, \quad j \geq 1$$
$$\Pr(D_{n+1} = j + 1 | D_n = j) = 1 - p, \quad j \geq 1$$
$$\Pr(D_{n+1} = 1 | D_n = 0) = 1.$$

This representation allows probabilities of imbalance to be calculated by recursion. Using the stationary probabilities of the Markov chain, limiting probabilities of imbalance can be calculated. For example, the probability of exact balance, when the total sample size is even, has the limit

$$\Pr(D_{2k} = 0) \to 2 - \frac{1}{p},$$

as $k \to \infty$. Using this fact, or by direct calculation, we can also find that

$$\Pr(D_{2k+1} = 1) \to \frac{2p - 1}{p^2},$$

as $k \to \infty$. One can use these results to compare, for example, BCD(2/3) to complete randomization. The asymptotic probability that the biased coin design will produce perfect balance or best possible balance is at least $1/2$. On the other hand, the probability that complete randomization will produce this level of balance approaches zero.

If one wanted to guess the next assignment under biased coin randomization, the best strategy is to pick the group with the fewest participants, or to pick either group with equal probability in the case of equal group sizes. In this case, the probability of a correct guess for assignment $n + 1$ is $\frac{1}{2}\Pr(D_n = 0) + p P(D_n > 0)$, which, using the previous results, approaches $1 - 1/4p$ as $n \to \infty$. This produces the following limiting property of the expected bias factor:

$$\frac{E[F]}{n} \to \frac{2p - 1}{4p}.$$

This means that the expected bias factor increases at the same rate as that of the permuted-block design, giving a greater potential for selection bias than the random allocation rule. When $p = 2/3$, the potential for selection bias is about the same in large samples as a permuted-block design with block size 6. F' is always 0 for the BCD, however, reflecting the fact that there is randomness in all BCD assignments.

5.3.2 Urn Randomization

A more flexible adaptive method of randomization that allows for the probability of treatment assignment to depend on the magnitude of imbalance is called *urn* randomization. There are two parameters that must be specified for urn randomization and we denote a particular choice $UD(\alpha, \beta)$. The procedure is equivalent to placing colored balls in an urn and drawing balls as follows. Start with α white balls and α red balls. A ball is drawn at random. If the ball is white, the first participant is assigned to treatment 1. Otherwise, the participant is assigned to treatment 2. The ball is then replaced and β balls of the opposite color are added to the urn. This is repeated for each participant until all participants are assigned treatment. Note that $UD(1, 0)$ is equivalent to complete randomization and $UD(\alpha, 1)$ is approximately complete randomization when α is large. Wei and Lachin (1988) describe $UD(0, 1)$ as having desirable properties (when $\alpha = 0$, a fair coin flip is used to begin).

Again, we consider the Markov chain described previously in the context of the biased coin design. After n assignments with $UD(\alpha, \beta)$, a total of βn balls have been added to the original 2α. If the imbalance is $D_n = j$, there must be $\alpha + \beta(n + j)/2$ balls of one color and $\alpha + \beta(n - j)/2$ of the other. The transition probabilities are now

$$\Pr(D_{n+1} = j - 1 | D_n = j) = \tfrac{1}{2} + \tfrac{\beta j}{2(2\alpha + \beta n)}, \ \ j \geq 1$$

$$\Pr(D_{n+1} = j + 1 | D_n = j) = \tfrac{1}{2} - \tfrac{\beta j}{2(2\alpha + \beta n)}, \ \ j \geq 1$$

$$\Pr(D_{n+1} = 1 | D_n = 0) = 1.$$

For example, the transition probabilities for $UD(0, 1)$ are $\tfrac{1}{2}(1 \pm j/n)$. These are the probabilities for complete randomization, multiplied by inflation/deflation factors corresponding to the amount of imbalance. This method guards against severe imbalance in any trial and gives better balance in small trials than complete randomization. For large trials, urn randomization eventually behaves like complete randomization. The following approximation holds for large n:

$$\Pr(D_n > j) \approx 2\Phi \left(-\frac{j + 0.5}{\sqrt{\frac{n(\alpha + \beta)}{3\beta + \alpha}}} \right).$$

Taking the case of $UD(0, 1)$, the probability of a large imbalance can be approximated by

$$\Pr(Q > R) \approx 2\Phi \left((1 - 2R)\sqrt{3n} \right).$$

This design can also be shown to achieve efficiency similar to that of the random allocation rule. In particular, $UD(0, 1)$ needs at most 4 more observations to give essentially the same efficiency as the random allocation rule, which is perfectly balanced (Wei and Lachin 1988).

The probability of making a correct guess of treatment assignment for participant $n + 1$ is

$$g_{n+1} = \frac{1}{2} + \frac{E[D_n]\beta}{2(2\alpha + \beta n)},$$

where $E[D_n]$ can be computed recursively using the transition probabilities and the property

$$\Pr(D_n = j) = \Pr(D_n = j \,|\, D_{n-1} = j - 1) \Pr(D_{n-1} = j - 1)$$
$$+ \Pr(D_n = j \,|\, D_{n-1} = j + 1) \Pr(D_{n-1} = j + 1).$$

It follows that $E[F] = \sum_{i=1}^{n} g_i - n/2$. Once again, as the sample size increases, urn randomization is similar to complete randomization and thus the potential for selection bias becomes increasingly small.

Again, we consider permutation tests. Under complete randomization, all assignment patterns in the reference set are equally likely. This is not the case for $UD(\alpha, \beta)$. In fact, certain assignment patterns may not be possible. For example, for $UD(0,1)$ any pattern that assigns the first two participants to the same treatment is impossible. These complications make the permutation distributions of test statistics more difficult to calculate. Consider a linear rank statistic under the $UD(\alpha, \beta)$. Let $V = \frac{1}{4} \sum_{i=1}^{n} b_i^2$, where

$$b_i = a_i - \bar{a} - \sum_{j=i+1}^{n} \frac{[2\alpha + (i-1)\beta]\beta(a_j - \bar{a})}{[2\alpha + (j-1)\beta][2\alpha + (j-2)\beta]}, \quad 1 \leq i < n$$

$$b_n = a_n - \bar{a}.$$

If this V is used as the variance term in (5.1), the resulting statistic will be asymptotically standard normal.

5.3.3 Play-the-Winner Rule

When a clinical trial is used to compare two treatments and one of the treatments is superior to the other, many participants are given an inferior treatment for the duration of the trial. One method, that can be used in an attempt to allocate the better treatment to a greater number of individuals, is called the *play-the-winner rule*. This rule was proposed by Zelen (1969) and can be applied in the case where the outcome is binary: "success" or "failure." The basic idea is the following: the first participant is assigned one of the two treatments, with equal probability given to each. If that participant's response is a success, the following participant is assigned to the same treatment. In the case of a failure, the other treatment is assigned. The following treatment assignments are made in the same way. Under this mechanism, the probability of a participant's allocation to any particular treatment depends on the (unknown) probability of success for each treatment. Assuming the trial stops immediately following a failure, it can be shown that the number of participants assigned to a treatment can be written as a sum of i.i.d. geometric random variables.

The method just described is called the *modified* play-the-winner rule. In practice, the delay between the time of the treatment assignment and the time the outcome is known is usually larger than the time between enrollment of consecutive subjects. In this situation, the method is equivalent to using a box and both black and orange balls. A success in the treatment 1 arm or a failure in the treatment 2 arm each lead to adding a black ball to the box. Otherwise, an orange ball is added. To assign treatment to a new participant, a ball is drawn without replacement from the box. A black ball indicates an assignment to treatment 1 and an orange ball indicates assignment to treatment 2. In addition, if there are no balls in the box, treatment assignment is determined by flipping a fair coin. The procedure stops when a fixed number of failures are observed in each group or when the predetermined sample size is reached. The properties of this method are essentially identical to those of the modified rule, but are easier to derive for the latter.

Clearly, treatment balance is not a goal of the play-the-winner rule. Balance is expected only if the treatments have the same effect. In fact, the degree of imbalance can be used to test for a difference between treatments.

To illustrate this, suppose one uses the play-the-winner rule and the trial is stopped when v failures have been observed on each treatment. Let N_1 and N_2 be the total number of patients assigned to treatments 1 and 2, respectively. Also, let p_1 and p_2 be the true probabilities of success for each treatment and let $q_i = 1 - p_i$, $i = 1, 2$. The joint distribution of N_1 and N_2 is

$$\Pr(N_1 = n_1, N_2 = n_2) = \binom{n_1 - 1}{v - 1}\binom{n_2 - 1}{v - 1}p_1^{n_1}p_2^{n_2}\left(\frac{q_1 q_2}{p_1 p_2}\right)^v$$

and the conditional distribution of N_1, given $N_1 + N_2 = N$, is

$$\Pr(N_1 = n_1 | N_1 + N_2 = N) = \frac{\binom{n_1-1}{v-1}\binom{N-N_1-1}{v-1}r^{n_1}}{\sum_{j=v}^{N-v}\binom{j-1}{v-1}\binom{N-j-1}{v-1}r^j},$$

where $r = p_1/p_2$. Under the null hypothesis that $p_1 = p_2$, this expression simplifies to

$$\Pr(N_1 = n_1 | N_1 + N_2 = N) = \frac{\binom{n_1-1}{v-1}\binom{N-N_1-1}{v-1}}{\binom{N-1}{2v-1}}.$$

An exact significance test is performed by summing these probabilities for all possible values of N_1 greater than or equal to the observed value. Zelen (1969) also shows that the approximate conditional mean and variance of N_1 are given by

$$\mu = E[N_1|N_1 + N_2 = N] \approx \frac{N}{2} + \frac{N(N - 2v)}{4(2v + 1)}\log r$$

$$\sigma^2 = \text{Var}(N_1|N_1 + N_2 = N) \approx \frac{N(N - 2v)}{4(2v + 1)}.$$

Thus, if the observed value of N_1 is n_1, an approximate $100(1-\alpha)\%$ confidence interval for r is

$$\exp\left\{[(n_1 - \mu)/\sigma^2] \pm z_{1-\alpha/2}/\sigma\right\}.$$

Potentially, one of the biggest problems with this procedure is the high susceptibility to selection bias. Recent outcomes determine subsequent treatment assignment. Thus, if an experimenter is unblinded to the outcomes, he/she may know the next treatment assignment exactly and may exercise judgment that could undermine the validity of the trial. In addition, because the randomization probabilities can change over time, a time trend in outcome can confound the treatment effect and bias its estimate. This confounding can magnify early random differences into spurious conclusions as follows (Karrison et al. 2003). Suppose that there is truly no difference between two treatments in terms of outcome, but that the probability of success increases over time for all patients. Suppose also that the success rate for the first treatment is initially slightly higher than for the second, by chance. The play-the-winner rule will then assign more patients to the first treatment. Success rates are improving and later patients are more likely to get the first treatment, so the difference in effect will be amplified. This will then lead to even more patients receiving the first treatment, increasing the difference, and so on. Realistic levels of time-outcome confounding can then generate spurious results. This is a drawback to the play-the-winner rule. Jennison and Turnbull (2000) show that bias due to time trend is obviated by randomizing patients in blocks with constant assignment probabilities within blocks and an analysis that accounts for them. They also show how increasing the block sizes when randomization proportions deviate from 0.5 can render the information contribution of the block identical, greatly simplifying the consequent analysis. In this way, the naive analysis that does not account for response-adaptivity can be correct. Simon et al. (1975) have also demonstrated that play-the-winner designs can actually require more participants than a simple fixed sample design.

A trial that used the play-the-winner rule to allocate treatments (also an example of some of the difficulties surrounding this rule) was the Michigan extracorporeal membrane oxygenator (ECMO) trial (Bartlett, Roloff, Cornell, Andrews, Dillon, and Zwischenberger 1985). Infants were assigned to either conventional therapy, including intensive ventilatory support, or to ECMO, an external system for oxygenating blood. The first infant was assigned to ECMO and survived. The second infant was assigned to conventional therapy and died. After this, nine more infants were assigned to ECMO, all survived, and the trial was stopped. Of course, the conclusion was made that ECMO was beneficial. The problem, however, is that the sickest patient was the one who happened to be assigned to conventional therapy. Ware (1989) argued that the results were not sufficient to justify use of ECMO.

Randomized Play-the-Winner Rule

A randomized play-the-winner rule was proposed by Wei and Durham (1978). Their goal was to modify the rule in a way that reduces the potential for selection bias. Starting with a box containing u black balls and u orange balls, a ball is drawn and replaced. If the ball is black, the first participant is assigned to treatment 1. If the ball is orange, treatment 2 is assigned. The procedure continues in this way until a participant's outcome is known. If the outcome is a success, an additional β balls of the color corresponding to that individual's treatment are added to the box, along with α balls of the opposite color, where $\alpha \leq \beta$. If the outcome was a failure, the same number of balls are added, but the colors of the balls are reversed. This is repeated each time an outcome is known and each additional assignment is made by drawing and replacing a ball. This procedure is similar to the urn design. The difference, however, is that balls are added each time an outcome, rather than a treatment assignment, is known. Furthermore, the color of the balls is determined by both the treatment assignment and the corresponding observed outcome.

It can be shown that the expected bias factor, in the absence of a time trend, has the following asymptotic property

$$\frac{E[F]}{n} \rightarrow \frac{(w-1)(p_1 - p_2)}{2(p_1 + p_2) + 2w(q_1 + q_2)},$$

where $w = \beta/\alpha$. The limit is increasing in w. This presents a trade off. When w is large, the rule behaves more like the non-randomized version, allowing for higher selection bias. On the other hand, when w is small, the method is approximately equivalent to complete randomization. In this case, the expected number of participants receiving each treatment is about the same, contrary to the original goal of assigning more *patients* to the superior treatment.

5.4 Covariate-Adaptive Randomization Procedures

Another category of adaptive randomization methods involves prognostic factors considered to be of interest. Such methods are referred to as *covariate-adaptive* methods. These procedures are used in an attempt to achieve balance with respect to these variables and make the treatment groups as comparable as possible. The reason for considering such methods is that, for example, in an "unlucky" randomization, a higher percentage of high-risk participants could be assigned to one of the treatment groups. Then, even if there is no true difference between treatments, an unadjusted statistical analysis might show otherwise. Here, two randomization procedures are presented: stratified randomization and the Pocock-Simon method. The first is well known and relatively easy to implement. While these methods are interesting in theory, the associated advantages may not outweigh the difficulties. There are exceptions to this that are mentioned in this section.

5.4.1 Stratification

The most common method used to enforce covariate balance is called *stratification*. The permuted-block design can be considered a special case of stratification, where individuals are stratified according to time or the order in which they entered the trial. Typically, however, the term "stratification" is used only when blocking is performed based on other attributes. The concept is simple; trial participants are grouped into strata based on factors of interest and a separate realization of the randomization rule is applied to each of these groups. A simple example is depicted in Figure 5.3. Within each stratum, one may use any randomization procedure that enforces balance; permuted blocks are the usual choice for randomization within strata. A discussion of stratification was given by Meier (1981) and some of his observations are presented here. Many of the concepts also apply to other forms of covariate-adaptive randomization.

There is wide agreement that stratification should be performed in the *analysis* stage of a clinical trial if it is present in the design. The issue that has been the subject of debate is whether or not allocation should be stratified. As

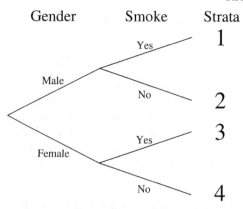

Figure 5.3 *Diagram of a simple example of stratification. There are 2 factors with 2 levels each: gender (male, female) and smoke (yes, no). This gives a total of $2 \times 2 = 4$ strata.*

mentioned previously, randomization alone should produce comparable groups and deviations from this are permitted under the theory of permutation tests. Also, no amount of stratification can achieve balance for *all* covariates.

One reason for stratification is that it reduces variance and thus increases precision of estimates. Another argument is that it makes within stratum analyses easier. One example of this might be the subgroup analysis of estimating the treatment effect by gender. A third reason related to the decision to stratify, which is probably the most common reason—also the most scientifically irrelevant—is public perception. Critics of particular clinical trials have been known to point out imbalances in covariates and claim that these represent "flaws" in the design and analyses of those trials. The fear of such criticism should not be considered adequate justification for stratification.

The increase in precision due to stratification is related to the precision gain achieved by treatment balance discussed in section 5.2.2. The conclusion is the same: only a high degree of imbalance will have a significant effect on the power of tests and efficiency of estimates. A problem can also arise when there are a large number of strata compared to the total sample size. This will lead to a large number of incomplete blocks, may decrease the precision, and thus can defeat the purpose that motivated stratifying in the first place.

This increase in precision alone, though small, may seem sufficient to make stratification a good choice of randomization scheme. One must also take into account, however, the additional administrative burden that stratification places on the clinical and data management centers. Stratification requires the collection of more data, and more data requires more collection, storage, management, etc. (see Chapter 6). Another problem may result from error in classification. It is not uncommon for individuals to be assigned to the wrong stratum. This may be due to a mistake or to ambiguity of the classification system. One must then decide how to include data for a misclassified individual when performing the analysis.

This additional burden, combined with the relatively minor benefit, makes stratified allocation a difficult procedure to recommend, although it is widely used. While it is true that the method helps validate analyses performed on subgroups that are pre-defined and part of the stratification, these analyses are not part of the principal question. The primary goal is to generate a valid test for overall treatment effect. Despite the fact that most of the arguments presented here suggest stratification is not recommended, there is a widespread agreement that a multicenter trial should use randomization stratified by clinic. This is not difficult to perform and classification errors are unlikely. Other variables that are known to be of great importance and have unambiguous classifications may possibly be used with care in a stratified randomization.

5.4.2 Pocock-Simon

Pocock and Simon (1975) developed a method with the primary goal of achieving balance with respect to a number of covariates in small studies. This approach could be considered an application of the biased coin design to stratification. The covariate values for individuals already assigned treatment, along with those of the next individual to be assigned treatment, are combined to calculate a score measuring imbalance. The treatment assignment that results in the lowest imbalance is given the highest probability.

To make this precise, suppose we have J factors that we would like to balance in K treatment groups. For each participant to be enrolled in a trial, let x_{jk} be the number of participants already assigned to treatment k who have the same level of factor j as the new participant. Thus, we will have an array of JK integers. Next, define

$$x_{jk}^t = \begin{cases} x_{jk}, & t \neq k, \\ x_{jk} + 1, & t = k \end{cases}$$

so that x_{jk}^t is the number of participants with the given level of factor j who would be in treatment group k if the new participant were assigned to group t. Next, letting $D(y_1, \ldots, y_K)$ be a function that measures the degree of imbalance among K non-negative integers, $d_{jt} = D(x_{j1}^t, \ldots, x_{jK}^t)$ is the imbalance with respect to factor j that would result if the new participant were assigned to treatment t. We then define a measure that combines imbalance across all J factors, $G_t = G(d_{1t}, \ldots, d_{Jt})$. This is calculated for each treatment and then the treatments are ranked according to these values. In other words, let $G_{(1)} = \min_t G_t$, etc., so that $G_{(1)} \leq G_{(2)} \leq \cdots \leq G_{(K)}$. Then, letting τ be the assigned treatment, assignment is based on probabilities

$$\Pr(\tau = (t)) = p_t, \text{ where } p_1 \geq p_2 \geq \cdots \geq p_K \text{ and } \sum p_t = 1.$$

This means that the treatment that leads to the lowest degree of imbalance is given the highest probability of assignment. Note that if there are tied values of G, either the ties should be randomly broken when the values are ordered or the corresponding probabilities should be equal.

The following are possible choices for D:

1. Range: the difference between the highest and lowest numbers. This is probably the most straightforward choice.

2. Variance: $D(y_1, \ldots, y_K) = \sum (y_k - \bar{y})^2 / (K - 1)$.

3. Upper Limit: e.g., $D(y_1, \ldots, y_K) = I(\text{Range} > U)$, for a defined limit U. The variance or another measure could also be used instead of the range.

For G, a reasonable choice is

$$G(d_1, \ldots, d_J) = \sum_{j=1}^{J} w_j d_j,$$

where, for each j, w_j is a weight reflecting the importance of factor j. For choosing the assignment probabilities, Pocock and Simon suggest letting $p_1 = p > 1/K$ and $p_t = (1 - p)/(K - 1)$, for $t = 2, \ldots, K$. They also suggest other formulas: one that gives K distinct values and another that additionally makes use of the $G_{(t)}$ values themselves.

Example 5.2. *Minimization.* Minimization is a specific, deterministic case of the Pocock-Simon method that was introduced earlier by Taves (1974). Suppose we have only two treatments and two factors: smoking status (Y/N) and gender (M/F). So $K = 2$ and $J = 2$. Suppose that we use the range as a measure of imbalance and that G is a weighted average with weights $w_1 = 2$ and $w_2 = 1$. Thus, the first factor is considered twice as important as the second. Formally,

$$G_t = w_1 |x_{11}^t - x_{12}^t| + w_2 |x_{21}^t - x_{22}^t| = 2|x_{11}^t - x_{12}^t| + |x_{21}^t - x_{22}^t|.$$

Now, if we let $p_1 = 1$ so that $p_2 = 0$, the allocation becomes deterministic and is called *minimization*. Suppose a female smoker enters the trial and the previous treatment assignments are broken down according to the table:

Tmt	Smoker Y	N	Gender M	F	Total
1	9	17	13	13	26
2	7	23	16	14	30

It is straightforward to use this table to compute the following values:

$$x_{11}^1 = 10 \quad x_{12}^1 = 7 \quad x_{21}^1 = 14 \quad x_{22}^1 = 14$$
$$x_{11}^2 = 9 \quad x_{12}^2 = 8 \quad x_{21}^2 = 13 \quad x_{22}^2 = 15$$

So, $G_1 = 2|10 - 7| + |14 - 14| = 6$ and $G_2 = 2|9 - 8| + |13 - 15| = 4$. Thus, the treatment assigned (with probability 1) is treatment 2. Notice that she is deterministically assigned to treatment 2, even though there are already more participants assigned to treatment 2 than to treatment 1. In addition, notice that the treatment 2 group already has more females than the treatment 1 group. Her assignment to treatment 2 emphasizes the fact that balancing for smoking status was deemed more important than balancing for gender. □

The method illustrated in this example (minimization) was used for treatment allocation in the Metoprolol CR/XL Randomised Intervention Trial in Congestive Heart Failure (MERIT-HF) (MERIT-HF Study Group 1999). A total of 3991 patients with chronic heart failure were randomized to either metoprolol CR/XL or placebo. The groups were balanced with respect to ten factors: site, age, sex, ethnic origin, cause of heart failure, previous acute myocardial infarction, time since last myocardial infarction (for those who had one), diabetes mellitus, ejection fraction (fraction of blood emptied by the heart during systole), and NYHA functional class (level of heart failure).

The Pocock-Simon method has advantages over a basic stratified randomization, but it still carries many of the same disadvantages. It is most useful in a small study with a large number of strata (Therneau 1993).

Another randomization scheme called *maximum entropy constrained balance randomization*, which is closely related to the Pocock-Simon method, was proposed by Klotz (1978). The method provides a criterion for selecting the assignment probabilities, which are allowed to be distinct for each individual. Specifically, one chooses p_k, $k = 1, \ldots, K$, to maximize the entropy,

$$H(p_1, \ldots, p_K) \equiv - \sum_{k=1}^{K} p_k \ln p_k,$$

subject to the constraint that

$$\sum_{k=1}^{K} G_k p_k \leq C(\eta) \equiv \eta G_{(1)} + \frac{1 - \eta}{K} \sum_{k=1}^{K} G_k.$$

The parameter η is a predetermined parameter between 0 and 1 that determines the amount of randomness in the allocation, 0 producing deterministic assignments and 1 assigning equal probabilities to all treatments. Good candidates for the measure of imbalance, G_k, are those described previously.

5.5 Summary and Recommendations

Selecting the randomization method that is to be used for a clinical trial should follow careful consideration of the goals of the study. There is no formula that gives the optimal choice from the available procedures. For large trials, many of the differences between procedures are not large enough to be consequential. Thus, the comparisons and suggestions given here apply mainly to trials with smaller sample sizes.

If one is interested in enforcing balance between treatment groups, the simple random allocation rule will achieve this goal, unless the total sample size is not reached. Permuted-block randomization will also provide perfect balance, even when a study ends prior to reaching enrollment goals, as long as the last block is full. With complete randomization, treatment imbalance in the number of participants is possible, but this possibility diminishes as $n \rightarrow \infty$ and significant imbalance is unlikely for even moderate sample sizes. The biased coin design enforces balance much better than complete randomization. The correction probability, however, is constant, so the probability of a particular treatment assignment depends only on whether or not there is imbalance, not on the magnitude of imbalance. Urn randomization goes further by allowing the correction probability to depend on the magnitude of imbalance. Urn randomization is much better than complete randomization at protecting against very high imbalance with small sample sizes.

While the only consequence of treatment imbalance is a reduction in power (or an increase in total sample size), even a small amount of selection bias can lead to erroneous conclusions. In addition, selection bias does not diminish with large sample sizes. One of the biggest advantages of using complete randomization is that there is no possibility of selection bias. In contrast, the random allocation rule has high potential for selection bias when participants enter the trial one at a time. Permuted-block randomization is more susceptible to selection bias than both the random allocation rule and complete randomization. Keeping block sizes unknown or using random block sizes helps to reduce the potential for certain kinds of selection bias. Also, it is much easier to randomize entire blocks at once than with the random allocation rule. This eliminates selection bias entirely. The biased coin design is susceptible to selection bias at a level similar to that of a permuted-block design. In terms of selection bias, the urn design is a good choice, as it is similar to complete randomization.

Recall that the preferred hypothesis test in an analysis of a randomized study is a permutation test. The calculation of the corresponding test statistic and its distribution must be based on the particular randomization procedure employed. For example, if permuted-block randomization is used and a test does not adjust for blocking, the size of the test may be incorrect. While the error in this situation is usually on the conservative side, this is difficult to guarantee or to check. In many cases, the value of an observed linear rank statistic is the same under several randomization methods, but each method provides a different estimate of variance. To further illustrate the importance of considering the randomization method used when performing an analysis, we give a simple example:

Example 5.3. Suppose we have the results for a clinical trial in which 12 participants enrolled. The treatment assignment to group 1 or 2 and the rank of the continuous response for each individual are known and are as in the following table.

Participant	1	2	3	4	5	6	7	8	9	10	11	12
Assignment	1	2	1	2	1	2	1	2	1	2	1	2
Rank	12	1	11	2	10	3	9	4	8	5	6	7

We wish to conduct a two-sided test of the hypothesis $H_0: \mu_1 = \mu_2$, where μ_i is the underlying mean response under treatment i. We use the Wilcoxon rank sum statistic: the sum of the ranks in group 1 minus n_1 times the average rank, 6.5. Thus, using the table, the observed value is $12+11+10+9+8+6-6\times6.5 = 17$. Now, suppose we do not know the randomization procedure used. The following table shows several randomization methods and the resulting p-value corresponding to the observed data.

Method	p-val
Random Allocation Rule	0.004
Complete	0.001
Permuted-Block $(m = 2)$	0.063
Permuted-Block $(m = 4)$	0.019
Permuted-Block $(m = 6)$	0.010
Biased Coin (BCD(2/3))	0.007
Urn Design (UD(0,1))	0.002

While most of the p-values shown are considered significant at conventional levels, this example clearly shows that the analysis depends heavily on the procedure used to assign treatment. □

The main disadvantage encountered when using adaptive randomization schemes is complexity. The calculations required for permutation tests are very difficult, perhaps impossible, in many adaptive settings. Some analyses can be performed through simulations. These are only approximations, however, and the accuracy of such approximations is not well known. In addition, the computational effort required can be significant. Another alternative is to invoke population model assumptions. These assumptions may be reasonable, but in most cases they cannot be tested.

Another disadvantage to using covariate-adaptive procedures, particularly the Pocock-Simon method, is that the actual random sequence used to allocate treatment cannot be entirely generated in advance. Even when using the play-the-winner rule, the next participant's assignment can usually be determined before they are enrolled. Covariate-adaptive methods require knowledge about several characteristics to generate the next treatment assignment. This can complicate the process of treatment assignment. Modern technology (e.g., IVRS, see Chapter 6) makes these schemes somewhat easier to implement.

The disadvantages of adaptive methods support the conclusion that fixed randomization procedures—and a few treatment-adaptive methods—are the preferred choice in most clinical trials. In trials where stratification is desired, clinical site should be one of the variables used. Further stratification should be kept to a minimum; only those characteristics that are known to play an important role should be included. The permuted-block method is the preferred choice in this setting. In an unstratified study, the permuted-block design is still a good choice, given that the trial is double-blinded. When there is concern that the blinding may be insufficient, complete randomization or an urn design should be used to reduce potential bias. The selection of an allocation procedure to be used in a study should depend on the particular study's constraints and objectives. The primary goal of randomization—to provide a guarantee of independence between treatment assignment and outcome—establishes the required foundation for causal inference. Any other goal (e.g., equal group sizes, covariate balance, etc.) is secondary.

5.6 Problems

5.1 Suppose you conduct a two-arm randomized clinical trial with a total sample size of 12. Assume the outcome is normal with constant variance and the test statistic to be used is the difference in sample means. As discussed in this chapter, the allocation that is balanced (6 in each group) is the most efficient. In this case, that means balanced allocation leads to the smallest variance of the test statistic. Suppose complete randomization is to be used.

   (a) What is the efficiency of balanced allocation vs. the allocation that gives 7 in one group and 5 in the other? (Efficiency, in this case, is defined as the variance of the test statistic for imbalance, divided by the same for balance.)

   (b) Make a table with a column for each possible allocation (including the balanced case). For each case, give the efficiency of the balanced allocation and the probability under complete randomization of realizing such an allocation.

   (c) What is the median efficiency of the balanced vs. unbalanced designs? What is the mean efficiency?

   (d) Make a conjecture about what might happen to the median efficiency as the sample size increases. Write a computer program to support your claim and show the results.

5.2 Suppose you are asked to help design a trial with three treatment groups: a placebo (P), a low dose of a drug (LD), and a high dose of the same drug (HD). The investigators are primarily interested in efficacy of the two dose levels, and not in comparing the two levels to each other. The hypotheses of interest are the following:

$$H_{01}: \mu_{LD} = \mu_P$$

and

$$H_{02}: \mu_{HD} = \mu_P,$$

where μ represents the mean reponse. You must determine the "optimal" proportion of the full sample that should be assigned to each group. The statistic to be used in each case is the difference in sample means between the corresponding groups. Assume that the outcomes are independent and normally distributed with known variance σ^2. The total sample size is fixed at n.

(a) Recall that for a single hypothesis test comparing two groups, the optimal allocation is to put half in each group. One advantage of this is that it minimizes the variance of the test statistic. If the investigators are interested only in estimating the two differences in means, what is the optimal proportion that should be assigned to each group?

(b) Which (if any) of the assumptions on the outcomes could be relaxed and still give the same result? Explain.

(c) Another reason for allocating half of the sample to each group in the single-hypothesis case is to maximize the power of the test. Suppose the investigators take this point of view and are only interested in showing efficacy of *either* treatment. In other words, the goal is to maximize the probability that at least one of the two null hypotheses is rejected, given that the alternatives are true (use $\mu_{LD} - \mu_P = 0.5\sigma$ and $\mu_{HD} - \mu_P = \sigma$). Assume that we reject either null hypothesis if the corresponding standardized difference in means is greater than 1.96. (Note: simulation may be helpful.)

5.3 Consider the example on page 166.

(a) Suppose the observed responses (from smallest to largest) were $\{1.16, 1.65, 1.89, 2.34, 2.37, 2.54, 2.74, 2.86, 3.04, 3.50, 3.57, 3.70\}$. Perform a t-test and compare the p-value to the table in the example.

(b) Suppose the randomization method used was permuted-block with 2 blocks of size 6. The p-value in the table for the correct analysis (taking the blocks into account) is .01, but the p-value calculated by ignoring blocks (random allocation rule) is .004. Discuss this in the context of the discussion at the end of Section 5.2.3.

5.4 Consider a stratified trial that uses the permuted-block design with block size 4 in each stratum. Let N_1 and N_2 be the number of subjects in each group at the end of the trial. If the trial stops before the last block is full (in any stratum) the overall treatment group sizes may not be balanced. Assume that each possible number (1, 2, 3, or 4) of subjects in the final block of each stratum has equal probability $(1/4)$.

(a) For one stratum (i.e., no stratification), give the exact distribution of $N_1 - N_2$. Calculate $\mathrm{Var}(N_1 - N_2)$ and $E|N_1 - N_2|$ (we know, by symmetry, that $E[N_1 - N_2] = 0$).

(b) Calculate $E|N_1 - N_2|$ exactly for the case of 2 strata by using the probabilities from part (5.4(a)). Repeat this procedure for 4 strata.

(c) Assume we can approximate the distribution of $N_1 - N_2$ with the normal distribution, using the variance calculated in part (5.4(a)) (for each stratum). Calculate $E|N_1 - N_2|$ for the cases of 1, 2, and 4 strata and compare your result with previous calculations.

(d) Approximate $E|N_1 - N_2|$ for the cases of 8, 16, 32, 64, 128, 256, 512, 1024, 2048, and 4096 strata.

(e) Compare these values to the case with no stratification from part (5.4(a)). Compare them to complete randomization when the total sample size is 100 ($E|N_1 - N_2| \approx 8.0$). Discuss.

5.5 For each of the randomization schemes described below, discuss the properties of the approach. Refer to topics presented in this chapter such as size of the reference set, balance, selection bias, and testing. What are your recommendations for the use of these methods? Assume a total sample size of 12.

(a) Suppose the experimental treatment is not yet available. The investigators start the trial anyway and assign the first 3 subjects to placebo. The random allocation rule will then be used for the next 6 subjects and the final 3 subjects will be assigned to the experimental treatment.

(b) It is determined that a trial will use complete randomization. The randomization sequence, however, will be generated entirely in advance and if the sequence happens to be severely imbalanced (defined as having 10 or more subjects in one group), another sequence will be generated until an acceptable one is found.

CHAPTER 6

Data Collection and Quality Control

Statisticians have multiple roles in the design, conduct, and analysis of randomized clinical trials. Before the trial starts, the statistician should be involved in protocol development. After the trial starts, the statistician may be involved in interim analyses. It is important that interim results reflect, as closely as possible, what is actually occurring at that time in the trial, despite the fact that the database will not yet have undergone the scrutiny usual in producing the final analysis dataset. The statistician usually plays a major role in the final analyses of trial data and in presenting these results to the broader scientific community.

Clearly, the success of a trial depends on the data that are collected. First and foremost, data must be collected that both answer the scientific questions of interest and satisfy regulatory requirements. The statistician must have sufficient grasp of the scientific questions and familiarity with the relevant outcome measures to ensure that the results are as unambiguous as possible. Statisticians are often in the unique position to anticipate data collection and analysis complications that might arise if particular outcome measures are selected. Second, the data collected need to be of sufficient quality that the integrity of the result is assured. The statistician must understand the data collection process and the limitations of the data collected in order to correctly characterize the results.

Two fundamental measures of data quality are *completeness* and *accuracy*. The manifestations of poor data quality are *bias* and increased variability. *Bias* is a systematic error that would result in erroneous conclusions given a sufficiently large sample (in small samples bias may be overwhelmed by variability). Increased variability decreases power for detecting differences between treatment groups and increases uncertainty in any treatment differences that are identified.

While missing data (incompleteness) decrease the effective sample size and thereby decrease power, the greater danger is the introduction of bias. Analytic issues involving missing data are dealt with in more detail in Chapter 11, so here we will only say that, except in very special circumstances, the bias introduced by missing data cannot be accounted for by analytic methods without strong, untestable, assumptions. At best its potential impact can only be quantified via sensitivity analyses.

Non-missing data can be inaccurate as a result of either random or systematic errors. Random errors can occur, for example, because the person transferring a value from a diagnostic instrument or source document to a data collection form misread the initial value. This kind of error is unlikely to introduce bias because it is not likely to be related to assigned treatment and, for numeric data for example, is probably as likely to increase as decrease the value. Conversely, bias may be introduced by a poorly calibrated instrument if the values it produces tend to be higher or lower than they should. While this kind of bias may skew the distributions of the values from a given clinical site, it is not likely to be treatment related and therefore should not introduce bias into treatment comparisons. The impact of errors in non-missing data is primarily that of increasing the variability of the responses.

The potentially increased variability introduced by inaccurate non-missing data must be considered in the light of the overall sampling variability. For example, the standard deviation for systolic blood pressure measurements repeated for the same subject is in the range of 8–$9 mmHg$, and the population standard deviation of systolic blood pressure measurements at a particular visit for all subjects enrolled in a trial may be 15–$20 mmHg$. Random transcription errors in at most, say, 5% of subjects are likely to increase this standard deviation by only a few percent and will have minimal impact on statistical inference. Typical error rates in clinical trials have been shown to be far less than 5%, probably well below 1%, and perhaps as low as 0.1% (Califf et al. 1997; Eisenstein et al. 2005). There appears to be little empirical evidence to support the extensive use of intensive quality control procedures used in many trials today.

In order to obtain high quality results from randomized clinical trials, close attention must be paid to the data collection process and to the design of data collection forms. The primary goal of the data collection process should be to minimize the potential for bias; hence, the first priority should be completeness. In this chapter, we discuss the process of planning for the collection of clinical trial data, specific issues that arise for selected types of clinical data, and issues regarding quality control. We will address problems that can occur in the data collection process and suggest strategies to help alleviate them.

6.1 Planning for Collection of Clinical Trial Data

Since data collection procedures are difficult to change once a study is underway, extensive planning should be undertaken before the first subject is screened. The planning process involves determining what data will be collected, what mechanisms will be used for data collection, and the design of data collection forms. We discuss each of these in turn.

6.1.1 Identification of Information Required

General Issues

The data collection processes should be driven by the safety and efficacy measures of interest, which in turn depend on the disease being studied, the nature of the intervention, anticipated side effects, and the specific questions outlined in the study protocol. To achieve the objectives of a clinical trial, data must be collected that directly address each of the questions posed in the protocol. Defining the relevant measures and corresponding analyses should be a collaborative effort among study sponsors, clinical investigators, and statisticians. These parties should jointly develop both the procedures for data collection and the specific content and format of the data collection instruments.

The statistician may be in a unique position to assess whether the data being collected will adequately address the questions posed in the protocol and will permit the analysis plan to be executed. Data must be collected and coded in a meaningful way. For example, "free text" (uncoded descriptive phrases) may provide information at the subject level, but is not readily analyzed.

One challenge that all trials face is determining how *much* data to collect. It is common to collect more data than is required by the protocol. There is often a temptation to collect "everything possible" in the event that unanticipated questions arise during the course of the trial. In general, however, data should not be collected that are not specifically called for. All data that are collected must be entered into the study database and subject to quality control. Extra data collection and processing burdens the investigators and participants, may draw attention away from crucial data, and adds to the costs of the sponsor.

The prudent strategy is to collect only what is required by the protocol. This will depend on the type of trial being designed. Early phase I trials, which tend to be small, may collect a large quantity of data for each subject in order to investigate possible adverse effects of the treatment. Later stage phase III trials, which tend to be much larger, may need to focus data collection on what is essential in order to keep costs and effort under control. Experience in a particular disease or treatment will guide not only the type, but also the amount of data that are necessary.

Before a clinical trial is opened for accrual, a data collection process must be developed. Investigators, in their anxiety to get a trial going and begin recruiting participants, may not have all of the data collection procedures worked out in advance. This can lead to incomplete or inconsistent data and has the potential to cause difficulties in the analysis of the data. Careful planning can minimize subsequent problems and enhance the overall integrity of the trial.

Given the fact that resources (time, money, personnel) are invariably limited, priorities should be established for different categories of data. Focusing resources on collecting and cleaning the most critical data, such as primary outcomes and serious adverse events, may be necessary.

Key Categories of Data

The study protocol defines the stages of trial participation—entry into the trial, treatment, and follow-up—and outlines the study tests and procedures to be performed and the outcomes to be assessed. The specific data elements collected should reflect the objectives specified in the protocol. A brief overview is given below, with further detail provided in Section 6.2.

Baseline data. Data collected prior to the start of treatment are referred to as *baseline* data.

Efficacy outcome data. *Efficacy outcome* data may be a simple accounting of survival status or the occurrence of a morbid event such as a heart attack, stroke, hospitalization, or cancer recurrence. Other outcome data may involve results of diagnostic scans or other complex measurements. In some areas of clinical study, potential outcomes must be reviewed and adjudicated by experts in the field. Data collection procedures must be developed that are appropriate to the type, complexity, and assessment frequency of the outcome measure.

Safety data. Safety data include both serious adverse events (SAEs), discussed in further detail in Section 6.1.2, and non-serious adverse events or toxicities. Regulatory reporting requirements for SAEs may influence both the process and content of data collection. Since potential adverse events frequently cannot be anticipated in advance, adverse event reporting may be more extensive than other categories of data collected.

Safety data also include laboratory data, based on serum or urine chemistry values, vital signs, or other physical measurements that are usually collected throughout the study according to a predetermined schedule.

Follow-up status. *Follow-up status* or *subject study status* refers to the status of the subject with respect to treatment and follow-up. For example, the subject may be currently on their assigned treatment, off treatment but still being followed, dead, or lost to follow-up. Depending on the nature of the trial, there may be other important categories.

External Factors Influencing Data Collection

Over and above the requirements of an individual protocol, there may be other factors that influence selection of the data to be collected. For example, there may be multiple concurrent trials for the same intervention in different populations or for similar populations in different geographic regions. As discussed in Chapter 1, approval of a new agent or indication by the U.S. Food and Drug Administration (FDA) often requires two trials demonstrating a positive beneficial effect. In these cases, the data collected for the related trials should be similar, if not identical.

Also, many trialists now attempt to combine all trials of the same intervention, or the same class of interventions, in order to obtain a more precise estimate of benefit and to investigate rare but important adverse events, especially SAEs. This type of analysis is often referred to as *meta-analysis*. In order to facilitate these analyses, it is desirable for data collection to conform to certain standards and be as comparable as possible for baseline, primary, and secondary outcomes, and for adverse events.

6.1.2 Mechanisms of Data Collection

Different categories of data lend themselves to different mechanisms of collection; descriptions of several such processes are described below. When planning a trial, consideration should be given to the advantages and disadvantages of various approaches, with logistics and careful specifications defined prior to trial initiation. In this section we describe several common data collection mechanisms and close with a discussion of data collection schedules.

IVRS

A common mechanism used for checking eligibility and randomizing subjects is an interactive voice response system or IVRS. A well-designed IVRS system is accurate, efficient, and allows subjects to be enrolled and/or randomized 24 hours a day from clinical sites anywhere in the world. Personnel from clinical sites interact with the IVRS via telephone, and once they have identified their site and provided required passwords, respond to a series of questions regarding a potential study participant. Eligibility and other selected baseline data can be collected immediately. Covariate-adaptive randomization procedures (see Section 5.4) can also be implemented using IVRS systems, and randomization can be easily stratified by region or other prespecified risk factors.

In addition, IVRS systems are often used for other aspects of trial management, including dose titration in a double-blind study, distribution and tracking of drug supplies or devices used for the intervention, and collecting participant information relating to early termination of treatment or follow-up.

There are many advantages to using an IVRS. First, the trial management personnel and the statistician have real-time accounting of recruitment progress, can monitor site or regional activity more effectively, and ultimately can terminate recruitment more efficiently. Second, having up-to-date information on the number and status of participants in the study, with computer-generated information on subject identifiers, treatment assignment, and the date of randomization, facilitates up-to-date monitoring of subject safety (see Chapter 10).

Clinical Case Report Forms (CRFs)

The traditional method of data collection involves entering data into a study-specific *case report form* (CRF) which is a series of paper forms or *CRF pages*, typically organized by the type of data being collected. For example, one page might be an eligibility checklist, another might collect information regarding a participant's medical history, and a third page, filled out at the time of study entry, might record data gathered during a physical exam. CRFs designed for clinical trials are typically distinct from the source documents, which are usually part of the general medical record. While paper CRFs are still common, electronic CRFs, in which the data are entered directly into a computer system, are now being used with increasing frequency. Basic principles of CRF design, discussed in more detail in Section 6.1.3, apply to either medium.

CRFs are typically completed at the clinical site by a study coordinator or members of the health care team. Completed pages may be collected in person by monitors from the coordinating center or they may be mailed, faxed, or submitted via the internet to a central location for inclusion in the study database. Depending on the technology used, the data may be scanned, keyed, or uploaded into the database using specialized software. Completed forms are subject to a variety of quality control procedures, outlined in more detail in Section 6.3, with queries sent back to the clinical site for clarification or correction of problems. It is important that the statistician be involved in the formulation of the quality control procedures, as this will affect the quality of both interim analyses and the final analysis at the completion of the trial.

Expedited Safety Reports

An adverse event (AE) is any undesirable experience associated with use of a medical product by a subject. The adverse event is *serious* (SAE) and should be reported to the FDA when the outcome is:

- death,
- life-threatening,
- hospitalization (initial or prolonged),
- disability,
- congenital anomaly, or
- requires intervention to prevent permanent impairment or damage.

While there is typically a CRF page designed to capture serious adverse events (SAEs), regulatory reporting requirements may dictate that an expedited system be set up to report these events to the IRB or the FDA with a minimum of delay.

Depending on the nature of the intervention, the study population, and the type of adverse experience, some or all SAEs may need to be reported by the investigator within 24 hours, with full documentation to follow within 15 days. Sponsors, especially for industry supported trials, often develop company-wide independent systems for SAE reporting and review. Reporting may initially be via telephone or FAX to the Safety Division of the organization rather than to the group responsible for data management of CRF data.

Although SAE reporting systems are primarily designed for clinical review of individual cases rather than aggregate analysis, there is an increasing acknowledgment that these data can and must be collected in a manner that allows them be used for multiple purposes. Frequently an SAE reporting system represents the most up-to-date source of information regarding serious outcomes such as mortality and, when linked via a unique subject ID to the assigned treatment group, can provide valuable information for interim monitoring of safety by an IRB or a Data Monitoring Committee.

Central/Reference Laboratories

Some categories of clinical trial data are generated at facilities that are external to the clinical site. Blood may be drawn, urine collected, or tissue samples taken and submitted to a local or central laboratory for analysis or review. Procedures such as ECGs or x-rays may be read and interpreted by a specially designated organization or committee of experts. Central laboratories may also have mechanisms for assisting in the management of trial participants, such as rapid feedback to clinical sites regarding abnormal test results. Usually, central laboratories have their own internal quality control, providing high quality data. Particularly for multicenter trials, use of central facilities is an excellent way to maintain standardization and quality.

Results of central analysis or review are often placed in an electronic file and sent to the coordinating center for inclusion into the study database, linking to other clinical data through the use of a consistent subject ID. The frequency, format, and content of the data transfer must be agreed upon in advance by the central laboratory, the trial sponsor, and the data management team. The trial statistician can play a key role in the planning process, helping to ensure that data are generated and stored in a way that will facilitate the planned analyses.

Endpoint Tracking and Adjudication

A specific type of external review that deserves special mention is the adjudication of potential efficacy outcomes. The study protocol will define the objectives of the trial, detailing the efficacy outcomes of interest.

Frequently there is an independent committee (endpoint classification committee or ECC) that will re-examine all events deemed by the site investigators to be study outcomes and determine whether or not these events meet the study definition for the specific outcomes. For example, an investigator may indicate that a subject has experienced a myocardial infarction; however, the endpoint adjudication committee may determine that this event does not meet the prespecified trial criteria. Typically there is a data management group designated to manage cases sent to the ECC for review. This group receives initial event reports from the clinical sites, requests detailed information from the site documenting the case, submits this information to the ECC for review, and enters the ECC final determination into the clinical database. Central to this process is usually an outcome tracking system that may be a simple spreadsheet or sophisticated database system. Even though it is generally unmonitored, the endpoint tracking database is often far more up-to-date than the clinical database, and, therefore, can be useful for interim monitoring of study endpoints.

Schedule of Data Collection and Submission

Data collection is usually organized around the visit schedule of the participants. Not all data are necessarily collected with the same frequency. For example, some laboratory data (from either serum or urine specimens) may be collected weekly for 6 weeks, then monthly for 6 months and finally every 6 months until the end of the trial. X-rays or ECGs may be performed annually, whereas information regarding adverse events and concomitant medication may be gathered at every clinic visit. The schedule of required visits, tests, and assessments is typically detailed in the study protocol.

In a multi-center trial, the protocol or data management plan also specifies the frequency with which CRF pages are to be submitted to the coordinating center for inclusion in the central database. In some cases there is a window specified relative to the study visit (e.g., within 2 weeks of the visit). For other trials, individual *clinical research associates* (CRAs) may visit clinical sites on a regular basis (e.g., quarterly) in order to monitor and collect outstanding CRF pages. In still other cases, data submission deadlines may be set to conform to planned interim analyses. In general, the goal is to minimize the time lag in data reporting, which is one of the benefits of using modern internet-based data collection systems.

Although not all data are needed immediately, certain categories of data must be kept as current as possible. SAEs should be reported expeditiously for regulatory reasons. For trials that are being monitored by a Data Monitoring Committee (DMC), information required for their consideration—for reviewing trial progress, participant safety, and assessing primary and secondary outcomes—must be as up-to-date as possible. DMCs cannot effectively carry out their responsibilities if key information is not available, hence the lag-time must be minimized between assessment and the availability of data for analysis. Tracking the timeliness of data flow can aide in ensuring that the database is current as well as in providing an assessment of how much information is available for a given report.

6.1.3 CRF Design and Review

The trial statistician, often representing the sponsor and the investigator's steering committee, should be involved in the design of the protocol and the data collection forms. In some trials, another statistician, unblinded to the results by treatment group, will conduct the interim analyses for presentation to the independent DMC. There is usually a third statistician who is a voting member of the DMC. While all three may have input into the data collection process, it is principally the trial statistician who is most closely involved in designing the CRF.

Form design must be a collaboration among clinicians, database managers, and statisticians. Statisticians must be assured that the data collected will be adequate to meet the objectives of the protocol, and they may have unique insights into analysis needs that may shape the design of the forms themselves. Special attention should be paid to the unique requirements for interim reports that depend on a database that is continually evolving and has not been fully cleaned or locked.

In this section, we discuss topics related to the design or review of CRFs, including general issues relating to structure, organization, and format. A more detailed discussion of selected types of clinical data will be covered in Section 6.2.

General Principles of Form Design

Well-designed forms are essential for meeting the goal of obtaining accurate, complete, and timely clinical trial data. Here we present a set of principles that are useful in developing and evaluating both paper CRFs and electronic data collection instruments.

First, the CRF must be clear and easy to use by different groups of people: those who fill them out, those doing data entry, and ultimately those who perform the data analyses. Although forms can be accompanied by separate instruction pages, it is preferable that they be self-explanatory with definitions included and possible responses clearly indicated.

The package should be logically organized, with the content of each individual page clearly laid out. Using the same style or format on all pages makes form completion easier for the clinical team and ultimately leads to better quality data. The CRF should be parsimonious, focused on data necessary for analysis. Collecting the same information on multiple pages should be avoided.

If possible, it is advisable to begin with a CRF that has been used for a previous study, making modifications and improvements based on prior experience and any specific requirements of the present study. Eventually, certain classes of CRFs can be perfected and used repeatedly. Familiarity with the format and content of a form increases the likelihood that the clinical team will complete it as intended, improving data quality and completeness and ultimately requiring that less time and effort be spent in quality control.

When a new CRF is created, it should be tested prior to implementation. While a draft version may appear perfectly clear to the designer, it may be confusing to those who must complete it or certain clinical realities may not have been anticipated. A modest amount of pre-study effort can save an enormous amount of time in the long run, as making changes to a CRF once a trial is underway can create both logistical and analytical problems.

Organization of the CRF

The structure of the CRF should be reviewed with respect to how the pages are organized. It is important to clearly specify when pages should be completed at the site and when the data are to be submitted for inclusion in the central database. Typically pages that are to be completed at the same time are grouped together (for example, information collected at screening, the randomization visit, the end of treatment visit, etc.). Individual pages should be clearly labeled and the flow should be logical.

Table 6.1 provides a basic categorization of CRF pages that might be used for a cardiovascular trial with clinical event endpoints. Further details regarding selected categories of clinical data can be found in Section 6.2.

Table 6.1 *CRF pages typical in cardiovascular studies and when they may be completed.*

Study Visit	Assessments Performed
Screening and baseline only	Inclusion criteria
	Exclusion criteria
	Demographics
	Tobacco and alcohol classifications
	Medical and surgical history
	Physical examination
	Baseline medications
	Randomization and first dose information
Both baseline and at selected follow-up visits	Weight and vital signs
	Cardiovascular assessment
	Quality of life (QOL) assessment
	ECG results
	Serum samples for laboratory testing
	Urinalysis
Assessment at each follow-up visit	Clinic visit and contact summary
	Compliance with intervention
	Adverse events
	Concomitant medications
	Hospitalizations
	Clinical endpoints (death, MI, stroke, etc.)
Study completion	Treatment termination
	Final physical examination
	Final assessments of QOL or cardiovascular status
	End of study date and subject status

While tests and procedures are typically organized by visit, certain types of follow-up data may be collected on a log-form, rather than a visit-oriented form. Examples include adverse events and concomitant medications. Log-forms have multiple rows, allowing for multiple entries, each with associated start and stop dates and relevant characteristics (severity, action taken, out-come for adverse events; dose, route of administration, indication for medica-tions). It may be useful for log-forms to include a check box for "none" so it can be clear that the data are not missing, but rather that the subject had nothing to report.

When data are being used for interim analyses, it is important to consider the submission schedule for different categories of information. If data on a log-form are not included in the central database until all rows on the page have been filled, none of the data on a partially filled page will be available for use in interim analyses. In a study where certain types of medications are of particular importance for interim monitoring, for example, it might be preferable to have check boxes at each visit to indicate whether or not the subject had taken that medication at any time since the last visit. Another way to increase data availability is to require that log-forms be submitted on a regular basis (e.g., quarterly), regardless of whether or not they have been filled.

Header Information

Each CRF page should have a clearly marked space for collecting *header in-formation*, with a consistent style used throughout. The header should clearly identify the study, the CRF page, the participant, and the visit associated with the data. Information contained in the header is critical for linking data for a given individual and visit, and is also important for tracking data flow and completeness.

Participants must be clearly identified on each page of the CRF, including the unique identifier assigned to that subject for the trial (screening number and/or randomization number). It may be advisable to include additional identifying information, such as clinical site and/or subject initials, that can help identify errors in recording subject IDs.

Each header should also include information about the relevant time point in the trial. Follow-up visits may be identified by a unique visit number in the database, or they may be organized by calendar date (or sometimes both). Provisions should also be made for information collected at unscheduled visits and at the end of the trial. An example of a case report form header in given in Figure 6.1.

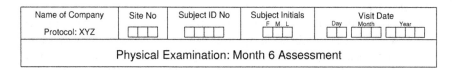

Figure 6.1 *Sample CRF page header.*

Form Layout

Clarity and simplicity should guide the process of developing or reviewing draft CRFs. The more complicated the form, the more likely it is to be misinterpreted. The flow of questions on each page should be clearly delineated, with unambiguous specification of which questions are to be filled out only when particular responses are given to previous questions (e.g., "packs per day" should be filled out if the response to "smoker?" is "yes"). Questions should be short and straightforward. Double-negatives should be avoided, and compound questions should be replaced with multiple, simple questions with appropriate skip conditions.

The amount of data to be collected on each page must be considered. There should be enough white space on the page to make it easy to read and follow; densely packed forms are hard to use. Minimizing the number of pages (or questions) is a worthy goal that should be accomplished by avoiding the temptation to collect data that will never be used. As emphasized before, each data element collected should have a purpose and be connected to questions outlined in the protocol.

Instructions to the investigators should be as concise and clear as possible, using uncomplicated language. The scope of the information to be entered on a given page should be made clear, especially if there is the potential for duplication of information. For example, if there is a CRF page dedicated to documenting use of a specific medication, the instructions provided for a more general concomitant medication page should indicate that the specific medication is excluded (and recorded elsewhere).

Item Formats and Content

Simplicity, clarity, and consistency in the style and content of CRF response fields will serve to enhance the quality of the data collected by minimizing errors and maximizing the completeness of the information. Getting it right the first time is important, as correction of errors is both time consuming and costly, and in some cases, errors can be difficult or impossible to detect.

Each response field should be reviewed in order to ensure that the format is clearly specified and is appropriate for the needs of data collection and analysis. The field type (character or numeric, categorized, or continuous) must be unambiguous. Except in specific circumstances, free text is not recommended. Care should be taken to ensure consistency in both style and content across all CRFs used in the trial.

Coded fields. Categorical data will typically have a limited number of response choices for a given question, either to be completed by checking an appropriate box or by filling in a blank with one of the responses provided. It is best if the style used is consistent within and across CRF pages.

Instructions should state clearly whether coded items are to be filled out by selecting a single response or by checking all that apply. If the instructions are to "select one," the options should be reviewed to ensure that the choices are both exhaustive and mutually exclusive. Coding conventions for similar response sets should be as consistent as possible across forms (e.g., 0 = No, 1 = Yes). It can be helpful for data review and analyses if numeric code values (1, 2, 3) are printed on the form next to the check boxes or labels (e.g., Mild, Moderate, Severe).

Consideration should be given to whether fields should be filled out as "check all that apply" or require a "Y/N" response for each response category. For example, on a medical history page, it is preferable to have an explicit designation that a given category does not apply (e.g., *History of CHF = N*) in order to distinguish between negative and missing responses. Figure 6.2 provides examples of different types of coded fields.

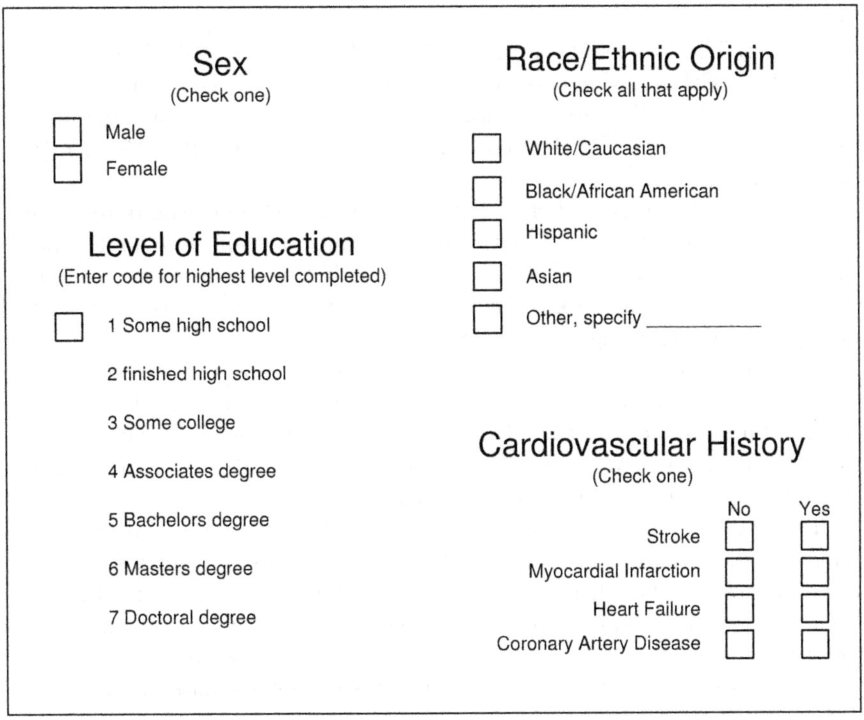

Figure 6.2 *Examples of different types of coded fields.*

Numeric fields. For continuous data, it may be helpful to provide boxes to indicate the number of digits expected, along with a preprinted decimal place, if appropriate.

It is important to clearly indicate how to handle data that can be measured using different units (e.g., weight in *kg* versus *lb*). There are several choices:

- require the data to be provided using a single standard unit

- provide different response fields for measurements using different units

- allow the respondent to provide a number and select between choices of units.

Text fields. Free form text responses should be used sparingly, as they do not lend themselves to statistical analysis. One situation where text *is* appropriate is in an "Other, specify _____" option of a multiple choice question. By soliciting the text prospectively, it may be possible to code a limited number of these responses at a later time.

Certain types of data (e.g., adverse events or medications) are often recorded at the clinical site as free form text and then subsequently coded at the coordinating center, either by trained individuals or though the use of an automated program. See Section 6.2.4 for further discussion of coding systems. If codes are to be entered on the CRF itself, adequate space should be provided adjacent to the text field.

Dates. The format of date fields should be clearly specified and should be consistent within and across forms. For international trials, it is advisable to use DD-MON-YYYY format (for example, 10-JUN-2006) in order to avoid confusing MM/DD/YY (United States convention) and DD/MM/YY (European convention).

There may be certain fields that allow for a portion of the date to be unknown. For example, the month and year may be sufficient for the date of initial diagnosis of a preexisting condition. If this is the case, it should be clearly indicated on the CRF how the unknown portion of the date is to be designated when filling out the form.

Missing data. As previously discussed, it is important to minimize the amount of missing data. However, when information is not available, the handling of missing data in the CRF should be clearly described. There are often guidelines given in the instructions for the entire CRF, though handling of certain questions may be specified at the item level.

Frequently, a distinction needs to be made between data that are missing, and a response that represents "unknown," "not done," "not applicable," or "not available." The distinction may affect whether or not the field is queried (e.g., a test that was not done is not going to yield any further information), and whether or not the data should be included as a separate category (e.g., cause of death evaluated as "unknown" versus "not yet entered").

Changes to CRFs During a Trial

In general, once a CRF for a given study is finalized, it ideally should not be modified during the course of the trial. Changes in CRFs cause confusion for the clinical team, require modifications to the structure and content of the database, and may adversely affect the ability to draw valid conclusions at the end of the trial. Making modifications mid-study has serious implications and every effort must be made to perfect the protocol and the CRF before the trial is launched. Taking short cuts initially with the hope of rectifying problems later is not an acceptable strategy.

Despite careful planning, there are circumstances in which a CRF may need to be modified during the course of a trial. There may be amendments to the study protocol that require additional visits, additional information to be obtained, or additional tests to be conducted. If additional information or visits are required, previous data for those variables may not be attainable retrospectively, hence the implications for data collection and analysis need to be considered before changes are made.

In some cases, questions (or entire forms) may be eliminated because the information proved not to be useful or because a particular test could not be implemented. Such changes would probably not be disruptive to the protocol or the analysis, but would require a modification of the CRF.

In other instances a code set may need to be refined based on review of responses given as "Other, specify _____." Amended CRFs should be annotated with a version number so that it is clear which pages were completed under which version of the CRF. Changes to coded categories may be necessitate the recoding of data collected using a previous version of the form.

Relationship Between the CRF and Database

There are many software systems used to collect, manage, and analyze data. Some database management systems are developed internally by the sponsor or a Contract Research Organization (CRO) and others are commercially available. Examples of the latter would include basic spreadsheets (e.g., Microsoft Excel), simple databases (e.g., Microsoft Access), and elaborate systems such as Oracle Clinical. The choice of system depends on the needs of the trial and the financial resources available. One feature that should be considered, however, is the ability to provide an audit trail of changes that were made to the database, by whom and when. This is especially important for industry-sponsored trials that are subject to regulatory auditing.

Typically, the structure of the CRF corresponds to the structure of the database, with different pages corresponding to different tables or datasets, and each question on the CRF represented by a variable (or column) in the dataset. A helpful practice is to create what is known as an *annotated CRF*, physically or electronically marking on blank forms the names of the underlying datasets, variables, and formats, or code tables. This documentation is not only useful within the data management group, but can assist statisticians in understanding the relationship between the CRF and the database.

For some categories of data (e.g., demographics) there will be one record in the database for each subject, whereas data collected over time may be stored as one record per subject per follow-up visit. Still other types of information may be recorded as one record per reported event for each subject (e.g., adverse events, clinical endpoints).

6.2 Categories of Clinical Data

The mechanisms for data collection and organization of CRF pages will depend on the nature of the particular data elements being collected. In this section we describe categories of data typical to clinical trials, highlighting issues that require consideration when formulating data collection mechanisms and procedures.

6.2.1 Subject Identification and Treatment Assignment

Every subject must be assigned a study code or number that uniquely identifies the individual within the trial, yet does not contain any information that would lead to identification outside the context of the study. Subject identification numbers (IDs) are often generated by an IVRS system as described in Section 6.1.2 and may be assigned at the time of initial screening or upon randomization into the trial. In some cases the subject ID is a composite of the site number and participant sequence number. It is critical, however, that, once assigned, this number be permanent—it should not change over time or if the participant moves and becomes active with a new clinical center. The subject ID must be used on all forms, specimens, and test results to allow all data for a given individual to be linked together for analysis.

Whether or not the clinical trial is a randomized study, it is very important that there be a date associated with the official entry of the subject into the study. If an IVRS system is being used, the date of randomization (or registration) can be automatically captured. All subjects who have been entered onto the study must be officially accounted for, even if no study treatment is ever given. The date of randomization marks the beginning of the follow-up period, and is used in calculations for time-to-event analyses. Clinical events and adverse events that take place prior to randomization are not counted. In general, the randomization should take place just prior to the initiation of the intervention. In some cases, however, the date of randomization and the start date of the intervention may differ. A long delay increases the likelihood that events will occur after randomization but prior to intervention, leading to complications for analysis and interpretation of trial results.

At randomization, each participant is assigned to a specific treatment group. In an open-label study, the treatment is known to investigators as well as participants and should be recorded on the CRF and become part of the database immediately. For a masked (double-blind) trial, the treatment group is usually not stored in the clinical database, but in a separate file that is carefully guarded and not released (except to an independent group responsible for interim analysis) until the database is locked at the end of the trial. A *randomization number* stored in the clinical database links the subject to the treatment assignment.

As will be discussed further in Section 6.3, checking that the randomization algorithm has been accurately implemented is an important quality control procedure to be carried out early in the study.

During the course of a study, information from an IVRS system may be the most up-to-date source of randomization date and treatment assignment. Except for subject ID and treatment assignment, however, IVRS data are not considered part of the official record of the trial. Hence, the information should ultimately be recorded in the CRF or otherwise incorporated into the central database, with reconciliations performed between the various systems, if necessary.

6.2.2 Screening and Baseline Information

Baseline data (collected at a screening or randomization visit) have a variety of uses including:

- Verifying eligibility
- Characterizing the study population
- Assessing baseline comparability of treatment groups
- Providing a starting point from which to measure change
- Defining subgroups for safety or efficacy analyses
- Modeling a response incorporating prognostic variables.

The data collection process begins with the screening of potential participants. The amount of information collected is dependent on the extent of the eligibility criteria specified in the protocol, factors that qualify an individual for participation in the trial (inclusion criteria) and those that preclude participation (exclusion criteria). These are collected in order to validate that study participants are eligible to participate.

Once the participant is deemed eligible and informed consent has been obtained, a more detailed assessment of the participant is performed with data captured on baseline forms. Standard components of baseline data are demographics (including gender, age, and ethnic background) and medical history. Medical history information may include any or all of the following:

- questions that serve to further characterize the disease under study (e.g., etiology of heart failure, breast cancer stage);
- co-existing conditions that may have an effect on the course of the disease or the effect of the intervention (e.g., diabetes for studies of cardiovascular disease);
- smoking status or history and alcohol consumption;
- assessments of medications that the participant is taking to treat their disease.

The eligibility criteria determine who can participate. The range of participants who actually consent to being in the trial, however, may be much narrower than allowed by the eligibility criteria. Appropriate selection of data to be collected at baseline allows the researchers to accurately characterize the population that has actually been included. In some cases, limited information is also collected on potential subjects who met the eligibility criteria but declined enrollment, in order to compare them with those who entered the trial.

As outlined in Table 6.1, baseline data include not only medical history information, but also results of physical examination and protocol-specific procedures, tests, or questionnaires. Frequently, these assessments are repeated at prespecified intervals throughout the study. Obtaining results prior to the start of treatment allows for analyses that adjust for individual baseline values, thus controlling for the variability among subjects prior to study start. These data will be most useful if measurements are gathered in a similar way pre- and post-treatment and preferably stored in datasets structured by follow-up date and/or visit number. For example there might be a single dataset for vital signs containing both pre- and post-treatment measurements. Note that the definition of the baseline value for use in the analysis should be specified in the analysis plan. It might be defined as the value measured at initial screening, the last one prior to the start of treatment, or the average of several measurements taken at different pre-treatment visits. Depending on the definition, the dates and times of assessment may need to be recorded in the database along with the visit code.

6.2.3 Follow-up Visits, Tests, and Procedures

Once the trial is underway, participants are typically scheduled for periodic visits to assess their progress. For follow-up visits that are required by the protocol, there should be an indication in the database of whether or not the visit was made. In some cases, a preprinted visit form will be completed, with an indication of either the date of the visit or the fact that the visit did not take place. This allows the clinical trial management to track visit compliance and timeliness.

Follow-up tests and procedures are often organized by visit, corresponding to a prespecified schedule outlined in the study protocol, with some assessments required at each visit and others performed at less-frequent intervals. Since adherence to the data collection schedule is important, compliance should be tracked by either the data management group or the statistician.

A wide range of data may be collected at follow-up visits. The protocol may require periodic assessment of weight and vital signs, safety monitoring of laboratory tests such as serum and urine chemistries, or tests of performance. Questionnaires, such as instruments to evaluate quality of life, may be administered at regular intervals. For some trials, the visit number is preprinted or manually entered on the CRF; however, either way it is advisable to include a visit (or assessment) date on the form as well. If more than one assessment is made within the time window for a given visit, the analysis plan should specify which measurements are to be used. Possibilities include the first visit, the last visit, or the one closest to the target visit date.

As discussed in Section 6.1.2, certain tests and procedures may be analyzed or reviewed centrally. Visits should be designated consistently between the CRF data and the data from central laboratories. In some cases, there may be a CRF page that contains limited information indicating which data are to be analyzed or reviewed centrally. If so, there should be fields in the database that allow the data analyst to link the CRF information to the data from the external source (for example, the sample ID number for a laboratory specimen).

Other data that are typically collected in an ongoing basis include information regarding adherence to the study treatment, adverse experiences (both serious and non-serious), concomitant non-study medications or interventions, and information regarding the primary and secondary outcomes. Each of these categories is addressed in more detail in the following sections.

6.2.4 Adherence to Study Treatment

The credibility of the results of a clinical trial relies on the extent to which the participants adhere to the intended course of treatment as outlined in the protocol—poor adherence to assigned treatment can leave the results of the trial open to criticism. Hence, it is necessary to collect data that enable a meaningful assessment of adherence to assigned treatment.

Minimally, the start and stop dates of treatment should be collected. Analyses of the timing of (premature) treatment withdrawal can aid in the interpretation of the final results.

Some studies call for "per protocol" analyses in addition to those performed according to the intention-to-treat principle. These analyses typically involve analyzing only those events (potential primary events or adverse events) that occur while the participant is complying with the intervention. We note that these analyses are vulnerable to bias and the results must be viewed cautiously. The biases inherent in these analyses are discussed in greater detail in Chapter 11.

Some interventions (for example, a surgical procedure or device implantation) involve a one-time administration of the treatment, and overall adherence is measured simply by the proportion of subjects receiving their assigned treatment. For drug treatments, the degree of compliance may be measured by the percent of pills taken based on the number prescribed, or the amount of the dose received as a function of the target dose.

6.2.5 Adverse Experiences

Assessing the safety of any new intervention is one of the most important tasks for a clinical trial. However, it is also the most challenging, because safety is multi-faceted and not easily defined.

As discussed in Section 6.1.2 there are regulatory requirements for rapid reporting of serious adverse events. In order to comply with regulations, most trial sponsors have developed a separate fast-track reporting system for SAEs. In addition to a brief description of the event (e.g., pneumonia), information collected usually includes the following:

- the reason the event qualifed as an SAE (Did it lead to hospitalization? Was it life-threatening?),

- the severity of the event (often coded on a scale of mild, moderate, severe),

- was the event thought to be related to the intervention (definitely, possibly, definitely not),

- the outcome of the event (Was it fully resolved? Were there lingering sequelae? Was it fatal?),

- modifications to the study treatment made as a result of the event (change in dose, temporary hold, permanent discontinuation).

There will also be a detailed narrative that describes treatment and follow-up of the adverse experience. Information collected in the SAE reporting system, particularly the coded fields, can be useful for interim safety monitoring.

While other adverse events (AEs) may not qualify as SAEs, they can still be relevant to the assessment of the risks and benefits of the intervention being tested. Thus, data on the occurrence of all AEs, especially those that are more severe or affect adherence, should be collected. Some AEs might be common to the disease being treated, some might be common to all assigned treatments, and some attributed to the new treatment. While prior studies might suggest what side effects are likely to be associated with the new intervention, many AEs are not sufficiently frequent to be seen in smaller studies. Thus, the AE reporting system must be prepared for both expected and the unexpected events. It is the latter that create challenges.

For adverse experiences that are anticipated based on a known side-effect profile of a drug, it may be most effective to present the participant with a checklist of potential toxicities to be reviewed at each follow-up visit. For example, a subject being treated for cancer might be asked if they had experienced any nausea and vomiting, peripheral neuropathy, or hair loss since the last visit, and if so, how severe it was. Some types of anticipated toxicities, such as decreases in white blood cell counts, might be abstracted by a data manager based on review of the local lab data and summarized according to objective criteria such as the Common Toxicity Criteria used in cancer clinical trials.

A common practice in industry-sponsored trials of new drugs is to ask the participant an open-ended question soliciting any complaints or problems they have experienced since the previous visit. These complaints are typically summarized with a brief phrase by the health professional, recorded on a log-form, and subsequently coded in a systematic way for analysis. A variety of hierarchical coding systems such as WHOART, SNOMED CT, and MedDRA have been developed and used over the years. Coding may either be performed by trained individuals or through the use of computer-based auto-encoding systems.

In recent years, there has been a movement towards creating a standard coding system that can be used worldwide. The MedDRA system (Medical Dictionary for Regulatory Activities) is considered the new global standard in medical terminology. This system allows for a detailed level of coding, and relates the detailed codes to broader high level terms and system organ classes (e.g., cardiac or gastrointestinal system). Table 6.2 illustrates the hierarchical nature of the MedDRA coding system focusing on the high level term of "heart failure."

Table 6.2 *A subset of the MedDRA coding system highlighting the high level term "Heart failure."*

System Organ Class	High Level Term	Preferred Terms
Cardiac system	Heart failures NEC	Cardiac failure acute
		Cardiac failure chronic
		Cardiac failure congestive
		Cardiogenic shock

For some purposes, the lower level detailed coding may be useful. For the purposes of comparing different treatment groups, however, this level of coding is likely to be too fine, since the frequency of the specific event may not be large enough to detect differences between groups. Examination of the system organ class or high level term may detect an AE signal, with the finer breakdown giving additional information. For some studies, preferred terms from different parts of the hierarchy may be combined based on specifications given in the protocol or questions posed by a monitoring committee (e.g., thrombotic events).

In addition to the classification of the event, the start and stop dates are usually recorded, along with a coded severity and the determination by the clinical investigator of whether the event might be related to the intervention. Although it is a standard component of AE reporting, the assessment of relatedness to treatment may not be meaningful. The primary treatment comparison of AE incidence should always be performed without regard to this assessment, even when the statistical analysis plan calls for a summary of treatment-related adverse experiences.

6.2.6 Concomitant Medications and Interventions

Another important question is whether the participants in the different treatment arms were treated comparably in all respects except for the interventions being tested. One aspect of this question is whether other interventions administered to subjects were similar. For example, it may be important to ascertain whether there are differences by assigned treatment in the use of particular non-study concomitant medications. If one group received more of a particular medication than the another, it may difficult to ascertain whether any differences in benefits and risks were due to the experimental intervention or to the ancillary treatments.

If it is known in advance what medications (or classes of medications) might be relevant, it might be advisable to explicitly ask the participant at each visit whether or not these medications are being taken (or have been taken since the previous visit). For example, in a trial of a new drug for congestive heart failure, documentation of the participants' use of other drugs in general classes such as beta-blockers, ACE inhibitors, and diuretics would likely be important. For a trial of anemia treatment, it might be helpful to ascertain whether or not subjects are receiving oral or intravenous iron supplementation.

In industry-sponsored trials of new drugs, it is common for information about *all* medications to be recorded, along with detailed information regarding start and stop dates, route of administration, dose, and indication. Recording and analyzing concomitant therapies, especially medications, can be time-consuming and challenging. There are many medications that may be relevant to the disease being studied, each having both generic and trade names. While standard coding systems do exist, such as the ATC (anatomic, therapeutic classification) system, they are complex because many drugs are used for multiple purposes (e.g., aspirin can be used for pain relief or for cardioprotective purposes). Furthermore, much of the data collected may rely on participant recall with exact dates unknown.

While clinicians often consider concomitant medication data to be important, it may be difficult to summarize. For example, in a recent trial, members of the DMC wanted to know whether there had been a change in the dose of concomitant diuretics that were being administered. Although dose, route, and frequency were collected, the varied treatments that fell into this category made the question impossible to answer except on the level of individual subjects.

6.2.7 Clinical Endpoints

As described in Section 2.5, the primary efficacy outcome in most long-term and some short-term trials is the occurrence of one or more of a predefined set of clinical events, usually analyzed using time-to-event (survival analysis) methods detailed in Chapter 7. One element of effective interim monitoring of such trials is an assessment of the reliability and timeliness of the endpoint data. As described in Section 6.1.2, some of the information in the endpoint tracking database, such as the dates on which critical steps in the adjudication process are completed, can be useful for this purpose. These include the date an event occurred, the date that the detailed information for the event was sent to the sponsor and to the endpoint adjudication committee, and the date on which adjudication was completed. This information can be summarized or displayed graphically to depict the endpoint data flow through the adjudication process. Steps where the process is delayed can be identified and procedures established to help alleviate problems.

The data that are available for interim analyses will be a mixture of events that have completed various stages of the adjudication process and so will include both confirmed and unconfirmed events. Given the delays in event adjudication, typically from 3 months to more than a year, adjudicated events usually comprise a relatively small fraction of all reported events, especially among those occurring most recently. While the primary interim analysis may be based solely on ECC-confirmed endpoint events, there are other useful analyses that can be performed that make use of all available data—endpoint tracking, investigator reports from the clinical database, and ECC confirmed (Cook 2000; Cook and Kosorok 2004). Analyses making use of all reported events are far more up-to-date than those using only confirmed events and have been shown to be quite reliable, despite using data that have not been subjected to rigorous monitoring.

These more complicated analyses require that events from all three sources have a common unique event identifier. This unique identifier should be assigned at the time of initial entry into the tracking database and communicated back to the site for entry onto the potential endpoint page of the CRF and also included in the material forwarded to the ECC for adjudication. Because event types and dates may be in error and corrected over time, it is usually difficult, if not impossible, to link events from the three sources using only subject ID, event type, and event date; hence, the unique event identifier is essential to this process.

6.2.8 Subject Treatment, Follow-up, and Survival Status

There is probably no category of data that has been the cause for as much confusion as subject follow-up status. The confusion arises from the failure to make a clear distinction between *withdrawal from assigned treatment* and *withdrawal from follow-up*. A common mistake in trials is to stop collecting follow-up data when the participant terminates their intervention. The usual rationale is that, if the participant is no longer receiving the intervention, they are not subject to either the benefits or the risks of the intervention. This rationale is inconsistent with the principles underlying randomized controlled trials, however. The reason for using randomized controlled trials is that by creating treatment arms that differ solely as a result of either chance or assigned treatment, the relative effect of the treatments under study can be ascertained. When follow-up is curtailed because subjects are no longer adhering to their assigned treatment, the subjects who remain in each group are probably not representative of the original treatment groups, and we have potentially introduced a third difference between groups—selection bias—defeating the purpose of performing a randomized trial at all. This bias can only be avoided by ensuring that, to the extent possible, all subjects are followed for the entire protocol defined period regardless of their adherence to assigned treatment.

Data capturing a subject's status are sometimes collected by an IVRS system in addition to the case report form. While the IVRS data may be available more rapidly for interim analyses, well-designed CRFs should collect subject status with respect to both the intervention and follow-up, usually with distinct pages designated to record "early treatment termination" and "study termination."

Early treatment termination refers only to withdrawal from the study intervention. Treatment may be withheld at various times, but it is most important to record if and when the termination becomes permanent. A field should be included in the CRF page indicating the date that the subject received their last treatment, and the reason(s) for treatment termination should be specified (either by selecting a single primary reason, or choosing all applicable reasons from a specified list). Possible reasons for early termination may include adverse event, subject request, physician discretion, or death. It is strongly recommended that there be a single CRF page designated for collecting information on permanent treatment discontinuation.

Study termination implies that the subject is no longer being followed. Typically, the only valid reasons for early study termination are death, withdrawal of consent, or loss to follow-up. A single CRF should be used to collect data on termination from study, including the end-of-study reason as well as the date of death or the date of last visit and/or contact.

Whether or not mortality is a designated study endpoint, the reporting of deaths is required by regulatory bodies, and this information is critical to the understanding of the safety of interventions. Many trials have a separate CRF specifically for death for recording, not only the date of the death, but also the presumed cause (e.g., fatal heart attack or stroke, death resulting from a specific type of cancer, or accidental death). Cause of death may also be adjudicated by the ECC.

In order to minimize the amount of censored survival data, the vital status of each participant should be recorded systematically at each scheduled visit. If a subject does not come to the clinic for their scheduled visit, the clinic should attempt to contact the subject to ascertain whether or not the participant is alive. All attempts should be made to ensure that information on a subject's outcome status is collected. If this is not possible, the subject may still allow information regarding survival status to be collected at the end of the trial. A brief discussion of censoring for subjects who are lost to follow-up appears in Section 11.3.4 on page 362.

6.3 Data Quality Control

It should be clear by this point that the analysis and conclusions drawn from any trial are only as good as the quality of the data collected. A well-designed CRF properly focused on the primary questions of the trial, along with procedures that ensure that data will be collected on all subjects to the extent possible, are the best guarantors of high quality data. As we have indicated, some degree of random error can be tolerated with an adequately powered trial, as long as it does not introduce bias. A good quality control program, however, can help to ensure that procedures are followed and that the opportunity for systematic errors to find their way into the database is minimized.

A data quality control program will have multiple components that depend on the source of data and mechanism for collection, as well as on the stage of the data management process. Some quality control measures apply during the data collection process itself; others are best implemented centrally at the data management center, while still others tend to be performed prior to data analysis.

6.3.1 QC During Data Collection and Entry

Typically, a system for data entry will have built-in checks to promote the collection of accurate data. At the simplest level, fields can be defined as either numeric or character and only valid data types can be entered. Most software systems also allow a limited code set to be defined and permit simple checks of allowable ranges for numeric data (e.g., height must be between 40 and 80 inches). More sophisticated systems can check for inconsistencies between different fields (e.g., dates out of sequence), alerting the individual entering the data to potential problems. Electronic CRFs can streamline the process by providing immediate feedback to the sites when entries are out of range or inconsistent, minimizing the requirement for subsequent queries.

When paper CRFs are submitted to a central office for data entry, there may be a system of double data entry in which different people enter the data with on-line comparison and reconciliation of the two entries. (Alternately, one person can enter the same data at two different times.)

In some multi-center trials, monitors are sent out to the sites on a regular basis to check and collect the study CRFs. Site-level monitoring compares data entered into the CRF with source documents and is a time-consuming, labor-intensive process. Electronic CRFs do not necessarily reduce the requirement for site monitoring since entries that pass through online edit checks may still be inconsistent with source documents. Some data, such as survival status, should be carefully checked; however not all data require the same level of quality control. For less critical data, simple entry checks may be adequate, not requiring source verification.

6.3.2 QC by the Data Management Center

Once information become part of the central database, either through electronic CRFs or entered from paper forms, more complex *edit programs* can be run against the database by the data management center. Programmed edit checks can identify missing data or information that is inconsistent between different forms or between similar forms collected at different times. Such programs often generate electronic *queries* that are then sent to the sites for data verification or correction. It is important that the database system have the capability of generating an audit trail of modifications to the data.

Another means of quality control is to apply data analysis tools to identify systematic errors that may have resulted from either inadequate data collection instruments or inadequate procedures at study sites. If certain fields in the database have generated a large number of queries, it might be advisable to examine the forms for clarity. Additional strategies might include examining variability between and within clinical sites or regions or looking for evidence of unexpected drifts over time.

Auditing

In the process of quality control of trial data, choices have to be made regarding the intensity of auditing. One approach, often used by industry sponsored trials, is to perform on-site, page by page, field by field, auditing of the CRF data against the source documents. Another approach, more often done by government sponsored trials, is to conduct central quality control using software and statistically based methods, accompanied by sample auditing of trial sites, and perhaps targeting key trial outcome measures. The first approach is significantly more costly and may not be cost-effective according to a review by Califf et al. (1997). Two examples follow in which the cost of intense auditing was as much as 30% of the total cost of the trial, yet had little or no effect on the final results.

In one case, a large multicenter randomized cardiovascular trial was conducted by an academic-based cooperative group to determine if a new intervention would reduce mortality and other morbidity in patients at risk for a heart attack (The GUSTO Investigators 1993). Prior to submission to regulatory agencies for approval, the sponsor of the trial conducted intense on-site monitoring. Analyses performed before and after the audit did not alter the numerical results in any appreciable way, even though some errors were discovered.

Another example is provided by a well publicized fraud case (Fisher et al. 1995). A large multicenter breast cancer trial was conducted by an academic cooperative group to determine which of two strategies was better, a standard radical mastectomy removing the entire breast or a modified breast sparing surgery followed by a chemotherapy of tamoxifen. One of the centers modified dates of six subjects during the screening process so that presumably the breast biopsy used to diagnose the cancer would not have to be repeated to be in compliance with the protocol. Although this anomaly was discovered and reported by the statistician, a controversy arose and an intense audit was conducted at several of the clinical sites (Califf et al. 1997). While the audit discovered errors, they were on average less than 0.1% of the data fields and there was no meaningful effect on the results. This experience, as well as others, suggests that perhaps standard statistical quality control of the incoming data, described elsewhere in this section, is adequate and cost-effective.

6.3.3 QC of External Laboratories and Review Committees

Central laboratories are another source of possible error. Most high quality laboratories have internal quality control procedures in which the same specimen may be submitted twice during the same day, or on different days, to ascertain reproducibility and variability. Results that fall outside those predetermined limits may require that the laboratory temporarily halt the process and recalibrate or correct the deficiencies.

Some trials have submitted duplicate specimens from a clinical site as an external check of reproducibility. In one study it was discovered that while a specific external group was the best research laboratory for a particular outcome, once the trial began, it could not handle large volumes required by the protocol (The DCCT Research Group: Diabetes Control and Complications Trial (DCCT) 1986). Statistical analyses of the data received from the laboratory early in the trial uncovered the lack of reproducibility and a change of laboratories was made.

Adjudication committees reviewing clinical endpoints often have a built-in process by which two reviewers provide an assessment of the event (e.g., cause of death), their assessments are compared, and a third person (or perhaps a larger group) discusses and resolves the discrepancies. For some studies, a subset of the clinical events are resubmitted through the entire process to evaluate the reliability of the process and to prompt further discussion and retraining if necessary.

6.3.4 QC by the Data Analysis Center

An independent Data Analysis Center (DAC) is responsible for producing interim analyses for the DMC and therefore has an interest in the completeness and quality of the data it receives—data that may not have been subjected to the final monitoring process. Before conducting any statistical analysis, the DAC statistician should perform a series of standard checks in order to clearly understand the quality of the available data. While the DAC does not have a direct role in the data collection and management process, the knowledge gained through this process can often be helpful to the data management center since the DAC is generally focused on those data quality issues that will have the greatest impact on the primary results of the trial. In this section we outline some of the processes that the DAC can employ to assess data quality and handle problems that are uncovered.

Verification of Treatment Assignments

In double-blind trials, the link between subject and treatment assignment is a critical piece of information that may need to be verified. There have been instances in which the DAC was provided the wrong version of the randomization schedule so that all treatment comparisons were completely invalid.

In many trials there is a known, expected biological response (for example, a decrease in serum cholesterol or an increase in the frequency of an adverse event such as diarrhea) that, when observed, provides evidence that the treatment assignments are correct. Conversely, if the expected biological response is not observed, this may suggest that the treatment assignments are incorrect. For studies with permuted-block randomization schemes that are stratified by, say, clinical site, the examination of consecutive enrolled subjects within sites may reveal that the randomization is not performing as expected and the link may be incorrect.

For studies using an IVRS, the IVRS should be able to provide the DAC with the actual treatment assignments, which should ensure that the assignments are correct.

Examination of Datasets

Examination of the transferred datasets is particularly important at the beginning of the trial in order to promote a better understanding of the variables and relationships among them. For subsequent data transfers, careful examination of the data can serve to either verify or correct assumptions about the data structure and is critical for identifying potential problems with the incoming data. Data checks may include any or all of the following:

- tabulations of coded data,
- cross-tabulations identifying relationships among key variables,
- range checks for numeric fields and dates,
- comparison between date fields to identify invalid sequences, or
- checks of conventions for recording missing data (for both numeric and character fields).

Particular attention should be paid to comparing critical information (such as death, date of death) from different sources. If gaps or inconsistencies in data fields are identified, the data management center can be alerted or queried. Careful examination can lead to more informed decisions regarding the appropriate algorithms to use for defining derived variables (e.g., which data source is most reliable for date of death).

Treatment of Missing, Erroneous, and Inconsistent Data

By their very nature, datasets used for interim analyses will contain information that is entered in error or not yet coded and some values will be missing. As the trial progresses, important inconsistencies and gaps in information will be identified and resolved, with the goal of producing a clean file by the time the final report is prepared. There are a variety of ways data problems can be handled for interim analyses. Possible actions include:

- deleting impossible values (e.g., age=0),
- recoding obviously incorrect units (temperature C = 98.4),
- hard-coding "fixes" to key data fields if the corrected value has been verified with the source and written documentation is available,

- including all outliers and relying on nonparametric analyses that are robust to extreme values, and

- defining algorithms and/or hierarchies for deriving variables for analysis.

It is important that analysis conventions be well-defined and documented in both the programs used in the data handing process and in a separated document. It can be helpful if these conventions also accompany the DMC report.

Interactions with the Data Management Center

It is helpful if guidelines and expectations for communication with the data management center are defined early in the trial. In many cases, there are quality control measures already in place at the data management center and problems identified by the DAC will ultimately be caught and dealt with at the source. Communication regarding classes of data problems (particularly early in the trial) can be helpful in assisting the data management center to implement additional checks. Problems identified by comparing data from different sources (e.g., death information from the safety database versus that recorded on the CRF) may be identified at the DAC much earlier than by the data management center. It is important to ascertain whether or not the data management center wants to be informed about data discrepancies. Sometimes it is advisable to simply provide limited information with no expectation of a response.

When communicating with the data management center about data anomalies, the following guidelines apply.

- Prioritize different types of problems, and focus on those most important to the analysis (e.g., information about endpoints or deaths).

- Be clear regarding the purpose of notification and whether or not a timely response is requested.

- Make sure that no potentially unblinding information is included in the communication.

- Maintain careful written and/or electronic documentation of questions and answers.

6.4 Conclusions

In this chapter, we have discussed elements of data collection and quality control with which the statistician must be engaged. Planning and testing of data collection procedures including the CRF is perhaps the most important task. If this is done carefully, the need for quality control and auditing at the conclusion of the trial will be decreased substantially. Using or developing standard data collection procedures is also important to minimize the requirement for retraining of clinical staff for each new trial. The formulation of definitions of fields and outcomes is part of the standardization process. Ongoing data quality control is necessary and now facilitated by most data management software. Thus, many errors can be detected quickly and corrections made to collection procedures as necessary. Sample auditing is probably more than adequate for most trials and 100 percent auditing should be used only for special circumstances.

CHAPTER 7

Survival Analysis

In many clinical trials, particular adverse events (more generally referred to as *failures*) such as death, hospitalization, or relapse are important outcomes for evaluation of therapy. Typically only a subset of subjects experiences an outcome event during the study, so the response for each subject can be viewed as having two components: an indicator of whether the event has been observed, and the time from randomization to the event, often referred to as the *failure time*. Because of the bivariate nature of the outcome, standard methods for analyzing either binary outcomes or continuous outcomes are inadequate. Specifically, the lengths of follow-up typically vary, usually depending on time of enrollment, so that the failure probabilities vary between subjects. Analyses that consider only the binary indicator of failure may be subject to bias and loss of efficiency. Furthermore, analyses that consider only the failure times are inadequate because failure times for subjects without events are unknown.

For mathematical convenience, and with no loss of generality, it is usually assumed that all subjects will fail given sufficient follow-up time. For subjects who are not observed to fail before the end of the study, the failure time is not known exactly, but instead is assumed only to be greater than the follow-up time. When this happens, the failure time is said to be (right) *censored* at the end of follow-up. The censoring event may be the end of the study, the subject withdrawing from the study, or some other event, after which the failure cannot be observed. This chapter presents some of the basic methods used in the analysis of censored survival data. This material should be considered introductory and the reader is encouraged to consult other texts such as Kalbfleisch and Prentice (1980), Cox and Oakes (1984), Lee (1992), Lawless (2003), and Fleming and Harrington (1991).

7.1 Background

The term *failure time* (or *survival time*; we will use the terms interchangeably even though the failure in question may not be fatal) refers to a positive-valued random variable measured from a common time origin to an event such as death or other adverse event. The true failure time may be unobserved due to a censoring event. Censoring can happen through several different mechanisms, which will be explained later in more detail.

Let T denote the failure time, with probability density function $f(t)$ and cumulative distribution function $F(t) = P(T \leq t) = \int_0^t f(u)du$. In this chapter we will assume that $F(t)$ is continuous on the positive real line, although for most results this assumption is not necessary. Associated with T is a *survivor function* defined as

$$S(t) = 1 - F(t) = P(T > t)$$

and a *hazard* function defined as

$$\lambda(t) = \lim_{h \to 0} \frac{\Pr\{T \in (t, t+h]|T > t\}}{h} = \frac{f(t)}{1 - F(t)} = \frac{f(t)}{S(t)}.$$

The hazard function, $\lambda(t)$, can be thought of as the conditional probability of failing in a small interval following time t per unit of time, given that the subject has not failed up to time t. Because $\lambda(t)$ is a probability per unit time, it is time-scale dependent and not restricted to the interval $[0, 1]$, potentially taking any non-negative value. We define *cumulative hazard*, $\Lambda(t)$, by

$$\Lambda(t) = \int_0^t \lambda(t)dt = \int_0^t \frac{f(u)du}{1 - F(u)} = -\log[1 - F(t)] = -\log S(t),$$

and so we have that $S(t) = \exp\{-\Lambda(t)\}$.

In general, there are three types of censoring that may be encountered: right, left, and interval censoring. In clinical trials, most failure time data is right censored, although occasionally interval censored data arises.

1. The failure time T is *right censored* if it is known only that $T > C$ for some known value C.

2. The failure time T is *left censored* if it is known only that $T < B$ for some known value B.

3. The failure time T is *interval censored* if it is known only that $B < T < C$ for some known values B and C.

As indicated previously, right censoring usually occurs when subject follow-up ends prior to the failure time. Interval censoring usually occurs when the failure cannot be observed at the time it actually happens, but only some time afterward, typically when an assessment can be made. For example, recurrence of tumors in cancer patients often requires an examination using sophisticated imaging tests such as CT or PET scans, which are to be done only periodically. When a tumor appears on follow-up scan but was not evident on the prior scan, all that is known is that the tumor developed some time between the two scans. Left censoring may occur if the tumor appears on the first scan after treatment, in which case all that is known is that the tumor began prior to the first scan. One can easily see that both right and left censoring are special cases of interval censoring; left censoring occurs when $-\infty = B < C < \infty$ and right censoring when $-\infty < B < C = \infty$. This chapter will deal only with right censored failure times. Interval censored or left censored data require more specialized methods and are beyond the scope of this book.

A key assumption that we will make is that for each subject, T and C are stochastically independent. If censoring is strictly administrative—the subject has reached a predetermined end of follow-up—then this condition will be automatically satisfied. Loss to follow-up, on the other hand, may be related to a subject's disease status, and hence not independent of T. Unfortunately, it is not possible to ascertain whether loss to follow-up is independent of T, since, by definition, when C is random, one can never observe both T and C, and so one is often forced to assume that if there is dependence between the censoring and failure times, it does not introduce bias into the analysis.

There are three primary questions of interest when considering failure time data in the clinical trial setting:

- estimation of $S(t)$,

- tests of the null hypothesis $H_0: S_1(t) = S_2(t)$, for all t where $S_\tau(t)$ is the survivor function for treatment group τ, and

- estimation of the effect of treatment or other covariates on the survival distribution.

Estimates of $S(t)$ are routinely shown graphically in summaries of study results and are used for informal comparisons between the study population and historical populations, or for visual comparisons of treatment groups. Formal assessments of the effect of treatment on primary and secondary outcomes are usually based on tests of hypotheses of the form of H_0 given above. Finally, regression models are often used to assess robustness of the observed treatment effects to potential baseline imbalances between treatment groups, to quantify the average effect of treatment, or assess consistency of effect across a range of baseline subgroups.

7.2 Estimation of Survival Distributions

The survival distribution $S(t)$ can be estimated using either a parametric or nonparametric approach. While nonparametric estimates are most commonly used, there are situations in which parametric estimates are useful. In what follows, both approaches will be considered. We begin with discussion of the parametric approach.

7.2.1 Parametric Approach

A *parametric* model is one in which the entire distribution of the failure time is uniquely determined by a finite number of parameters. In principle, any distribution on the positive real line can be used as a failure time distribution; however, there are only a limited number of distributions that are commonly used in practice.

The Exponential Model

The simplest parametric model is the *exponential* model. Often the exponential distribution is used at the design stage because sample size and power can be easily calculated using the exponential distribution. Under the exponential model, the hazard function, $\lambda(t)$, is constant over the positive real line and the distribution is characterized by this value, $\lambda(t) = \lambda > 0$. That the hazard function does not depend on t is equivalent to saying that the exponential distribution is "memoryless", by which we mean that $\Pr\{T > t | T > t_0\} = \Pr\{T > t - t_0\}$. That is, if we know that a subject has survived event-free to time t_0, then the probability of surviving to a future time t depends only on the difference $t - t_0$ and T effectively "forgets" the length of the initial event-free interval. This property makes the exponential distribution useful for studies involving chronic diseases in which the disease risk is not expected to change over the course of the study. Conversely, for acute conditions, where risk is initially high, but decreases shortly thereafter, the exponential distribution will not be appropriate. See Cook (2003) for an example of a study that was designed using an exponential model when the true hazard function was decreasing with time. Following is a catalogue of important quantities associated with the exponential distribution.

$$
\begin{aligned}
\lambda(t) &= \lambda > 0 \\
\Lambda(t) &= \int_0^t \lambda(u)du = \lambda t \\
S(t) &= \exp(-\Lambda(t)) = e^{-\lambda t} \\
f(t) &= -\frac{d}{dt}S(t) = \lambda e^{-\lambda t} \\
E(T) &= \frac{1}{\lambda} \\
\mathrm{Var}(T) &= \frac{1}{\lambda^2}.
\end{aligned}
$$

Maximum Likelihood Estimation for Exponential Data

Parameters in parametric models are most often estimated using the method of *maximum likelihood* (see Appendix A.2 for an overview of maximum likelihood estimation). Suppose that $t_1, t_2, \ldots, t_n$ are an i.i.d. sample from an exponential distribution with parameter λ. First, we suppose that there is no censoring so that all subjects are observed to fail. The likelihood for λ is

$$
L = L(\lambda) = \prod_1^n f(t_i) = \prod_1^n \lambda \exp(-\lambda t_i).
$$

The log-likelihood is

$$
\log(L) = \sum_{i=1}^n \log(\lambda) - \lambda t_i.
$$

The maximum likelihood estimate of λ, $\hat{\lambda}$, is the value of λ that maximizes L or $\log(L)$ and that we obtain by solving

$$
U(\lambda) = \frac{\partial}{\partial \lambda}\log(L) = \sum_{i=1}^n \frac{1}{\lambda} - t_i = 0.
$$

The function $U(\lambda)$ is known as the *score function* (see Appendix A.2). Hence, if $t_. = \sum t_i$ is the total observation time, $\hat{\lambda} = n/t_.$ which is simply the total number of subjects (or events) divided by the total observation time.

If we do not observe all subjects to fail, so that the failure time for subject i is censored at time c_i, let $y_i = \min(t_i, c_i)$, then the likelihood for subjects observed to fail is the same as above, while the likelihood for subjects not observed to fail is the probability of reaching time y_i without failing, $S(y_i)$. If we let δ_i be the indicator of failure for subject i, i.e.,

$$\delta_i = \begin{cases} 1 & \text{if subject } i \text{ fails} \\ 0 & \text{if not.} \end{cases}$$

Then the likelihood can be written:[1]

$$
\begin{aligned}
L &= \prod_1^n f(y_i)^{\delta_i} S(y_i)^{1-\delta_i} \\
&= \prod_1^n (\lambda \exp(-\lambda y_i))^{\delta_i} \exp(-\lambda y_i)^{1-\delta_i} \\
&= \prod_1^n \lambda^{\delta_i} \exp(-\lambda y_i).
\end{aligned}
$$

If $\delta_. = \sum_{i=1}^n \delta_i$ is the total number of observed events, then we may write the log-likelihood as

$$\log(L) = \delta_. \log(\lambda) - \lambda y_..$$

The score function is

$$U(\lambda) = \frac{\delta_.}{\lambda} - y_.$$

and L is maximized by solving $U(\lambda) = 0$ to obtain

$$\hat{\lambda} = \delta_./y_. = \frac{\text{total events}}{\text{total person years exposure}}.$$

The Fisher information (Appendix A.2) is $\mathcal{I}(\lambda) = E\delta_./\lambda^2$. Note, however, that $E_\lambda \delta_.$ and, therefore, $\mathcal{I}(\lambda)$ depends on the length of follow-up, and hence on the censoring distribution. We can, however, estimate $E_\lambda \delta_.$ conditional on the observed total follow-up time, $y_.$, by $E_\lambda \delta_. = \lambda y_.$ so that $\mathcal{I}(\lambda) \approx y_./\lambda$. Finally, the sampling variance of $\hat{\lambda}$ can be estimated by

$$\text{Var}(\hat{\lambda}) = \frac{1}{\mathcal{I}(\hat{\lambda})} \approx \frac{\delta_.}{y_.^2}.$$

Now suppose we wish to test $H_0 : \lambda = \lambda_0$ for some given $\lambda_0 > 0$. The

---

[1] To be mathematically precise, L does not correspond to the product of density functions in the usual sense (i.e., with respect to Lebesgue measure). If C_i represent censoring times (that may be random variables, provided that they are independent of the y_i), however, L is the product of Radon-Nykodym derivatives of the CDF's of the y_i with respect to Lebesgue measure plus point masses at the U_i. One sometimes calls this a *generalized density function*.

likelihood ratio statistic (Appendix A.3) is

$$
\begin{aligned}
2\log\frac{L(\hat{\lambda})}{L(\lambda_0)} &= 2(\delta.\log(\hat{\lambda}) - \hat{\lambda}y. - \delta.\log(\lambda_0) + \lambda_0 y.)\\[2mm]
&= 2(\delta.\log\frac{\delta.}{y.} - \delta. - \delta.\log(\lambda_0) + \lambda_0 y.)\\[2mm]
&= 2(\delta.\log\frac{\delta.}{\lambda_0 y.} - (\delta. - \lambda_0 y.)).
\end{aligned}
$$

Note that if $\delta.$ is equal to its expected value under H_0, $\lambda_0 y.$, then the LR statistic is zero. The Wald test statistic (Appendix A.3) is

$$
\frac{(\hat{\lambda} - \lambda_0)^2}{\mathrm{Var}\hat{\lambda}} = \frac{(\delta./y. - \lambda_0)^2}{\delta./y.^2} = \frac{(\delta. - \lambda_0 y.)^2}{\delta.},
$$

and the score test statistic (Appendix A.3) is

$$
\frac{U(\lambda_0)^2}{\mathcal{I}(\lambda_0)} = \left(\frac{\delta.}{\lambda_0} - y.\right)^2 \frac{\lambda_0}{y.} \approx \frac{(\delta. - \lambda_0 y.)^2}{\lambda_0 y.}.
$$

Note that both the Wald and score tests involve the observed $\delta.$ minus its expectation under H_0, given $y.$, $\lambda_0 y.$. For the Wald test, however, the variance (derived from $\mathcal{I}(\lambda)$) is evaluated at the MLE $\hat{\lambda}$, while for the score test, the variance is evaluated at λ_0. The LRT does not directly involve $\mathcal{I}(\lambda)$, but simply uses the log-likelihood evaluated at both $\hat{\lambda}$ and λ_0.

Example 7.1. Suppose we have the following failure times ($^+$ indicates censored observations).

$$9, 13, 13^+, 18, 23, 28^+, 31, 34, 45^+, 48, 161^+$$

We have that $\delta. = 7$ and $y. = 423$, so $\hat{\lambda} = 0.016$. Suppose we wish to test $H_0: \lambda = .03$. Under H_0, $E_{\lambda_0}\delta. = .03 \times 423 = 12.7$. The LR statistic is $2(7\log 7/12.7 - (7 - 12.7)) = 3.05$. The Wald test statistic is $(7 - 12.7)^2/7 = 4.62$ while the score statistic is $(7 - 12.7)^2/12.7 = 2.55$. In this case, because the variance of $\delta.$ under H_0 is larger than when $\lambda = \hat{\lambda}$, the score statistic is smaller than the Wald statistic. The LR statistic is between the score and the Wald statistics. In large samples, the three statistics will generally be quite close together.   □

   The primary advantage of the exponential distribution is that it is simple, and many quantities involving the survival distribution can be calculated directly, resulting in relatively simple formulas. On the other hand, because it relies on the strong assumption that the hazard function is constant, it often does not adequately represent observed data. The exponential distribution can be generalized to create other parametric families of distributions. Here we briefly discuss the *gamma*, *Weibull*, and *log-normal* families.

1. The *gamma* distribution is defined by two parameters commonly referred to as *shape* and either *scale* or *rate*. The rate or scale parameters are re-

ciprocals of one another so either one can be used to specify the distribution. Properties related to the shape of the distribution such as skewness $(E(T - \mu)^3/\sigma^{3/2}$ where $\mu = ET$, and $\sigma^2 = \mathrm{Var}T)$ and kurtosis $(E(T - \mu)^4/\sigma^4 - 3)$ are determined by the shape parameter. We will let α denote the shape parameter and λ the rate parameter. The corresponding scale parameter is $1/\lambda$. The gamma distribution has density

$$f(t) = \frac{\lambda^\alpha}{\Gamma(\alpha)} t^{\alpha-1} e^{-\lambda t}, \text{ for } \alpha > 0, \lambda > 0,$$

where $\Gamma(\cdot)$ is the ordinary gamma function. The mean and variance are

$$E(T) = \frac{\alpha}{\lambda} \text{ and } \mathrm{Var}(T) = \frac{\alpha}{\lambda^2}.$$

Note that the exponential distribution is the special case of the gamma distribution for which $\alpha = 1$. The cumulative distribution function can be written in terms of the *incomplete gamma function*, $\gamma(\alpha, x) = \int_0^x s^{\alpha-1} e^{-s} ds$ as

$$F(t) = \gamma(\alpha, \lambda t)/\Gamma(\alpha),$$

so that

$$S(t) = 1 - \gamma(\alpha, \lambda t)/\Gamma(\alpha)$$

and

$$\lambda(t) = \frac{\lambda^\alpha t^{\alpha-1} e^{-\lambda t}}{\Gamma(\alpha) - \gamma(\alpha, \lambda t)}.$$

2. Another common parametric family is the *Weibull* family. Similar to the gamma family, the Weibull family is a two-parameter generalization of the exponential distribution characterized by shape and rate/scale parameters. The distribution is most easily defined by the survivor function

$$S(t) = e^{-(\lambda t)^\alpha}, \tag{7.1}$$

where $\alpha > 0$ is the shape parameter, and $\lambda > 0$ is the rate parameter. For technical reasons, software that fits parametric models will often parameterize the Weibull distribution in terms of the scale, $1/\lambda$, and $\log(\alpha\lambda)$. Again, the Weibull distribution with $\alpha = 1$ is the exponential distribution. We have

$$\begin{aligned}
\Lambda(t) &= (\lambda t)^\alpha \\
\lambda(t) &= \alpha\lambda(\lambda t)^{\alpha-1} \\
f(t) &= \lambda(t)S(t) = \alpha\lambda(\lambda t)^{\alpha-1} e^{-(\lambda t)^\alpha}.
\end{aligned}$$

(Note that the *parameter*, λ, on the right hand side should not be confused with the *function*, $\lambda(t)$, on the left hand side.) The mean and variance of T are:

$$E(T) = \frac{1}{\lambda}\Gamma(1/\alpha + 1)$$

and

$$\mathrm{Var}(T) = \frac{1}{\lambda^2}(\Gamma(2/\alpha + 1) - \Gamma(1/\alpha + 1)^2)$$

3. The failure time, T, follows the *log-normal* distribution if $\log T$ is normally distributed. Hence, the log-normal distribution is characterized by the mean, μ, and variance, σ^2, of the corresponding normal distribution, so that $\log T \sim N(\mu, \sigma^2)$. Thus, we have that

$$S(t) = 1 - \Phi\left(\frac{\log t - \mu}{\sigma}\right)$$

where $\Phi(\cdot)$ is the cumulative distribution function for the standard normal distribution. The density function is

$$f(t) = \phi\left(\frac{\log t - \mu}{\sigma}\right)/\sigma t$$

where $\phi(\cdot)$ is the probability density function for the standard normal distribution. The mean and variance of the log-normal distribution are

$$E(T) = e^{\mu + \sigma^2/2}$$

and

$$\text{Var}(T) = e^{2\mu + \sigma^2}\left(e^{\sigma^2} - 1\right).$$

As with the exponential distribution, parameter estimates for each of these families can be derived using maximum likelihood. In general, closed-form solutions do not exist except for the exponential distribution. The form of the likelihood is similar to that of the exponential case,

$$L(\theta) = \prod_{i=1}^{n} f(y_i)^{\delta_i} S(y_i)^{1-\delta_i},$$

where θ is the vector of model parameters that depend on the parametric family. The derivatives of the log-likelihood are straightforward, although often complicated computationally.

7.2.2 Nonparametric Approach

Nonparametric approaches do not require assumptions regarding the functional form of the failure time distribution. If the data are uncensored, so that all failure times are observed exactly, then the survivor function, $S(t)$, can be estimated easily as the proportion of subjects surviving to time t. Equivalently, $\hat{S}(t) = 1 - \hat{F}(t)$ where $\hat{F}(t)$ is the *empirical distribution function* for the observed failure times. When observations are censored, however, other approaches are required.

One of the earliest procedures for estimating survival distributions is known as the *actuarial* or *life table* approach. This method is commonly used in settings where data for large numbers of subjects are summarized as tables of subjects at risk and dying during a set of predefined time intervals. For ease of discussion, we will assume that the failure under consideration is death.

Suppose that we have a series of intervals denoted $\mathcal{I}_1, \mathcal{I}_2, \ldots, \mathcal{I}_K$, where

$\mathcal{I}_k = [\tau_{k-1}, \tau_k)$ for a sequence of times $0 = \tau_0 < \tau_2 < \cdots < \tau_K$. For each interval, let

- n_k be the number alive at the beginning of $\mathcal{I}_k$,

- d_k be the number dead during $\mathcal{I}_k$,

- and w_k be the number withdrawal during $\mathcal{I}_k$.

We estimate $S(t)$ as a sequence of conditional probabilities:

$$
\begin{aligned}
S(\tau_k) &= \Pr(T > \tau_k) \\
&= \Pr(T > \tau_1)\Pr(T > \tau_2|T > \tau_1)\cdots\Pr(T > \tau_k|T > \tau_{k-1}) \\
&= p_1 \cdots p_k
\end{aligned}
$$

where $p_k = \Pr(T > \tau_k|T > \tau_{k-1})$. Each p_k is the probability of survival in a given interval, given that the subject is alive at the start of the interval. If there is no withdrawal during interval $\mathcal{I}_k$, this probability can be estimated by the proportion of subjects starting an interval who do not die during the interval:

$$
\hat{p}_k = \frac{n_k - d_k}{n_k} = 1 - \frac{d_k}{n_k}.
$$

If subjects have withdrawn during the interval, we assume that, on the average, those who withdraw are at risk for half the interval. Therefore the "effective sample size" for the interval $\mathcal{I}_k$ is $n'_k = n_k - w_k/2$ and

$$
\hat{p}_k = 1 - \frac{d_k}{n'_k}.
$$

Hence,

$$
\hat{S}(\tau_k) = \prod_{l=1}^{k} \hat{p}_l = \prod_{l=1}^{k}\left(1 - \frac{d_l}{n'_l}\right).
$$

Rather than calculating the variance of $\hat{S}(\tau_k)$ directly, it is easier to calculate the variance of $\log \hat{S}(\tau_k) = \sum_{l=1}^{k} \log \hat{p}_l$. Assuming that $d_k \sim \text{Binomial}(n'_k, 1 - p_k)$ and that the number of events in disjoint intervals are uncorrelated,

$$
\text{Var}(\sum_{l=1}^{k} \log \hat{p}_l) = \sum_{l=1}^{k} \text{Var}(\log \hat{p}_l).
$$

Using the delta method (Appendix A.1),

$$
\begin{aligned}
\text{Var}(\log \hat{p}_k) &\approx (\frac{d}{dp_k}\log p_k)^2 \text{Var}[\hat{p}_k] \\
&= \left(\frac{1}{p_k}\right)^2 \frac{p_k(1 - p_k)}{n'_k} \\
&= \frac{1 - p_k}{n'_k p_k}.
\end{aligned}
$$

Therefore, we can use the estimate

$$\widehat{\mathrm{Var}}[\log \hat{S}(\tau_k)] = \sum_{l=1}^{k} \frac{1 - \hat{p}_l}{n'_l \hat{p}_l} = \sum_{l=1}^{k} \frac{d_l}{n'_l(n'_l - d_l)}.$$

Again, by the delta method, $\mathrm{Var}[e^X] \approx e^{2E[X]}\mathrm{Var}[X]$, so

$$\mathrm{Var}\hat{S}(\tau_k) \approx S^2(\tau_k) \sum_{l=1}^{k} \frac{1 - p_l}{n'_l p_l}.$$

Hence, we use

$$\widehat{\mathrm{Var}}(\hat{S}(\tau_k)) = \hat{S}^2(\tau_k) \sum_{l=1}^{k} \frac{d_l}{n'_l(n'_l - d_l)}.$$

This variance estimate is known as *Greenwood's formula*.

Example 7.2. Suppose that we have data from the first four columns of the following table.

k	τ_k	n_k	d_k	w_k	n'_k	$1 - \hat{p}_k$	$\hat{p}_k$	$\hat{S}(\tau_k)$	$\widehat{\mathrm{SE}}(\hat{S}(\tau_k))$
1	1	126	47	19	116.5	0.40	0.60	0.60	0.045
2	2	60	5	17	51.5	0.10	0.90	0.54	0.048
3	3	38	2	15	30.5	0.07	0.93	0.50	0.051
4	4	21	2	9	16.5	0.12	0.88	0.44	0.060
5	5	10	0	6	7.0	0.00	1.00	0.44	0.060

The five right most columns are derived from the others using the formulas previously defined. For example,

$$\hat{S}(\tau_2) = \hat{p}_1 \cdot \hat{p}_2 = \left(1 - \frac{47}{116.5}\right)\left(1 - \frac{5}{51.5}\right) = .54$$

$$\hat{\mathrm{Var}}(\hat{S}(\tau_2)) = (.54)^2 \left(\frac{47}{116.5(116.5 - 47)} + \frac{5}{51.5(51.5 - 5)}\right) = .0023.$$

$\square$

7.2.3 The Kaplan-Meier Estimator

The actuarial estimate (or a variation of it) is the only available nonparametric estimate when data are provided as a summary table as in the previous section. When failure times are known for individual subjects, this estimator can be improved upon. The *Kaplan-Meier* or *product-limit* estimate is obtained from the actuarial estimator by increasing the number of intervals, $\mathcal{I}_i$, so that the lengths of the intervals shrink to zero. As the length of each interval shrinks, the proportion of subjects withdrawing in each interval will also shrink to zero, so we only need to consider the number at risk at the start of each interval and the number of deaths within each interval. Also, because the actuarial estimator does not change over intervals in which there are no deaths, we only need to consider the intervals containing at least one death. Finally, as the interval lengths shrink to zero, each distinct death time will appear in a distinct interval. Thus, the data can be reduced to the set of distinct failure times and the number of subjects at risk and number of deaths at each failure time.

So, we let $t_1, t_2, \ldots, t_K$ be the set of distinct failure times. For each failure time, let n_k be the number of subjects at risk and d_k the number of deaths at time t_k. The conventional assumption is that, in the event of tied failure and censoring times, the censoring time is considered to be later than the failure time. Thus, n_k is the number of subjects with both censoring time and failure time on or after time t_k.

Then the Kaplan-Meier estimate of $S(t)$ is

$$\hat{S}(t) = \prod_{k:t_k \leq t} (1 - \frac{d_k}{n_k}).$$

Note that if $d_k > 1$, so we have tied failure times at t_k, we may randomly break the ties by adding small perturbations to the t_k (and assuming that all censored observations occur *after* the last of the failure times) and achieve the same estimate. To see this, note that the contribution to $\hat{S}$ from time t_l is

$$(1 - \frac{1}{n_k})(1 - \frac{1}{n_k - 1})(1 - \frac{1}{n_k - 2}) \cdots (1 - \frac{1}{n_k - d_k + 1})$$

$$= \frac{(n_k - 1)}{n_k} \frac{(n_k - 2)}{(n_k - 1)} \frac{(n_k - 3)}{(n_k - 2)} \cdots \frac{(n_k - d_k)}{(n_k - d_k + 1)}$$

$$= \frac{n_k - d_k}{n_k}$$

$$= 1 - \frac{d_k}{n_k}.$$

Furthermore, if there is no censoring, the Kaplan-Meier estimate reduces to the empirical distribution function. This follows because, in this case, the number at risk at any failure time is the total sample size minus the number of prior events. If k' is the largest value of k such that $t_k \leq t$, then

$$\hat{S}(t) = \left(1 - \frac{d_1}{n}\right)\left(1 - \frac{d_2}{n - d_1}\right) \cdots \left(1 - \frac{d_{k'}}{n - d_1 - d_2 \cdots - d_{k'-1}}\right)$$

$$= \left(\frac{n - d_1}{n}\right)\left(\frac{n - d_1 - d_2}{n - d_1}\right) \cdots \left(1 - \frac{n - d_1 - d_2 - \cdots - d_{k'}}{n - d_1 - d_2 \cdots - d_{k'-1}}\right)$$

$$= \frac{n - d_1 - d_2 - \cdots - d_{k'}}{n}$$

$$= 1 - \frac{d_1 + d_2 + \cdots + d_{k'}}{n}$$

$$= 1 - \frac{\text{number dead prior to time } t}{\text{total number subjects}}.$$

The variance estimate of $\hat{S}(t)$ is identical to that for the actuarial estimate and we again arrive at Greenwood's formula:

$$\widehat{\mathrm{Var}}(\hat{S}(t)) = \hat{S}^2(t) \sum_{k:t_k \leq t} \frac{d_k}{n_k(n_k - d_k)}.$$

Example 7.3. Using the data from Example 7.1, we construct the following table.

t_k	n_k	d_k	$\hat{p}_k$	$\hat{S}(t_k)$	$\widehat{\mathrm{SE}}(\hat{S}(t))$
9	11	1	10/11	10/11 $= 0.91$	0.09
13	10	1	9/10	9/11 $= 0.82$	0.12
18	8	1	7/8	63/88 $= 0.72$	0.14
23	7	1	6/7	27/44 $= 0.61$	0.15
28	6	0	6/6	27/44 $= 0.61$	0.15
31	5	1	4/5	27/55 $= 0.49$	0.16
34	4	1	3/4	81/220 $= 0.37$	0.16
45	3	0	3/3	81/220 $= 0.37$	0.16
48	2	1	1/2	81/440 $= 0.18$	0.15

Estimates of $S(t)$ for this example are plotted in Figure 7.1. The 95% pointwise confidence band is derived for the Kaplan-Meier estimate of $S(t)$ using the standard error computed using Greenwood's formula and applied to $\log(\hat{S}(t))$. The result was then transformed back to the original scale. Computation of the confidence band on the log scale is more reliable than directly using the standard errors above. We call the confidence band *pointwise* because for each time, t, there is a 0.95 probability that the band contains the true value of $S(t)$. The probability that $S(t)$ is contained with the band for *all* values of t is less than 0.95. *Simultaneous* confidence bands can be constructed with the property that the band contains $S(t)$ for all t within the range of the data with a specified probability (Fleming and Harrington 1991). □

Example 7.4. Figure 7.2 shows cumulative mortality, $F(t) = 1 - S(t)$, for the two treatment arms of the BHAT (Beta-Blocker Heart Attack Trial Research Group 1982) study. Note that the jumps in the estimated survivor functions are quite small for the first 30 months or so, after which the number of subjects at risk, n_k, is small and each death results in larger jumps. This behavior is typical, and often provides a visual clue regarding the reliability of the estimates at large times. Frequently, the curves exhibit erratic behavior at the most extreme times and these portions of the curves should be interpreted cautiously. In the primary publication of BHAT, the survival plot was truncated at 36 months. □

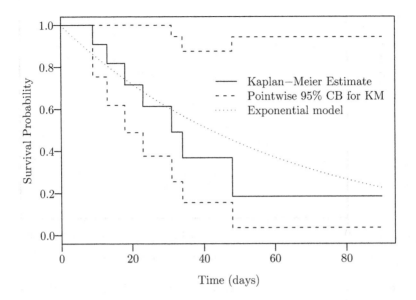

Figure 7.1 *Estimated survival from data in Example 7.1.*

7.3 Comparison of Survival Distributions

The goal of most randomized trials with survival outcomes is to make direct comparisons of two survival curves. The most general form of the null hypothesis is $H_0\colon S_1(t) = S_2(t)$ for all $t > 0$, although in practice we can only test this hypothesis over the range of the observed failure times. Tests of this hypothesis can be *parametric*—under an assumed parametric model—or nonparametric in which case the forms of $S_1(t)$ and $S_2(t)$ may be completely unspecified. We begin with parametric methods.

7.3.1 Parametric Methods

The simplest parametric test is based on the exponential model. If we assume that the observations in both groups are exponential, with possibly different rate parameters, λ_1 and λ_2, H_0 is equivalent to $H_0\colon \lambda_1 = \lambda_2$. The most straightforward test of H_0 is based on the Wald test. The Wald test is usually applied to the log of the hazard rate, in part because the sampling distribution of $\log \hat{\lambda}_\tau$ is better approximated by the normal distribution than is that of $\hat{\lambda}_\tau$.

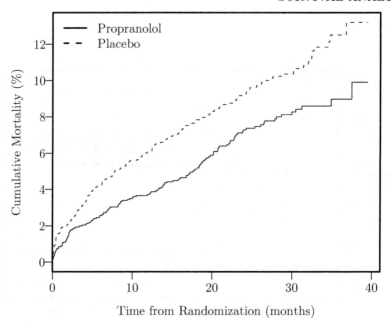

Figure 7.2 *Cumulative mortality from BHAT (Beta-Blocker Heart Attack Trial Research Group 1982).*

Note that by the delta-method, $\widehat{\text{Var}}\hat{\lambda}_\tau = 1/d_\tau$. Under H_0,

$$Z = \frac{\log \hat{\lambda}_1 - \log \hat{\lambda}_2}{\sqrt{\widehat{\text{Var}}\log \hat{\lambda}_1 + \widehat{\text{Var}}\log \hat{\lambda}_2}} \sim AN(0, 1)$$

where $AN(0, 1)$ indicates that the distribution of the statistic is asymptotically normal with mean zero and variance one.

Example 7.5. The 6–Mercaptopurine in Acute Leukemia trial was conducted to determine the effect of 6–Mercaptopurine versus placebo on length of complete remission for patients who had undergone steroid therapy (Freireich et al. 1963). The sequential phase of the trial was stopped after 21 pairs of subjects were entered and followed until at least one member of each pair relapsed. The results for these 42 subjects are below ($^+$ indicates censored observations).

Active 6^+, 6, 6, 6, 7, 9^+, 10^+, 10, 11^+, 13, 16, 17^+, 19^+, 20^+, 22, 23, 25^+, 32^+, 32^+, 34^+, 35^+

Control 1, 1, 2, 2, 3, 4, 4, 5, 5, 8, 8, 8, 8, 11, 11, 12, 12, 15, 17, 22, 23

If the active group is group 1 and the control group is group 0, we have $\hat{\lambda}_1 = 9/359 = 0.025$ and $\hat{\lambda}_0 = 21/182 = 0.115$. Also, $\widehat{\text{Var}}\hat{\lambda}_1 = 1/9 = 0.111$ and

$\widehat{\text{Var}}\hat{\lambda}_0 = 1/21 = 0.047$. The test statistic for $H_0: \lambda_1 = \lambda_0$ is

$$Z = \frac{\log 0.115 - \log 0.025}{\sqrt{.111 + .047}} = 3.83.$$

Thus, the observed difference in survival between those given 6–MP and those on control is statistically significant at level 0.0001 and we conclude that the active treatment reduced the recurrence rate.   □

The score test of H_0 can be obtained as follows. Let $\alpha = \log \lambda_1$ and $\beta = \log \lambda_1/\lambda_0$. H_0 is equivalent to $H_0: \beta = 0$. The log-likelihood is $\log L = d_1\alpha - e^\alpha y_1 + d_0(\alpha + \beta) - e^{\alpha+\beta}y_0$ and the score vector becomes

$$U(\alpha, \beta) = \begin{pmatrix} d_1 - e^\alpha y_1 + d_0 - e^{\alpha+\beta}y_0 \\ d_0 - e^{\alpha+\beta}y_0 \end{pmatrix}.$$

Under H_0, we assume that $\beta = 0$, and the MLE for α is $\hat{\alpha} = \log(d_1 + d_0)/(y_1 + y_0)$.

$$U(\hat{\alpha}, 0) = \begin{pmatrix} 0 \\ d_0 - \hat{\lambda}_0 y_0 \end{pmatrix}$$

where $\hat{\lambda}_0$ is the estimate of the common hazard rate under H_0. The Fisher information matrix is

$$I(\hat{\alpha}, 0) = \begin{pmatrix} \hat{\lambda}_0(y_1 + y_0) & \hat{\lambda}_0 y_0 \\ \hat{\lambda}_0 y_0 & \hat{\lambda}_0 y_0 \end{pmatrix}.$$

The test statistic is

$$U(\hat{\alpha}, 0)^T I^{-1} U(\hat{\alpha}, 0) = (d_0 - \hat{\lambda}_0 y_0)^2 \left(\frac{1}{\hat{\lambda}_0 y_1} + \frac{1}{\hat{\lambda}_0 y_0} \right) \sim \chi_1^2.$$

Example 7.6. Returning to the 6–MP acute leukemia example, the common hazard rate, $\hat{\lambda}_0 = 30/541 = 0.055$. The score test becomes:

$$\begin{aligned} U(\hat{\alpha}, 0)^T I^{-1} U(\hat{\alpha}, 0) &= (21 - 0.055 \times 182) \times \left(\frac{1}{0.055 \times 359} + \frac{1}{0.055 \times 182} \right) \\ &= 17.76 \end{aligned}$$

Note that the score test is slightly larger than the square of the Wald test $(3.83^2 = 14.68)$.   □

7.3.2 Nonparametric Methods

Two primary nonparametric approaches to testing $H_0: S_1(t) = S_0(t)$ for all t are tests based on ranks and *Mantel-Haenszel* type tests. More recently, tests formulated using counting processes provide a unified framework for studying the asymptotic properties of these tests. We consider counting process techniques to be beyond the scope of this book and will not consider them here.

Since the two approaches yield similar tests, we consider only Mantel-Haenszel type tests.

Suppose that we have two groups and let $t_1, t_2, \ldots$ be the set of distinct failure times for the two groups combined. For a given failure time t_j, we have

$$
\begin{aligned}
d_{j0}, d_{j1} &= \text{number events in groups } 0, 1 \text{ respectively} \\
n_{j0}, n_{j1} &= \text{number at risk in groups } 0, 1 \text{ respectively}
\end{aligned}
$$

We may consider the 2×2 table:

	Dead	Alive	Total
Group 1	d_{j1}	$n_{j1} - d_{j1}$	n_{j1}
Group 2	d_{j0}	$n_{j0} - d_{j0}$	n_{j0}
	$d_{j.}$	$n_{j.} - d_{j.}$	$n_{j..}$

If we consider this table to have arisen by tabulating events occurring within the interval $[t_j, t + \Delta t)$, then we have, conditional on $n_{j\tau}$, that $d_{j\tau}$ has, approximately, a binomial distribution with mean $E d_{j\tau} = n_{j\tau} \lambda_\tau(t_j) \Delta t$ where $\lambda_\tau(t_j)$ is the hazard function for group τ at time t_j. The difficulty with these binomial distributions is that they depend on the unknown hazard functions, $\lambda_0(t_j)$ and $\lambda_1(t_j)$, and the arbitrary increment Δt.

This difficulty can be alleviated by considering the distribution of d_{j1} conditional on the ancillary statistic $d_{j.}$.

The joint distribution (conditional on $n_{j\tau}, \tau = 0, 1$) of d_{j0} and d_{j1} is

$$
\begin{aligned}
p(d_{j0}, d_{j1}) &= \binom{n_{j0}}{d_{j0}} \binom{n_{j1}}{d_{j1}} (\lambda_0(t_j)\Delta t)^{d_{j0}} (1 - \lambda_0(t_j)\Delta t)^{n_{j0} - d_{j0}} \\
&\quad \times (\lambda_1(t_j)\Delta t)^{d_{j1}} (1 - \lambda_1(t_j)\Delta t)^{n_{j1} - d_{j1}} \\
&\approx \binom{n_{j0}}{d_{j0}} \binom{n_{j1}}{d_{j1}} \lambda_0(t_j)^{d_{j0}} \lambda_1(t_j)^{d_{j1}} \Delta t^{d_{j.}}.
\end{aligned}
$$

The *conditional* (on $d_{j.}$) distribution is

$$
\begin{aligned}
p(d_{j0}, d_{j1} | d_{j.}) &= \frac{p(d_{j0}, d_{j1})}{\sum_{u=0}^{d_{j.}} p(u, d_{j.} - u)} \\
&\approx \frac{\binom{n_{j0}}{d_{j0}} \binom{n_{j1}}{d_{j1}} \lambda_0(t_j)^{d_{j0}} \lambda_1(t_j)^{d_{j1}} \Delta t^{d_{j.}}}{\sum_{u=0}^{d_{j.}} \binom{n_{j0}}{u} \binom{n_{j1}}{d_{j.} - u} \lambda_0(t_j)^u \lambda_1(t_j)^{d_{j.} - u} \Delta t^{d_{j.}}} \\
&= \frac{\binom{n_{j0}}{d_{j0}} \binom{n_{j1}}{d_{j1}} \psi^{d_{j1}}}{\sum_{u=0}^{d_{j.}} \binom{n_{j0}}{u} \binom{n_{j1}}{d_{j.} - u} \psi^{d_{j.} - u}}, \quad (7.2)
\end{aligned}
$$

where $\psi = \lambda_1(t_j)/\lambda_0(t_j)$. The distribution defined by (7.2) is known as the *non-central hypergeometric* distribution and does not depend on the underlying hazard, but only on the hazard ratio ψ.

The null hypothesis $H_0: \lambda_1(t) = \lambda_0(t)$ for all t is equivalent to $H_0: \psi = 1$.

When this holds, (7.2) simplifies as

$$p(d_{j0}, d_{j1}|d_{j\cdot}) = \frac{\binom{n_{j0}}{d_{j0}}\binom{n_{j1}}{d_{j1}}}{\binom{n_{j0}+n_{j1}}{d_{j\cdot}}}$$

and this distribution is known as the (central) *hypergeometric* distribution. Under H_0 we have that the conditional mean of d_{j1} is

$$E[d_{j1}|n_{j1}, n_{j0}, d_{j\cdot}] = \frac{d_{j\cdot}}{n_{j\cdot}}n_{j1}$$

and its variance is

$$\text{Var}[d_{j1}|n_{j1}, n_{j0}, d_{j\cdot}] = \frac{d_{j\cdot}(n_{j\cdot} - d_{j\cdot})n_{j1}n_{j0}}{n_{j\cdot}^2(n_{j\cdot} - 1)}.$$

If the true underlying hazard is uniformly larger (or smaller) in group 1 than in group 0, then we expect that d_{j1} will be systematically larger (or smaller) than its expected value under H_0. In particular, this holds when we have proportional hazards ($\lambda_1(t)/\lambda_0(t) \neq 1$ does not depend on t). This suggests that the test statistic,

$$U = \sum_j d_{j1} - \frac{d_{j\cdot}}{n_{j\cdot}}n_{j1}, \tag{7.3}$$

which is the overall sum of the observed number of events minus its conditional expectation under H_0, is a measure of the degree to departure from H_0 suggested by the data. A formal test of H_0 requires that we compare U to its standard error under H_0.

First we note that the d_{j1} are not independent over the observed failure times; however, it can be shown that they are uncorrelated. Hence, we may use the following test statistic:

$$\frac{\left(\sum_j d_{j1} - E[d_{j1}]\right)^2}{\sum_j \text{Var}(d_{j1})} \sim \chi_1^2$$

This test is usually known as the *log-rank* test or *Mantel-Haenszel* test (Mantel 1966).

We also note that, since the distribution of the test statistic is derived under H_0 without reference to a particular alternative hypothesis, the log-rank test is valid for any alternative hypotheses including those for which the proportional hazards assumption does not hold, i.e., $\lambda_1(t)/\lambda_0(t)$ is not constant. It can be shown, however, that the log-rank test is optimal for proportional hazards alternatives, but it has lower power than other tests against non-proportional hazards alternatives. If we desire higher power for particular non-proportional hazards alternatives, the test can be modified to improve power by replacing the sum in (7.3) by a weighted sum, with weights chosen to optimize the test for the alternatives of interest.

In general, any test of the form

$$\frac{\left(\sum_j w_j(d_{j1} - E[d_{j1}])\right)^2}{\sum_j w_j^2 \text{Var}(d_{j1})} \sim \chi_1^2$$

where the weights, w_j, are correctly chosen (e.g., independent of treatment) is a valid test of the null hypothesis. The case $w_j = 1$ for all j gives the ordinary log-rank test. The case $w_j = n_{j.}$ is known as the *Gehan-Wilcoxon* test. Using this test statistic, early failures receive higher weight than later failures, and thus the test will be more sensitive to differences between the two groups that occur early in the follow-up period. One drawback of the Gehan-Wilcoxon test is that the weights depend on the extent of follow-up; with less follow-up, the size of the risk set decreases more quickly and hence gives relatively lower weight to failures occurring at later times than would be the case with more extensive follow-up, even though the underlying hazard functions do not change.

One family of weight functions, the G^ρ ("G-rho") family (Harrington and Fleming 1982), uses $w_j = \hat{S}(t_j)^\rho$, where $\hat{S}(t_j)$ is the Kaplan-Meier estimate of aggregate survival, ignoring treatment group. When $\rho = 0$, we have the ordinary log-rank test. The case $\rho = 1$ is known as the *Peto-Peto-Wilcoxon* test. Greater flexibility can be provided by choosing values of ρ between 0 and 1. Similar to the Gehan-Wilcoxon test, for $\rho > 0$, failures early in follow-up, when $\hat{S}(t)$ is larger, receive more weight than later failures when $\hat{S}(t)$ is small. Unlike the Gehan-Wilcoxon test, however, the weights do not depend on the extent of follow-up, except to the degree that the precision in $\hat{S}(t)$ is affected.

Example 7.7. Returning to the 6–MP example, there are 17 distinct failure times. At the first failure time, day 1, we have the table

	Dead	Alive	Total
Active	0	21	21
Control	2	19	21
	2	40	42

Here, $d_{11} - Ed_{11} = 0 - 2 \times 21/42 = -1$, $\text{Var}(d_{11}) = 2 \times 19 \times 21 \times 21/42^2/41 = .488$. At the second failure time, day 2, we have $d_{21} - Ed_{21} = 0 - 2 \times 21/40 = -1.05$, and $\text{Var}(d_{21}) = 2 \times 38 \times 21 \times 19/40^2/38 = .486$. Continuing, we have $\sum_{j=1}^{17} d_{j1} - Ed_{j1} = 9 - 19.3 = -10.3$, and $\sum_{j=1}^{17} \text{Var}(d_{j1}) = 6.25$. Thus, the chi-square statistic for the log-rank test of H_0 is

$$\frac{\left(\sum_j d_{j1} - E[d_{j1}]\right)^2}{\sum_j \text{Var}(d_{j1})} = \frac{(-10.3)^2}{6.25} = 16.8,$$

which is similar to the score test under the exponential model.   □

Example 7.8. In the BHAT example, there were 138 and 188 deaths in the propranolol and placebo groups, respectively. The expected numbers under the null hypothesis are 164.4 and 161.6 respectively. Note that 138 - 164.4 = -26.4 = -(188-161.6), so the difference between observed and expected is the same in absolute value, regardless of which group is chosen as group 1. The variance of the difference is 81.48. Note that this is approximated quite closely by $d_{..}/4 = (138 + 188)/4 = 81.5$. This approximation works well when the sample sizes and censoring patterns are the same in the two groups, which is usually the case in randomized trials with 1:1 randomization schemes. The log-rank chi-square statistic is $26.4^2/81.5 = 8.52$ ($p = 0.0035$), so we have strong evidence of the beneficial effect of propranolol on mortality in this population.   □

7.4 Regression Models

While randomized controlled trials are designed primarily as hypothesis testing instruments, testing is usually accompanied by estimation of the effect of assigned treatment, often adjusted for the effects of baseline covariates. Parameter estimation requires that we specify a model for the association between the covariate and the risk of failure. A fully parametric model is one in which the entire survival distribution is determined by a finite number of parameters. A semiparametric model is one in which there is an explicit model for the relative effect of the covariates; however, the hazard function is either unspecified or specified by infinitely many parameters. We begin with parametric models.

7.4.1 Parametric Models

A parametric regression model is a model for which we specify the functional form of the relationship between the failure time distribution and one or more covariates. The parameters involved are estimated from the data. While this can be done quite generally, we will restrict attention to models in which a parameter, μ, is a linear function of the covariates. That is, letting $\mathbf{z} = (z_1, z_2, \ldots, z_p)^T$ be a vector of covariates and $\beta = (\beta_1, \beta_2, \ldots, \beta_p)^T$ a vector of unknown coefficients, we assume that

$$\mu = \beta^T \mathbf{z} = \sum_{i=1}^{p} \beta_i z_i.$$

There are various choices for the parameter μ. For example,

(1) $\mu = E[T]$

(2) $\mu = \log E[T]$

Note that because $E[T] > 0$, for (1), we need to constrain β so that the predicted $\hat{\mu}$ is positive for all values of $\mathbf{z}$ to which it will be applied. For μ defined by (2), μ takes values over the whole real line and no constraint is necessary. For simplicity, we consider only (2).

If the data are exponential, $E[T] = 1/\lambda$, so (2) becomes $\log \lambda = -\beta^T \mathbf{z}$. For the latter we have

$$S(t; \mathbf{z}) = e^{-\exp(-\beta^T \mathbf{z})t},$$

where we write "$(t; \mathbf{z})$" to emphasize the dependence on both time and the covariate, $\mathbf{z}$. For the Weibull model, given in equation (7.1), it is common to let $\mu = -\log \lambda = \log E(T) - \log \Gamma(1/\alpha + 1)$. Then we have

$$S(t; \mathbf{z}) = e^{-\exp(-\alpha \beta^T \mathbf{z})t^\alpha}.$$

This model can be viewed as a *proportional hazards* model because the hazard ratio for two different values of the covariate $\mathbf{z}$,

$$\lambda(t; \mathbf{z}_1)/\lambda(t; \mathbf{z}_2) = e^{-\alpha \beta^T (\mathbf{z}_1 - \mathbf{z}_2)},$$

does not depend on t. It can also be viewed as an *accelerated failure time* model because, for a fixed reference value $\mathbf{z}_0$, the effect of the covariate is to re-scale the time *variable* by a factor of $e^{-\beta^T (\mathbf{z} - \mathbf{z}_0)}$, so that $S(t; \mathbf{z}) = S(e^{-\beta^T (\mathbf{z} - \mathbf{z}_0)} t; \mathbf{z}_0)$.

In general, the parameter β and any shape/scale parameters and their asymptotic covariances are estimated using maximum likelihood.

7.4.2 Semiparametric Models

The most commonly used models for estimation of treatment and covariate effects are semiparametric models. These are models for which a feature of the distribution, usually the hazard ratio $\lambda(t; z)/\lambda_0(t)$ where $\lambda_0(\cdot)$ is the *baseline hazard function*, is specified parametrically, while the rest of the distribution (e.g., the baseline hazard function, $\lambda_0(\cdot)$) is left unspecified, or defined nonparametrically. While the form of the hazard ratio can be quite general, computationally and conceptually it is easiest to consider the case in which the hazard ratio does not depend on t. The resulting model is the *Cox proportional hazards* model (Cox 1972; Kalbfleisch and Prentice 1980).

So, let $T_1, T_2, \ldots, T_n$ be the true (potentially unobserved) survival times and $C_1, C_2, \ldots, C_n$ the corresponding (potentially unobserved) censoring times where $(T_1, \ldots, T_n)$ and $(C_1, \ldots, C_n)$ are independent. Now let (Y_1, δ_1), $\ldots$, (Y_n, δ_n) be the observed times, $Y_i = T_i \wedge C_i$, $\delta_i = I(T_i \leq C_i)$ be the event indicators, and $\mathbf{z}_i = (\mathbf{z}_{i1}, \ldots, \mathbf{z}_{ip})^T$ be the explanatory covariate. Under the Cox proportional hazard model, we assume

$$\lambda(t; \mathbf{z}) = \lambda_0(t) e^{\beta^T \mathbf{z}} \tag{7.4}$$

where $\lambda_0(t)$ is the *baseline hazard function*. For two individuals with covariates $\mathbf{z}_1$ and $\mathbf{z}_2$ respectively,

$$\frac{\lambda(t; \mathbf{z}_1)}{\lambda(t; \mathbf{z}_2)} = \frac{\lambda_0(t) e^{\beta^T \mathbf{z}_1}}{\lambda_0(t) e^{\beta^T \mathbf{z}_2}} = e^{\beta^T (\mathbf{z}_1 - \mathbf{z}_2)}$$

hence the hazard functions for the two groups are proportional and the ratio is independent of the baseline hazard. The baseline hazard $\lambda_0(t)$ is often considered a *nuisance* parameter, in which case $\lambda(t; \mathbf{z})$, or equivalently $S(t; \mathbf{z})$, is not of interest.

We begin by noting that the parameter β in equation (7.4) has the following interpretations.

1. If z is binary, for example, $z = 1$ if sex is female (F) and $z = 0$ if sex is male (M), we have

$$e^\beta = \frac{\lambda(t; z = F)}{\lambda(t; z = M)}$$

   so β is the log-hazard ratio for females versus males.

2. If z is a continuous variable, then β represents the log-hazard ratio for subjects whose covariate values differ by one unit. If z represents subject age, then this is the log hazard ratio for subjects one year apart in age.

$$e^\beta = \frac{\lambda(t; z = z_0 + 1)}{\lambda(t; z = z_0)}.$$

   In this case, one year of age is unlikely to have a meaningful effect on risk and it may be preferred to report $10 \times \beta$, the log-hazard ratio corresponding to a 10 year increase in age.

3. If we have a categorical variable with c levels, we can parameterize using $c - 1$ indicator variables, using one category as the *reference* category. For example, suppose we have three types of lung cancer patients: adenocarcinoma, large cell, and *other*. Using *other* as the reference category, we create variables z_1 and z_2, defined by other ($z_1 = 0$, $z_2 = 0$), adenocarcinoma ($z_1 = 0$, $z_2 = 1$), and large cell ($z_1 = 1$, $z_2 = 0$). The coefficients β_1 and β_2 represent log hazard ratios as follows:

$$e^{\beta_1} = \frac{\lambda(t; \text{large})}{\lambda(t; \text{other})} \text{ and } e^{\beta_2} = \frac{\lambda(t; \text{adeno})}{\lambda(t; \text{other})}.$$

   The coefficients β_1 and β_2 represent the log-hazard ratios for large-cell and adenocarcinoma patients respectively versus other patients.

Now suppose that we have two covariates: treatment, z_1 (taking values zero and one), and a baseline characteristic, z_2, such as age, diagnostic category, or the result of a laboratory test. We can also include multiple baseline characteristics, but for simplicity we restrict attention to a single characteristic.

A general model using these covariates is

$$\log \lambda(t; \mathbf{z}) = \log \lambda_0(t) + \beta_1 z_1 + \beta_2 z_2 + \beta_3 z_1 z_2, \tag{7.5}$$

so that β_1 and β_2 represent main effects for treatment and z_2 respectively and β_3 represents an interaction between treatment and z_2. For a fixed value of z_2, the hazard ratio for $z_1 = 1$ versus $z_1 = 0$ is

$$\frac{\lambda(t; z_1 = 1, z_2)}{\lambda(t; z_1 = 0, z_2)} = e^{\beta_1 + \beta_3 z_2},$$

so that β_1 represents the log-hazard ratio for treatment when $z_2 = 0$ (which may be implausible, such as age=0) and β_3 represents the change in the log-hazard ratio for treatment per unit change in z_2 (this is often referred to as *effect modification*).

If we assume that the effect of treatment as measured by the hazard ratio is independent of baseline characteristics, then we have that $\beta_3 = 0$. We have the following general principles.

- If z_1 represents treatment and $z_2, z_3, \ldots, z_p$ represent other baseline covariates, then the model

$$\log \lambda(t; z) = \log \lambda_0(t) + \beta_1 z_1 + \beta_2 z_2 + \beta_3 z_3 + \ldots + \beta_p z_p \qquad (7.6)$$

  implies that, for all values of $z_2, z_3, \ldots, z_p$, the effect of treatment on the hazard is constant, and β_1 represents the hazard ratio for treatment *adjusted for* $z_2, z_3, \ldots, z_p$. In randomized trials, imbalances in baseline characteristics can only arise by chance, and the hazard ratio estimated from model (7.6) will likely be quite similar to that estimated without baseline covariates.

  We note, however, that if model (7.6) is correct, then, in general, the adjusted model for treatment will no longer be a proportional hazards model. On the other hand, unless the baseline covariate effects are quite large, the induced non-proportionality will be quite small and the proportional hazards assumption should be adequate. There are examples, however, when departures from proportionality create difficulties (Sloan et al. 1999).

- The test for interaction between treatment and a baseline covariate correspond to the test of the null hypothesis $H_0: \beta_3 = 0$ where β_3 is defined by equation (7.5). This hypothesis may be tested using either the Wald, score, or likelihood-ratio tests as described in Section 7.4.4.

- If equation (7.4) fails, the estimate of β_1 from equation (7.6) can still be interpreted as an average covariate-adjusted log-hazard ratio, and, therefore, can be a useful summary measure. The coefficient, β_3, for the interaction term in equation (7.5), on the other hand, depends strongly on the model assumptions. Rejection of the null hypothesis $H_0: \beta_3 = 0$ should not necessarily be interpreted as evidence that the treatment effect varies as a function of the baseline covariate. For example a more general form of model (7.4) is

$$\lambda(t; \mathbf{z}) = \lambda_0(t) g(\beta^T \mathbf{z}) \qquad (7.7)$$

  for a monotone function $g(\cdot) > 0$. If for some $g(\cdot)$, we have $\beta_3 = 0$ the interaction is called *removable* because its presence relies on the choice of the functional form, $g(\cdot)$.

  If, however, the interaction is such that in model (7.5) for some values of z_2 we have $\beta_1 + \beta_3 z_2 < 0$ and for others $\beta_1 + \beta_3 z_2 > 0$, then the interaction is *qualitative* (or *non-removable*) and cannot be removed by judicious choice of $g(\cdot)$, although such interactions are quite rare.

7.4.3 Cox Partial Likelihood

Inference for the Cox proportional hazards model is based on the *partial* or *conditional* likelihood, which, although it is not a likelihood in the usual sense, for our purpose, it has many of the properties of an ordinary likelihood. The partial likelihood is derived by considering each distinct failure time separately, conditioning on both the set of observed covariate values for subjects at risk at the given time and the number of observed failures. The argument is similar to that of section 7.3.2 for the log-rank statistic. The partial likelihood is the product of the conditional likelihoods from the distinct failure times. Because the data from successive failure times are not independent, multiplication of the conditional likelihoods does not yield a true likelihood; however, using martingale methods (Fleming and Harrington 1991), it can be shown that inference based on the partial likelihood is correct. We begin by deriving the partial likelihood for the case in which there are no tied failure times.

Suppose that $t_1, t_2, \ldots, t_n$ are the distinct failure times. Let R_j be the set of all subjects at risk at time t_j, and r_j be the number at risk. Suppose that we have a single covariate and z_{j1} is the covariate value and λ_{j1} is the hazard for the subject failing at time t_j, and $z_{j2}, z_{j3}, \ldots, z_{jr_j}$ and $\lambda_{j2}, \lambda_{j3}, \ldots, \lambda_{jr_j}$ the covariate values for the remaining subjects in R_j. We have the following table at time t_j:

dead	alive	covariate	hazard
1	0	z_{j1}	$e^{z_{j1}}\lambda_0(t_j)$
0	1	z_{j2}	$e^{z_{j2}}\lambda_0(t_j)$
0	1	z_{j3}	$e^{z_{j3}}\lambda_0(t_j)$
$\vdots$	$\vdots$	$\vdots$	
0	1	z_{jr_j}	$e^{z_{jr_j}}\lambda_0(t_j)$
1	$r_j - 1$		

The conditional likelihood for this table can be derived as follows. Pick exactly one subject from the set R_j according to the probability that they will fail in small interval around t_j. These probabilities have the form $e^{z_l}\lambda_0(t_j)\Delta t$, and the conditional probability that the table above is the one chosen, given that there is exactly one failure, is

$$\frac{e^{z_{j1}\beta}\lambda_0(t_j)\Delta t}{\sum_{l=1}^{r_j} e^{z_{jl}\beta}\lambda_0(t_j)\Delta t} = \frac{e^{z_{j1}\beta}}{\sum_{l=1}^{r_j} e^{z_{jl}\beta}}.$$

Note that the conditional likelihood does not depend on the underlying hazard function.

The partial log-likelihood is the sum of the log conditional likelihoods for all failure times,

$$\log L = \sum_j \left(z_{j1}\beta - \log \sum_{l=1}^{r_j} e^{z_{jl}\beta} \right).$$

In the case where there are ties, the exact partial likelihood is more complex, and computationally prohibitive in large samples. Two common approximations are the Breslow approximation,

$$\log L \approx \sum_j \left(s_j \beta - d_j \log \sum_{l=1}^{r_j} e^{z_{jl}\beta} \right),$$

and the Efron approximation,

$$\log L \approx \sum_j \left(s_j \beta - \sum_{k=1}^{d_j} \log \left[\sum_{l=1}^{r_j} e^{z_{jl}\beta} - \frac{(k-1)}{d_j} \sum_{l \in D_j} e^{z_{jl}\beta} \right] \right),$$

where D_j is the set of indices for the subjects failing at time t_j and $s_j = \sum_{l \in D_j} z_{jl}$.

7.4.4 Estimation and Testing

Using the Breslow approximation, the score statistic is

$$
\begin{aligned}
U(\beta) &= \frac{\partial}{\partial \beta} L(\beta) \\
&= \sum_j s_j - d_j \frac{\sum_{l=1}^{r_j} z_{jl} e^{z_{jl}\beta}}{\sum_{l=1}^{r_j} e^{z_{jl}\beta}} \\
&= \sum_j s_j - d_j \bar{z}_j,
\end{aligned}
$$

where $\bar{z}_j$ is a weighted mean of the covariate values for the subjects at risk at time t, weighted by the hazard ratios $e^{z_{jl}\beta}$. Hence the MLE, $\hat{\beta}$, satisfies an equation of the form observed $-$ expected $= 0$.

The Fisher information is

$$
\begin{aligned}
I(\beta) &= -\frac{\partial}{\partial \beta} U(\beta) \\
&= \sum_j d_j \frac{\sum_{l=1}^{r_j} z_{jl}^2 e^{z_{jl}\beta}}{\sum_{l=1}^{r_j} e^{z_{jl}\beta}} - d_j \left(\frac{\sum_{l=1}^{r_j} z_{jl} e^{z_{jl}\beta}}{\sum_{l=1}^{r_j} e^{z_{jl}\beta}} \right)^2 \\
&= \sum_j d_j \frac{\sum_{l=1}^{r_j} (z_{jl} - \bar{z}_j)^2 e^{z_{jl}\beta}}{\sum_{l=1}^{r_j} e^{z_{jl}\beta}}.
\end{aligned}
$$

Point estimates of $\hat{\beta}$ along with standard errors are computed in the usual way, along with the usual battery of tests: score, Wald, and likelihood ratio.

Now consider the special case in which we have a single binary covariate, taking values zero or one. Suppose we wish to test $H_0: \beta = 0$ using the score test. Then s_j is the number of subjects failing at time t_j with covariate value 1, which in the notation in section 7.3.2 is d_{j1}. Also, under H_0 the hazard ratios $e^{z_{jl}\beta}$ are identically equal to one and $\bar{z}_j$ is simply the proportion of subjects at risk for which $z = 1$, which, again in the notation in section 7.3.2, is $E[d_j] = n_{j1}/n_{j\cdot}$. Therefore,

$$
\begin{aligned}
U(0) &= \sum_j s_{j1} - d_j \bar{z}_j \\
&= \sum_j d_{j1} - d_j n_{j1}/n_{j\cdot}.
\end{aligned}
$$

The Fisher information becomes

$$
\begin{aligned}
I(0) &= \sum_j d_j \frac{\sum_{l=1}^{r_j} z_{jl}^2 e^{z_{jl}\beta}}{\sum_{l=1}^{r_j} e^{z_{jl}\beta}} - d_j \left(\frac{\sum_{l=1}^{r_j} z_{jl} e^{z_{jl}\beta}}{\sum_{l=1}^{r_j} e^{z_{jl}\beta}} \right)^2 \\
&= \sum_j d_j \left(\frac{n_{j1}}{n_{j\cdot}} - \frac{n_{j1}^2}{n_{j\cdot}^2} \right) \\
&= \sum_j \frac{d_j n_{j1} n_{j2}}{n_{j\cdot}^2}.
\end{aligned}
\tag{7.8}
$$

Hence, the score test reduces essentially to the log-rank test of section 7.3.2. Note that the Fisher information based on the Breslow approximation differs from the hypergeometric variance by a factor of $(n_{j\cdot} - 1)/(n_{j\cdot} - d_{j\cdot})$, which is one in the event that there are no ties, but otherwise may be slightly larger than one.

Example 7.9. Revisiting the BHAT example, the estimate of the log hazard ratio from the Cox proportional hazards model is $\beta = -0.326$, corresponding to a hazard ratio of $\exp(-.326) = .722$. The standard error of β obtained from the Fisher information matrix is 0.112, so the Wald test yields a chi-square statistic of 8.45 which is quite close to that of the log-rank test in Example 7.8.

We can also consider the effect of baseline covariates on death and compute the hazard ratio for treatment adjusted for baseline covariates. Table 7.1 summarizes the model that includes treatment, age, and sex. We see that the adjusted log hazard ratio for treatment changes from -0.326 to -0.317 (a clinically and statistically insignificant difference), the effect of age is quite large (HR = 1.58 for a 10 year increase in age), and the effect of sex is not significant by either Wald test or likelihood ratio test.

Table 7.1 *Cox proportional hazards model for BHAT. Treatment is coded as 1=propranolol, 0=placebo, and sex is coded as 1=female, 0=male. The likelihood ratio chi-square for the model without the sex term is 51.0 (2 df).*

	β	se(β)	Z	p-value
Treatment	-0.3172	0.11212	-2.829	0.0047
Age	0.0463	0.00738	6.269	<0.0001
Sex	-0.0711	0.14986	-0.474	0.64

Likelihood ratio chi-square: 51.2 (3 df) p <0.001

Next we consider the effect of race, which is coded with four levels: "White", "Black", "Asian", and "Other." We note from Table 7.2 that there is a highly significant difference between "Black" and "White" ($p < 0.001$); however, more appropriate is a simultaneous test of the effect of race, which cannot be achieved using coefficients in Table 7.2 without knowledge of the full covariance matrix. Instead, the likelihood ratio test can be constructed by using the difference in the likelihood ratio chi-square statistics between the model containing only treatment and age and the model with treatment, age, and race: $64.7 = 51.0$ with 3 degrees of freedom $p = 0.033$.   □

Table 7.2 *Cox proportional hazards model for BHAT. **Treatment** is coded as 1=pro-pranolol, 0=placebo, reference category for **race** is "White."*

	β	se(β)	Z	p-value
Treatment	-0.312	0.112	-2.781	0.0054
Age	0.047	0.007	6.432	< 0.001
Race				
Black	0.633	0.160	3.962	< 0.001
Asian	-0.128	0.504	-0.254	0.80
Other	0.178	0.581	0.306	0.761

Likelihood chi-square: 64.7 (5 df) $p < 0.001$

7.4.5 Estimation of the baseline hazard Λ_0

In the case where we have no ties, we can estimate the baseline hazard function, $\Lambda_0(t)$, as follows. Given $\hat{\beta}$ from Cox-model, $\hat{S}_0(t) = \prod_{t_j \leq t} \hat{\alpha}_j$ (see Kalbfleisch and Prentice (1980)) where

$$\hat{\alpha}_j = \left(1 - \frac{e^{\hat{\beta} z_j}}{\sum_{R_j} e^{\hat{\beta} z_l}} \right)^{e^{\hat{\beta} z_j}}.$$

We also have

$$\hat{\Lambda}_0(t) = \log \hat{S}_0(t).$$

In the case where we have ties, the Breslow estimate of $\Lambda_0(t)$ is

$$\hat{\Lambda}_0(t) = \sum_{t_i \leq t} \frac{d_i}{\sum_{R_i} e^{\hat{\beta} z_j}}.$$

7.4.6 Residuals

Similar to ordinary linear regression, examination of residuals can be useful in assessing model assumptions and fit. In the setting of the Cox proportional hazards model, however, the definition of the residuals is not as clear. Four commonly used types of residuals for Cox proportional hazards models are

Martingale: The Martingale residuals are defined as $\hat{M}_i = \delta_i - \hat{\Lambda}_0(t_i)\exp(\hat{\beta}z_i)$ where δ_i is the outcome for subject i (0 or 1) and $\hat{\Lambda}_0(t_i)$ is the baseline cumulative hazard at the end of observation for subject i. This residual is the difference between the outcome and its expected value, given the length of follow-up.

Deviance: $d_i = \text{sign}(\hat{M}_i)\sqrt{2[-\hat{M}_i - \delta_i \log(\delta_i - \hat{M}_i)]}$. The sum of the squares of the deviance residuals is twice the log-partial likelihood ratio $2(\log L(\hat{\beta}) - \log L(0))$.

Score: $(z_i - \bar{z}(t_i))\delta_i - \sum_{j:s_j \leq t_i}(z_i - \bar{z}(t_i))e^{\hat{\beta}z_i}d_j / \sum_{l \in R_j} e^{\hat{\beta}z_l}$ where $t_1, t_2, \ldots$ are the distinct failure times and $\bar{z}(s) = \sum_{l \in R_j} z_l e^{\hat{\beta}z_l} / \sum_{l \in R_j} e^{\hat{\beta}z_l}$. The sum of the score residuals is the score function $U(\hat{\beta})$ and hence is zero.

Schoenfeld: Schoenfeld residuals are defined for each event and have the form $z_j - \bar{z}(t_i)$. The Schoenfeld residuals are useful for identifying departures from the proportional hazards assumption.

See Wei (1984), Therneau, Grambsch, and Fleming (1990), Grambsch and Therneau (1994), and Grambsch, Therneau, and Fleming (1995) (and others) for procedures making use of residuals for diagnosing lack of fit in proportional hazards models.

7.5 Composite Outcomes

Recall the discussion in Chapter 2 regarding the composite failure-time outcomes (Section 2.5.2). There we presented a simple example of how mortality and nonfatal events interact to make interpretation of the result for the nonfatal event difficult. In this section we make the discussion more precise by defining the quantities of potential interest.

Statistically, the primary conclusion of the trial will be based on the results of a test of a hypothesis of the form $H_0 : \mu_0 = \mu_1$ where μ_j is a parameter of interest for treatment group $j, j = 0, 1$. Now suppose that we have a single type of nonfatal event. Let X be the time of the nonfatal event, and Y the time of death from any cause. Note that for subjects who die prior to experiencing the nonfatal event, we consider X to be undefined. There are several parameters upon which the primary statistical inference could potentially be based.

- $\lambda_N(t)$ is the hazard function at time t for the nonfatal event in the case where there is no competing risk of death. In the case where death is a competing risk, however, this quantity is not defined, and therefore can neither be estimated nor used to construct a valid assessment of treatment effect.

- $r(t) = \lim_{h \to 0} \Pr\{X \in (t, t+h] | X > t, Y > t\}/h$ which is known as the *cause specific hazard function* and is similar to the usual hazard function;

it differs in that it is conditional on the subject being alive at time t in addition to not having experienced the nonfatal event before time t.

- $\lambda_C(t)$ is the hazard function for the composite outcome of event-free survival, i.e., the hazard function for the earliest of the death time or the nonfatal event time.

Ideally, we could use $\lambda_N(t)$ as the parameter of interest for assessing the effect of treatment on the nonfatal outcome. Unfortunately because this quantity is not defined when death is a competing risk, alternative approaches are required.

The quantity $r(t)$ is always well defined and it, or the effect of treatment on it, can be easily estimated using either standard parametric or nonparametric estimates by treating death as a censoring mechanism. Because $r(t)$ is defined to be conditional on survival, we do not require the assumption that mortality constitutes "non-informative censoring." Similarly, the usual log-rank (or weighted log-rank) test can be used for testing hypotheses regarding the effect of treatment on this function. Note, however, that because subjects are required to be alive at time t, an effect of treatment on mortality will also affect the value of $r(t)$ even when there is no direct effect of treatment on the nonfatal outcome, similar to that seen in Table 2.5. Unfortunately, it is common practice for estimates of $r(t)$ to be used as estimates of the effect of treatment on the nonfatal outcome, apparently under the mistaken assumption that $\hat{r}(t) = \hat{\lambda}_N(t)$.

Since it combines fatal and nonfatal events, $\lambda_C(t)$, or associated treatment effects, can be estimated directly using standard methods (parametric or nonparametric) and the log-rank tests are valid tests of the effect of treatment on the event-free survival without additional assumptions regarding the association between fatal and nonfatal events.

The primary difficulty with using the composite outcome lies in its clinical interpretation. Strictly speaking, the assessment of the treatment effect on the composite must be interpreted as exactly that—attempts to decompose the effect into separate effects on the fatal and nonfatal components cannot be formally made on statistical grounds. Consequently, it is not possible to make statements regarding the independent effect of treatment on the nonfatal component without appealing to external factors such as clinical judgment or mechanistic biological models.

See the recommendations given in Section 2.5.2 for further discussion.

7.6 Summary

Survival analysis may be the most widely applied analytic approach in the analysis clinical trial data, certainly in disease areas such cancer and cardiology. The techniques described in this chapter are widely understood and accepted. The primary point of contention regards censored observations. Administrative censoring, i.e., censoring resulting from a subject reaching a predetermined study end, usually satisfies the required conditions that it be independent of outcome. Time trends in the underlying risk, so that baseline risk varies with time of enrollment, can induce a dependence leading to bias in Kaplan-Meier estimates; however, in randomized trials, there should be no corresponding bias in the hypothesis tests of interest.

A larger concern regards censoring which is not independent of outcome. Loss to follow-up may be both outcome and treatment dependent, so assessment of study discontinuation rates are important. Even when the rates are comparable among treatment groups, there is no guarantee, however, that when rates are high that bias has not been introduced. Sensitivity analyses such as those described in Chapter 11 (see Scharfstein, Rotnitzky, and Robins (1999), for example) can be helpful in understanding the potential impact of early study discontinuation. In the case of survival outcomes, the analysis is much more complex than the simple example we present.

A common source of dependent censoring (although we prefer the term "truncation" following Frangakis and Rubin (2002)) is death from causes not included in the outcome of interest. Frequently, especially in cardiology, deaths from non-cardiovascular causes are excluded from the primary outcome with the expectation that the treatment will have no effect, and therefore such deaths serve to dilute the observed difference, requiring a larger sample size. While this rationale is appealing, there are methodological difficulties because, as we have pointed out, the parameter of interest is no longer a hazard rate in the usual sense, but the additional condition that subjects be alive at the a specified time is imposed (see page 227). Since we cannot statistically rule out the possibility of a complex interaction between treatment, death, and the outcome of interest, these comparisons are inherently problematic. More troubling are secondary analyses of nonfatal components in which subjects are "censored at death." While these analyses will almost certainly be requested by investigators in many settings, one should always keep in mind that there are potential biases lurking in the background.

7.7 Problems

7.1 Show that the exponential distribution is "memoryless", i.e., if T has an exponential distribution, $\Pr\{T > t | T > t_0\} = \Pr\{T > t - t_0\}$.

7.2 Suppose that we have 20 patients, 10 per treatment group, and we observe the following survival times:

$$A: \quad 8+, 11+, 16+, 18+, 23, 24, 26, 28, 30, 31$$
$$B: \quad 9, 12, 13, 14, 14, 16, 19+, 22+, 23+, 29+$$

where the '+' indicates a censored observation.

(a) Compute and plot the Kaplan-Meier estimate of survival for the combined group and for each treatment group.

(b) Test equality of treatments using the log-rank test and the Gehan-Wilcoxon test.

7.3 Recall that one way of computing the expectation of a positive random variable is by integrating one minus the cumulative distribution function. When dealing with a survival time T, this means

$$E[T] = \int_0^\infty S(t)dt.$$

This is sometimes referred to as the *unrestricted mean life*. One quantity often used to estimate this mean is obtained by using the Kaplan-Meier estimate for S, giving the total area under the Kaplan-Meier curve.

(a) Show that, in the absence of censoring, the unrestricted mean life estimate is equal to the sample mean.

(b) Calculate the unrestricted mean life estimate for the combined group data from the previous exercise.

(c) What would happen if you tried to calculate the estimate for group B only?

CHAPTER 8

Longitudinal Data

Longitudinal data arise when an outcome variable such as pulmonary function, exercise testing, or quality of life is measured repeatedly over time. Standard approaches such as ordinary least squares (OLS) assume that errors are independent and identically distributed (i.i.d.). For longitudinal (or repeated measures) data, the i.i.d. assumption breaks down because individual observations are naturally associated with larger groups or *clusters*—two data points taken from one cluster will likely be more similar to one another than two data points taken from different subjects. Usually the clusters comprise repeated observations from individual subjects, although there can be other types of clusters such as clinical trial sites, schools, and geographical regions. In this chapter we will discuss a number of ways to model this correlation and account for it in assessing treatment differences. While the techniques discussed in this chapter can be easily adapted to other types of clustering, we will assume throughout that clusters correspond to subjects.

To motivate our approaches to longitudinal data, we begin with a simple, straight-line, regression model with independent errors

$$y_j = \beta_1 + \beta_2 \, t_j + e_j$$

where $j = 1, \ldots, n$ and n is the number of observations. Here β_1 is the intercept and β_2 is the slope. It is convenient to write the model in matrix form,

$$\boldsymbol{y} = \boldsymbol{X}\boldsymbol{\beta} + \boldsymbol{e}$$

where $\boldsymbol{X}$ is an n by 2 matrix with a column of 1's and a column of the t_j values. If we assume the errors are i.i.d. with mean zero, the familiar OLS estimator for $\boldsymbol{\beta}$ is

$$\hat{\boldsymbol{\beta}} = (\boldsymbol{X}^T \boldsymbol{X})^{-1} \boldsymbol{X}^T \boldsymbol{y}.$$

Of course, the model for the expectation function (the expected value of the right hand side of any regression equation) can be more complex (e.g., a higher order polynomial). As long as the expectation function is a linear function of the parameters and the errors are i.i.d. with zero mean, the OLS estimator is appropriate.

As we have noted, if multiple observations are collected from each subject, and a single expectation function is used for all subjects, the errors will usually not be i.i.d.—they will be correlated within subjects. This requires a more complex error term. Consider the model:

$$y_{ij} = \beta_1 + \beta_2 \, t_{ij} + \delta_{ij}$$

where $i = 1, \ldots, m$ and m is the number of subjects. We can write this in matrix form as:

$$\boldsymbol{y}_i = \boldsymbol{X}\boldsymbol{\beta} + \boldsymbol{\delta}_i$$

Here the δ_{ij} are not assumed to be i.i.d. within subject and a more complex correlation structure is required to model the within-subject correlation. Models of this type are called *population average* models and are discussed in Section 8.5. The term *population average* is used because the expectation function includes only parameters that are common to all subjects ($\boldsymbol{\beta}$). The most common method for estimating the parameters in population average models is generalized least squares.

The model we will discuss to begin in this chapter is the *subject-specific* model

$$y_{ij} = \beta_{i1} + \beta_{i2}\, t_{ij} + e_{ij}$$

or in matrix form

$$\boldsymbol{y}_i = \boldsymbol{X}\boldsymbol{\beta}_i + \boldsymbol{e}_i.$$

The term *subject-specific* is used because the parameters ($\boldsymbol{\beta}_i$) in the expectation function vary by subject. This allows the fitted values to vary from subject to subject which means it may be still acceptable to assume the e_{ij} are i.i.d.. The subject-specific model is described in detail in Section 8.2. There are a number of approaches to estimating parameters in this model including two-stage/OLS estimation (Section 8.3) and random-effect/maximum-likelihood estimation (Section 8.4).

In the remaining portion of this chapter, we describe an alternative to maximum likelihood estimation called restricted maximum likelihood (Section 8.6), standard errors and testing (Sections 8.7 and 8.8), additional levels of clustering (Section 8.9), and the impact of various types of missing data on the interpretation of the estimates (Section 8.11).

8.1 A Clinical Longitudinal Data Example

Smith et al. (1989) report the results of a study of 169 women aged 35-65, randomly assigned to either placebo and calcium supplementation treatment. Bone mineral content (BMC) was measured at several locations in the arm of each subject 11 times: at 3 month intervals the first year and 6 month intervals for the next 3 years. The primary outcome measure was the average rate of change of BMC during follow-up. The goal of the trial was to determine if calcium supplementation would prevent or decrease bone loss. If we assume that BMC changes linearly with time in each treatment group, two statistical models that we could use are:

$$\text{BMC} = \beta_0 + \beta_1 t + \beta_2 z + \beta_3 tz + \epsilon \tag{8.1}$$

and

$$\text{BMC} = \beta_0 + \beta_1 t + \beta_3 tz + \epsilon, \tag{8.2}$$

where β_0, β_1, β_2, and β_3 are model parameters, t is time from randomization, z is an indicator treatment ($z = 0$ for subjects assigned placebo and $z = 1$ for subjects assigned calcium supplementation), and ϵ is a mean zero random error term. Note that in each model, β_3 is the time-treatment interaction and represents the difference in slopes between the two treatment groups and, therefore, the hypothesis of interest is $H_0: \beta_3 = 0$.

The difference between these models is that model (8.1) contains a main effect for treatment whereas model (8.2) does not. In model (8.1), β_2 represents the mean difference at $t = 0$ between treatment groups and any differences at baseline are due to random variation. Because the trial is randomized, the population mean BMC at $t = 0$ must be the same for the two groups. Assuming that the model is correct (linear change in BMC with time), including a main effect term is unnecessary and may reduce power for comparison of slopes by a small amount. Fitzmaurice, Laird, and Ware (2004) and Thisted (2006) suggest that in randomized trials, model (8.2) should be preferred to (8.1) solely on the grounds that it is more efficient. We recommend the use of (8.2) for another, arguably more important, reason. If model (8.2) is correct, i.e., BMC changes linearly with time in each treatment group, $\hat{\beta}_3$, the estimate of β_3 obtained using the methods in this chapter is unbiased. On the other hand, if the true relationship between BMC and time is non-linear in a treatment dependent way, fitting model (8.1) may yield an estimate of β_2 which is biased away from zero, and the interpretation of the estimates of β_3 will be unclear. As we will argue using a simple example, model (8.2) is more robust to departures from linearity, and should be preferred on that basis. While one might argue that when model (8.2) does not fit the observed data a more suitable model should be used, unfortunately, the statistical tests for treatment benefit should be prespecified and not dependent on observed data. If the original model assumptions are shown to be incorrect after data are collected, supplementary analysis using more appropriate models can be performed; however, the prespecified analysis carries the most weight, and, therefore, should be as robust as possible against departures from assumptions.

We illustrate using the simple, hypothetical responses shown in Figure 8.1(a) (for the sake of the example, we show population means and ignore random error). In this example, the placebo subjects decline linearly while the responses for the treated subjects remain constant during the first time interval, then decline. Because model (8.1) has both a main effect and time-treatment interaction, it can be fit by estimating the slopes and intercepts separately for each group. For the placebo group the response is linear so the best line fits the data exactly (dashed line). The treated subjects do not decline linearly (so neither (8.1) nor (8.2) actually fits the data) and the "best line" is shown by the solid line. In this example the intercept for the line fit to the treated group is not the baseline value and the slopes of the best lines fit to each group separately are the same. That is, the time-treatment interaction is zero, despite there being a clear effect of treatment. Because the model assumptions are

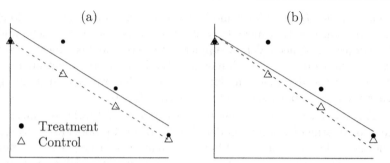

Figure 8.1 *Longitudinal data for which equation (8.1) does not hold. The symbols represent the true population means, the solid line represents the fitted line for Treatment, and the dashed line represents the fitted line for Control. Fitted lines in panel (a) are based on model (8.1) and in (b) are based on model (8.2).*

violated, the difference between groups is captured not by the time-treatment interaction, but by the main effect for treatment; i.e., the difference between the intercepts for the "best lines" fit to each group which is also the mean difference between groups over time.

Conversely, by fitting model (8.2) to these data, we force the intercepts for each line to be the same and, therefore, the treatment difference is captured, albeit crudely, by the time-treatment interaction, $\hat{\beta}_3$. Figure 8.1(b) shows the same data with lines representing the fitted model (8.2). While admittedly neither line fits the data very well and the common intercept doesn't have an obvious interpretation, the estimated difference in slopes, $\hat{\beta}_3$, represents, to some degree, the difference between groups in the average rate of change over the follow-up period and this difference can be used for a valid test of $H_0: \beta_3 = 0$. That is, under H_0, $E[\hat{\beta}_3] = 0$ for model (8.2), even if the change over time is not linear, provided that the follow-up times are the same in each group. Thus, in addition to being more efficient, model (8.2) is more robust to departures from the model assumptions and is preferable in practice.

8.2 The Subject-specific Model

To illustrate the model and some of the computations involved with longitudinal data we will use a very simple (non-clinical trial) example described in Grizzle and Allen (1969). Ramus (jaw bone) height of 20 boys was measured at 8, 8.5, 9, and 9.5 years of age. The goal of this analysis is to establish a normal growth curve for use by orthodontists. We will start with a subset of 3 boys (listed in Table 8.1 and plotted in Figure 8.2) to illustrate some models and methods.

For simplicity, we will initially assume that each subject has observations at the same set of time points $t_1, \ldots t_n$. Here $t_1 = 8$, $t_2 = 8.5$, $t_3 = 9$, and $t_4 = 9.5$

Table 8.1 *Ramus height of 3 boys measured at 8, 8.5, 9, and 9.5 years of age.*

Subject	Age	Ramus Height
2	8.0	46.4
2	8.5	47.3
2	9.0	47.7
2	9.5	48.4
8	8.0	49.8
8	8.5	50.0
8	9.0	50.3
8	9.5	52.7
10	8.0	45.0
10	8.5	47.0
10	9.0	47.3
10	9.5	48.3

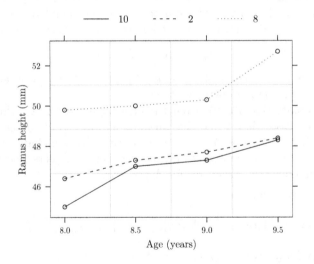

Figure 8.2 *Ramus height of 3 boys measured at 8, 8.5, 9, and 9.5 years of age.*

for each boy. It seems reasonable to assume a (straight line) linear model for the responses from the ith subject: $y_{ij} = \beta_{i1} + \beta_{i2} t_j + e_{ij}$, $j = 1, 2, 3, 4$, $i = 1, 2, 3$ where y_{ij} is the jth observation on the ith subject and t_j is the jth time point (assumed to be the same for all subjects), e.g., $y_{13} = 47.7$ (mm) and $t_{32} = 8.5$ (years). We also assume that $E[e_{ij}] = 0$. The models for all of the observations for subject i are

$$
\begin{aligned}
y_{i1} &= \beta_{i1} + \beta_{i2}\, t_1 + e_{i1} \\
y_{i2} &= \beta_{i1} + \beta_{i2}\, t_2 + e_{i2} \\
y_{i3} &= \beta_{i1} + \beta_{i2}\, t_2 + e_{i2} \\
y_{i4} &= \beta_{i1} + \beta_{i2}\, t_4 + e_{i4}.
\end{aligned}
$$

These can be rewritten in matrix form as

$$
\begin{bmatrix} y_{i1} \\ y_{i2} \\ y_{i3} \\ y_{i4} \end{bmatrix}
= \beta_{i1} \begin{bmatrix} 1 \\ 1 \\ 1 \\ 1 \end{bmatrix}
+ \beta_{i2} \begin{bmatrix} t_1 \\ t_2 \\ t_3 \\ t_4 \end{bmatrix}
+ \begin{bmatrix} e_{i1} \\ e_{i2} \\ e_{i3} \\ e_{i4} \end{bmatrix},
$$

or equivalently

$$
\boldsymbol{y}_i =
\begin{bmatrix} 1 & t_1 \\ 1 & t_2 \\ 1 & t_3 \\ 1 & t_4 \end{bmatrix}
\begin{bmatrix} \beta_{i1} \\ \beta_{i2} \end{bmatrix}
+ \boldsymbol{e}_i = \boldsymbol{X}_i \boldsymbol{\beta}_i + \boldsymbol{e}_i,
$$

where the design matrix $\boldsymbol{X}_i$ is the same for all i. We will keep the subscript, i, for generality. Now that we have notation for the complete error vector for subject i we can write down a more complete distributional assumption:

$$
\boldsymbol{e}_i \sim \mathcal{N}(\boldsymbol{0}_4, \sigma^2 \boldsymbol{\Lambda}_i(\boldsymbol{\phi}))
$$

where $\boldsymbol{0}_4$ is a 4 by 1 vector of zeros and $\boldsymbol{\Lambda}_i(\boldsymbol{\phi})$ is a 4 by 4 correlation matrix that depends on the parameter vector $\boldsymbol{\phi}$.

The possibility that $\boldsymbol{\Lambda}_i(\boldsymbol{\phi})$ is not the identity matrix makes this a *general linear model*. Note that while the variance parameter vector $\boldsymbol{\phi}$ is common among subjects, the subscript i on the matrices $\boldsymbol{\Lambda}_i$ is included to allow for the situation where the observation times vary over subjects (more details to follow). Some possible structures for $\boldsymbol{\Lambda}_i(\boldsymbol{\phi})$ are:

- General correlation matrix

$$
[\boldsymbol{\Lambda}_i(\boldsymbol{\phi})]_{hk} = [\boldsymbol{\Lambda}_i(\boldsymbol{\phi})]_{kh} =
\begin{cases}
\phi_{hk} & \text{for } h \neq k \\
1 & \text{for } h = k
\end{cases}
$$

where $[\boldsymbol{\Lambda}_i(\boldsymbol{\phi})]_{hk}$ is the h, k entry of $\boldsymbol{\Lambda}_i(\boldsymbol{\phi})$.

- Independence

$$
\boldsymbol{\Lambda}_i(\boldsymbol{\phi}) = \boldsymbol{I}_{4\times 4}
$$

where $\boldsymbol{I}_{4\times 4}$ is the 4×4 identity matrix.

- Equal correlation (*compound symmetric*, or *exchangeable*)

$$
\boldsymbol{\Lambda}_i(\boldsymbol{\phi}) =
\begin{bmatrix}
1 & \phi & \phi & \phi \\
\phi & 1 & \phi & \phi \\
\phi & \phi & 1 & \phi \\
\phi & \phi & \phi & 1
\end{bmatrix}.
$$

- Toeplitz (for equally spaced time points)

$$\mathbf{\Lambda}_i(\phi) = \begin{bmatrix} 1 & \phi_1 & \phi_2 & \phi_3 \\ \phi_1 & 1 & \phi_1 & \phi_2 \\ \phi_2 & \phi_1 & 1 & \phi_1 \\ \phi_3 & \phi_2 & \phi_1 & 1 \end{bmatrix}.$$

- AR(1) (*auto-regressive* 1) correlation for equally spaced observations

$$\mathbf{\Lambda}_i(\phi) = \begin{bmatrix} 1 & \phi & \phi^2 & \phi^3 \\ \phi & 1 & \phi & \phi^2 \\ \phi^2 & \phi & 1 & \phi \\ \phi^3 & \phi^2 & \phi & 1 \end{bmatrix}$$

or, in general

$$[\mathbf{\Lambda}_i(\phi)]_{hk} = \phi^{|h-k|}.$$

- General AR(1) correlation

$$[\mathbf{\Lambda}_i(\phi)]_{hk} = \phi^{|t_h - t_k|},$$

or equivalently

- Exponential correlation

$$[\mathbf{\Lambda}_i(\phi)]_{hk} = e^{\phi|t_h - t_k|}.$$

8.3 Two-stage Estimation

One of the simplest and most intuitive methods for estimating the parameters in the subject-specific linear model is two-stage estimation.

Stage 1 Fit the model for each subject separately. If we assume the observations within each subject are independent $(\mathbf{\Lambda}_i(\phi) = \mathbf{I})$ then

$$\hat{\boldsymbol{\beta}}_i = (\mathbf{X}_i^T \mathbf{X}_i)^{-1} \mathbf{X}_i^T \mathbf{y}_i.$$

For the Ramus height data the coefficients from each fit are the intercept and the slope. We have two numbers summarizing the data for each subject (an intercept and a slope) rather than the original 4 (ramus height at each of 4 time points).

Stage 2 Analyze the estimated coefficients. The most common second stage analysis is to calculate means and standard errors of the parameters calculated in the first stage. Other options include calculating the area under the curve, and the value of the curve or its derivatives at prespecified times. In this case we calculate the means:

Intercept	age
33.41667	1.706667

and use them to plot an estimated "typical" or "average" growth curve (Figure 8.3). We can also calculate standard errors and test hypotheses of

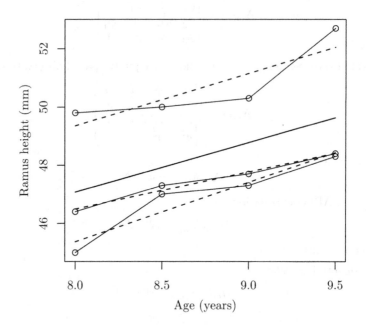

Figure 8.3 *Ramus height of 3 boys. The dashed lines correspond to subject fits. The light solid lines connect each subject's data points and the heavy solid line corresponds to the mean estimated coefficients:* $33.417 + 1.707$Age.

interest. The standard errors of the means of the coefficients are correct since they rely only on the independence of the estimates from different boys.

If the data are likely to be serially correlated (after all we are assuming a general linear model), there are two options

1. Assume a specific correlation structure (e.g., AR(1)) and find maximum likelihood estimates,[1] $\hat{\beta}_i$, $\hat{\sigma}_i$, and $\hat{\phi}_i$ for each subject. The log-likelihood for subject i has the multivariate normal (MVN) form

$$-\log(|\sigma_i^2 \Lambda_i(\phi_i)|) - (y_i - X_i\beta_i)^T [\sigma_i^2 \Lambda_i(\phi_i)]^{-1} (y_i - X_i\beta_i).$$

(For a matrix A, $|A|$ is the determinant of A.) We have added a subscript i to the variance parameters σ and ϕ since model fitting is done separately for each subject. Because there is only one observation at each time for each subject, a parsimonious correlation structure must be used—the general

[1] See Appendix A.2 for a discussion of likelihood inference.

correlation matrix has too many parameters to estimate in the first stage of two-stage estimation.

The maximum likelihood estimator for $\boldsymbol{\beta}_i$ has a closed form (given $\hat{\sigma}_i$ and $\hat{\boldsymbol{\phi}}_i$):

$$\hat{\boldsymbol{\beta}}_i = (\boldsymbol{X}_i^T(\hat{\sigma}_i^2\boldsymbol{\Lambda}_i(\hat{\boldsymbol{\phi}}_i))^{-1}\boldsymbol{X}_i)^{-1}\boldsymbol{X}_i^T(\hat{\sigma}_i^2\boldsymbol{\Lambda}_i(\hat{\boldsymbol{\phi}}_i))^{-1}\boldsymbol{y}.$$

This is also the generalized least squares (GLS) estimate. Furthermore, conditional on $\hat{\sigma}_i$ and $\hat{\boldsymbol{\phi}}_i$,

$$\mathrm{Var}(\hat{\boldsymbol{\beta}}_i) = (\boldsymbol{X}_i^T(\hat{\sigma}_i^2\boldsymbol{\Lambda}_i(\hat{\boldsymbol{\phi}}_i))^{-1}\boldsymbol{X}_i)^{-1}.$$

2. Ignore the correlation structure and assume independence. Note that in this case,

   - some efficiency is lost (relative to an estimation procedure that assumes the *correct* correlation structure),
   - estimates of $\boldsymbol{\beta}_i$ are unbiased, and
   - standard errors for $\hat{\boldsymbol{\beta}}_i$ are not correct, but this is not a problem because they are not used in the next stage.

The second option is what is commonly used because assuming the wrong correlation structure can result in poor performance because additional variance parameters need to be estimated (Carroll and Ruppert 1988).

The two-stage estimation method requires that reliable estimates of $\hat{\beta}_i$ can be obtained. In cases for which insufficient data are available for some subjects to reliably estimate $\hat{\beta}_i$ the two-stage method may not perform well.

8.3.1 Combined Estimation

In the two-stage analysis, even if we assume that observations within subjects are correlated $(\boldsymbol{\Lambda}_i(\boldsymbol{\phi}_i) \neq \boldsymbol{I})$, we do not pool information across subjects to estimate variance parameters. It may be better to obtain pooled estimates of the parameters in $\boldsymbol{\Lambda}_i$ assuming they are the same for all subjects. We start by writing our individual (subject-specific) models as one large regression model.

$$\begin{bmatrix} \boldsymbol{y}_1 \\ \boldsymbol{y}_2 \\ \boldsymbol{y}_3 \end{bmatrix}_{3n \times 1} = \begin{bmatrix} \boldsymbol{X}_1 & \boldsymbol{0} & \boldsymbol{0} \\ \boldsymbol{0} & \boldsymbol{X}_2 & \boldsymbol{0} \\ \boldsymbol{0} & \boldsymbol{0} & \boldsymbol{X}_3 \end{bmatrix}_{3n \times 3p} \begin{bmatrix} \beta_1 \\ \beta_2 \\ \beta_3 \end{bmatrix}_{3p \times 1} + \begin{bmatrix} e_1 \\ e_2 \\ e_3 \end{bmatrix}_{3n \times 1}$$

or

$$\boldsymbol{y} = \mathrm{Diag}(\boldsymbol{X}_1, \boldsymbol{X}_2, \boldsymbol{X}_3) \begin{bmatrix} \beta_1 \\ \beta_2 \\ \beta_3 \end{bmatrix} + \boldsymbol{e} \tag{8.3}$$

where

$$\boldsymbol{e} \sim \mathcal{N}(\boldsymbol{0}, \sigma^2 \mathrm{Diag}(\boldsymbol{\Lambda}_1(\boldsymbol{\phi}), \boldsymbol{\Lambda}_2(\boldsymbol{\phi}), \boldsymbol{\Lambda}_3(\boldsymbol{\phi}))).$$

Note that the correlation parameters ϕ no longer have a subscript i because we are assuming they are common across subjects.

Case I: $\Lambda_i = I$

Since Equation 8.3 has the form of a standard linear regression, we can estimate the vector of β_i's using OLS (Ordinary Least Squares). The OLS calculation gives us:

$$\left(\begin{bmatrix} X_1 & 0 & 0 \\ 0 & X_2 & 0 \\ 0 & 0 & X_3 \end{bmatrix}^T \begin{bmatrix} X_1 & 0 & 0 \\ 0 & X_2 & 0 \\ 0 & 0 & X_3 \end{bmatrix} \right)^{-1}$$

$$= \begin{bmatrix} (X_1^T X_1)^{-1} & 0 & 0 \\ 0 & (X_2^T X_2)^{-1} & 0 \\ 0 & 0 & (X_3^T X_3)^{-1} \end{bmatrix}.$$

So

$$\begin{bmatrix} \hat{\beta}_1 \\ \hat{\beta}_2 \\ \hat{\beta}_3 \end{bmatrix} = \begin{bmatrix} (X_1^T X_1)^{-1} & 0 & 0 \\ 0 & (X_2^T X_2)^{-1} & 0 \\ 0 & 0 & (X_3^T X_3)^{-1} \end{bmatrix} \begin{bmatrix} X_1^T & 0 & 0 \\ 0 & X_2^T & 0 \\ 0 & 0 & X_3^T \end{bmatrix} y$$

$$= \begin{bmatrix} (X_1^T X_1)^{-1} X_1^T & 0 & 0 \\ 0 & (X_2^T X_2)^{-1} X_2^T & 0 \\ 0 & 0 & (X_3^T X_3)^{-1} X_3^T \end{bmatrix} \begin{bmatrix} y_1 \\ y_2 \\ y_3 \end{bmatrix}$$

$$= \begin{bmatrix} (X_1^T X_1)^{-1} X_1^T y_1 \\ (X_2^T X_2)^{-1} X_2^T y_2 \\ (X_3^T X_3)^{-1} X_3^T y_3 \end{bmatrix}.$$

So, under independence, the OLS estimates of the β_is are the same, whether we do the estimation individually or as one large regression problem. The estimate for the only variance parameter is

$$\hat{\sigma} = (y - \hat{y})^T (y - \hat{y})/(nM - pM)$$

where

$$\hat{y} = \begin{bmatrix} X_1 \hat{\beta}_1 \\ X_2 \hat{\beta}_2 \\ X_3 \hat{\beta}_3 \end{bmatrix}.$$

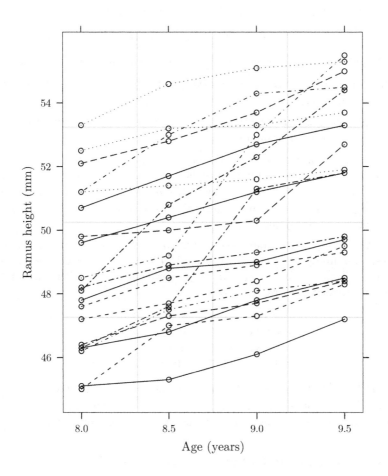

Figure 8.4 *Ramus height of all 20 boys.*

Case II: $\Lambda_i(\phi) \neq \boldsymbol{I}$

For these data we can start by assuming a general variance-covariance structure because the number of unique time points is low compared to the number
of individuals. Just as in the case where we assumed independence, we can
estimate $\boldsymbol{\beta}_i$, σ, and ϕ using maximum likelihood. The log-likelihood has the
MVN form

$$\sum_{i=1}^{M} -\log(|\sigma^2 \boldsymbol{\Lambda}_i(\phi)|) - (\boldsymbol{y}_i - \boldsymbol{X}_i \boldsymbol{\beta}_i)^T (\sigma^2 \boldsymbol{\Lambda}_i(\phi))^{-1} (\boldsymbol{y}_i - \boldsymbol{X}_i \boldsymbol{\beta}_i)$$

where M is the number of subjects (Laird and Ware 1982).

Once again, the maximum likelihood estimator for $\boldsymbol{\beta}_i$ (given $\hat{\sigma}$ and $\hat{\phi}$) has a closed form that is also the general least squares estimate:

$$\hat{\boldsymbol{\beta}}_i = (\boldsymbol{X}_i^T[\hat{\sigma}^2\boldsymbol{\Lambda}_i(\hat{\boldsymbol{\phi}})]^{-1}\boldsymbol{X}_i)^{-1}\boldsymbol{X}_i^T[\hat{\sigma}^2\boldsymbol{\Lambda}_i(\hat{\boldsymbol{\phi}})]^{-1}\boldsymbol{y}_i \qquad \text{for all } i$$

and, conditional on $\hat{\sigma}$ and $\hat{\boldsymbol{\phi}}$, $\text{Var}(\hat{\boldsymbol{\beta}}_i) = (\boldsymbol{X}_i^T[\hat{\sigma}^2\boldsymbol{\Lambda}_i(\hat{\boldsymbol{\phi}})]^{-1}\boldsymbol{X}_i)^{-1}$. Note that

- Standard errors for $\hat{\boldsymbol{\beta}}_i$ are only asymptotically correct since we are conditioning on knowing $\hat{\sigma}$ and $\hat{\boldsymbol{\phi}}$ when we don't.

- Complex correlation structures can be estimated since the data from subjects are pooled to estimate $\boldsymbol{\phi}$.

- We still have only estimates of the parameters for the individual curves and not the "typical" curve. One option is to use the fitted values corresponding to the mean of the $\hat{\boldsymbol{\beta}}_i$ as the typical curve. We know the (asymptotic) $\text{Var}(\hat{\boldsymbol{\beta}}_i)$ for all i, so we can calculate the (asymptotic) $\text{Var}(\text{Mean}(\hat{\boldsymbol{\beta}}_i))$, since the mean is a linear function.

For the entire Ramus data set the mean coefficients from the two-stage analysis (assuming independence) are $[33.7475, 1.866]^T$. From the combined maximum likelihood analysis (assuming general correlation with constant variance) the correlations are

$$\begin{bmatrix} 1.00 & -0.94 & -0.34 & 0.88 \\ -0.94 & 1.00 & 0.02 & -0.72 \\ -0.34 & 0.02 & 1.00 & -0.69 \\ 0.88 & -0.72 & -0.69 & 1.00 \end{bmatrix}.$$

$\hat{\sigma} = 0.271$ and the mean estimated parameters are $[33.7466, 1.866]^T$. The estimated intercept is very close to the estimate assuming independence and the slopes from the two models are identical to the precision shown.

8.4 The Random-effects, Subject-specific Model

For the subject-specific model we begin by proposing a model with the same form for each subject. In a random-effects, subject-specific model some or all of the parameters are assumed to have a probability distribution in the population of subjects. The assumed variance-covariance parameters along with any fixed effects (parameters in the expectation function) are typically estimated using either maximum likelihood or restricted maximum likelihood. Fixed effects can be thought of as the means of the random effects although (as described in what follows) it is possible to construct the model so that it includes fixed effects with no corresponding random effect.

8.4.1 The Model

If we assume a linear model for the data for each subject, the subject-specific model (with common variance parameters) is

$$\boldsymbol{y}_i = \boldsymbol{X}_i\boldsymbol{\beta}_i + \boldsymbol{e}_i, \quad i = 1, \ldots, M$$

$$e_i \sim \mathcal{N}(0, \sigma^2 \mathbf{\Lambda}_i(\boldsymbol{\phi})).$$

A natural additional assumption (random effects) is that the parameters $\boldsymbol{\beta}$ have a distribution among the population of subjects, say $\boldsymbol{\beta}_i = \boldsymbol{\beta} + \boldsymbol{b}_i$, where the random effects, $\boldsymbol{b}_i \sim \mathcal{N}(\mathbf{0}, \boldsymbol{D})$, represent the difference between the typical parameter values, $\boldsymbol{\beta}$, (the fixed effects) and the parameter values for subject i, $\boldsymbol{\beta}_i$. The complete model is:

$$\boldsymbol{y}_i = \boldsymbol{X}_i(\boldsymbol{\beta} + \boldsymbol{b}_i) + \boldsymbol{e}_i, \quad i = 1, \ldots, M$$

$$\boldsymbol{b}_i \sim \mathcal{N}(\mathbf{0}, \boldsymbol{D}_{p \times p}) \quad \boldsymbol{e}_i \sim \mathcal{N}\left(\mathbf{0}, \sigma^2 \mathbf{\Lambda}_i(\boldsymbol{\phi})\right).$$

Multiplying out we get $\boldsymbol{y}_i = \boldsymbol{X}_i \boldsymbol{\beta} + \boldsymbol{X}_i \boldsymbol{b}_i + \boldsymbol{e}_i, i = 1, \ldots, M$.

To make this model more general we allow the design matrix for the random effects to differ from the design for the fixed effects, $\boldsymbol{y}_i = \boldsymbol{X}_i \boldsymbol{\beta} + \boldsymbol{Z}_i \boldsymbol{b}_i + \boldsymbol{e}_i$, $i = 1, \ldots, M$, where $\boldsymbol{Z}_i$ is a $n \times q$ design matrix. This is useful when some parameters vary in the population and some do not. We know that since $\boldsymbol{b}_i$ is a length q MVN random variable then $\boldsymbol{Z}_i \boldsymbol{b}_i$ is a length n MVN random variable with distribution $\boldsymbol{Z}_i \boldsymbol{b}_i \sim \mathcal{N}\left(\mathbf{0}, \boldsymbol{Z}_i \boldsymbol{D} \boldsymbol{Z}_i^T\right)$ and it follows that

$$\boldsymbol{Z}_i \boldsymbol{b}_i + \boldsymbol{e}_i \sim \mathcal{N}\left(\mathbf{0}, \boldsymbol{Z}_i \boldsymbol{D} \boldsymbol{Z}_i^T + \sigma^2 \mathbf{\Lambda}_i(\boldsymbol{\phi})\right).$$

This allows us to write

$$\begin{aligned} \boldsymbol{y}_i &= \boldsymbol{X}_i \boldsymbol{\beta} + \boldsymbol{Z}_i \boldsymbol{b}_i + \boldsymbol{e}_i \\ &= \boldsymbol{X}_i \boldsymbol{\beta} + \boldsymbol{\delta}_i \end{aligned}$$

where $\boldsymbol{\delta}_i \sim \mathcal{N}(\mathbf{0}, \boldsymbol{\Sigma}_i(\boldsymbol{\alpha}))$ and $\boldsymbol{\Sigma}_i(\boldsymbol{\alpha}) = \boldsymbol{Z}_i \boldsymbol{D} \boldsymbol{Z}_i^T + \sigma^2 \mathbf{\Lambda}_i(\boldsymbol{\phi})$, or, equivalently,

$$\boldsymbol{y}_i \sim \mathcal{N}(\boldsymbol{X}_i \boldsymbol{\beta}, \boldsymbol{\Sigma}_i(\boldsymbol{\alpha})) \tag{8.4}$$

where $\boldsymbol{\alpha}$ is the vector containing all the variance parameters: $\sigma, \boldsymbol{\phi}$, and the unique entries in $\boldsymbol{D}$.

Equation 8.4 is the population average (or marginal) model for the data derived from the subject-specific (or conditional) random-effects model. See Section 8.5 for further discussion of these two modeling points of view. We can also derive the marginal density of $\boldsymbol{y}_i$ as

$$p(\boldsymbol{y}_i) = \int p(\boldsymbol{y}_i | \boldsymbol{b}_i) \, p(\boldsymbol{b}_i) \, d\boldsymbol{b}_i$$

where $\boldsymbol{y}_i | \boldsymbol{b}_i \sim \mathcal{N}(\boldsymbol{X}_i \boldsymbol{\beta} + \boldsymbol{Z}_i \boldsymbol{b}_i, \sigma^2 \mathbf{\Lambda}_i(\boldsymbol{\phi}))$, $\boldsymbol{b}_i \sim \mathcal{N}(\mathbf{0}, \boldsymbol{D})$ and $\boldsymbol{y}_i \sim \mathcal{N}(\boldsymbol{X}_i \boldsymbol{\beta}, \sigma^2 \mathbf{\Lambda}_i(\boldsymbol{\phi}) + \boldsymbol{Z}_i \boldsymbol{D} \boldsymbol{Z}_i^T)$.

8.4.2 Estimation for the Random-Effects Model

We estimate the fixed effects, $\boldsymbol{\beta}$, and the variance components, $\boldsymbol{\alpha}$, by maximizing the marginal log-likelihood which has the form

$$\sum_{i=1}^{M} -\log(|\boldsymbol{\Sigma}_i(\boldsymbol{\alpha})|) - \boldsymbol{r}_i(\boldsymbol{\beta})^T [\boldsymbol{\Sigma}_i(\boldsymbol{\alpha})]^{-1} \boldsymbol{r}_i(\boldsymbol{\beta})$$

where $r_i(\boldsymbol{\beta}) = \boldsymbol{y}_i - \boldsymbol{X}_i\boldsymbol{\beta}$.

Since the $\boldsymbol{b}_i$ do not enter into the marginal likelihood, alternative estimates must be defined. Typically, the best linear unbiased predictor (BLUP) is used where "best" in this case means that it minimizes the squared error of prediction (or loss), $\sum_{i=1}^{M}(\boldsymbol{y}_{i\text{true}} - \hat{\boldsymbol{y}}_i)^T(\boldsymbol{y}_{i\text{true}} - \hat{\boldsymbol{y}}_i)$. The BLUP for $\boldsymbol{b}_i$ can be shown to be

$$\hat{\boldsymbol{b}}_i = \hat{\boldsymbol{D}}\boldsymbol{Z}_i^T\boldsymbol{\Sigma}_i^{-1}(\hat{\boldsymbol{\alpha}})(\boldsymbol{y}_i - \boldsymbol{X}_i\hat{\boldsymbol{\beta}}) \tag{8.5}$$

See McCulloch and Searle (2001) Chapter 9, Section 4 for more details on $\hat{\boldsymbol{b}}_i$. This estimator can also be derived as the posterior mode of the distribution of $\boldsymbol{b}_i$ if we think of the random-effects model as an empirical Bayes model.

8.4.3 Example: Ramus Height Data

For the Ramus Height example we use the model $\boldsymbol{y}_i = \boldsymbol{X}_i\boldsymbol{\beta} + \boldsymbol{Z}_i\boldsymbol{b}_i + \boldsymbol{e}_i$, $\boldsymbol{e}_i \sim \mathcal{N}(\boldsymbol{0}, \sigma^2\boldsymbol{I})$, and $\boldsymbol{b}_i \sim \mathcal{N}(\boldsymbol{0}, \boldsymbol{D})$, where

$$\boldsymbol{X}_i = \boldsymbol{Z}_i = \begin{bmatrix} 1 & 8.0 \\ 1 & 8.5 \\ 1 & 9.0 \\ 1 & 9.5 \end{bmatrix}$$

and we assume that $\boldsymbol{D}$ is unstructured. Fitting this model yields estimates $\hat{\boldsymbol{\beta}} = [33.7475, 1.8660]^T$, identical to the estimate from the two-stage model, and $\hat{\sigma} = 0.4398$.

8.4.4 Marginal Versus Conditional Models

We return to the subset of 3 subjects from the complete data to illustrate the difference between the marginal and the conditional model. The parameter estimates for the fixed effects, $\hat{\boldsymbol{\beta}}$, can be used to construct marginal fitted values and marginal residuals. The top panel of Figure 8.5 shows the marginal fitted values, $\boldsymbol{X}_i\hat{\boldsymbol{\beta}}$, as the heavy solid line and the residuals associated with those fitted values for one subject as vertical dotted lines. These residuals correspond to the marginal errors, $\boldsymbol{y}_i - \boldsymbol{X}_i\boldsymbol{\beta}$, which have variance $\boldsymbol{\Sigma}_i(\boldsymbol{\alpha})$. They also have high serial correlation since (in this example) a subject's data vectors tend to be either entirely above the marginal fitted values or entirely below.

The bottom panel of Figure 8.5 shows the conditional (subject-specific) fit, $\boldsymbol{X}_i\hat{\boldsymbol{\beta}} + \boldsymbol{Z}_i\hat{\boldsymbol{b}}_i$, for the same subject as a heavy dashed line. The conditional residuals, $\boldsymbol{y}_i - (\boldsymbol{X}_i\hat{\boldsymbol{\beta}} + \boldsymbol{Z}_i\hat{\boldsymbol{b}}_i)$, which, in the fit to the complete data were assumed to be independent, are shown as vertical dotted lines. These residuals do not show the very high positive serial correlation of the marginal residuals.

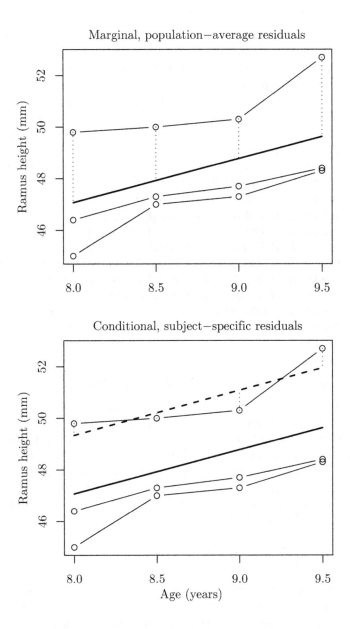

Figure 8.5 *Marginal and conditional residuals. In both panels the heavy solid line corresponds to the marginal or population average fitted values $\boldsymbol{X}_i\hat{\boldsymbol{\beta}}$ and the lighter lines connect the data points for each of the three subjects. In the top panel the dotted lines are the marginal residuals, $\boldsymbol{y}_i - \boldsymbol{X}_i\hat{\boldsymbol{\beta}}$. In the bottom panel one of the subject-specific fitted curves is shown as a heavy dashed line and the dotted lines are the corresponding conditional residuals, $\boldsymbol{y}_i - (\boldsymbol{X}_i\hat{\boldsymbol{\beta}} + \boldsymbol{Z}_i\hat{\boldsymbol{b}}_i)$.*

8.4.5 Serial Conditional Correlation

When we looked at the residuals from the first stage of the two stage estimation of the ramus data, we found substantial correlations. Since they do not seem to follow any simple structure such as AR(1), we might fit a general, subject-specific correlation structure.

If we are only interested in the estimate of the mean parameters, there is little difference between this model (general $\boldsymbol{\Lambda}_i$) and the first model, assuming conditional independence. However, the random-effects variance matrices $\hat{\boldsymbol{D}}$ are very different. The fitted coefficients $\hat{\boldsymbol{\beta}}+\hat{\boldsymbol{b}}_i$ for the two models are shown in Figure 8.6. These plots give some evidence supporting the general conditional correlation model since it is more plausible that the coefficients in (b) arise from a bivariate normal distribution than those in (b).

The standardized conditional residuals, $\boldsymbol{y}_i - [\boldsymbol{X}_i\hat{\boldsymbol{\beta}} + \boldsymbol{Z}_i\hat{\boldsymbol{b}}_i]$, divided by their estimated standard errors, are shown for the two models in Figure 8.7. The fitted curves, $\boldsymbol{X}_i\hat{\boldsymbol{\beta}}+\boldsymbol{Z}_i\hat{\boldsymbol{b}}_i$, for the two models are shown in Figures 8.8 and 8.9.

Notice that the slopes are quite similar among subjects for the general conditional correlation model. We might wish to refit this model with a random effect solely for the intercept. This fit results in very little change in the log-likelihood from the model with random slope. (See the first three lines in Table 8.2 for statistics assessing the overall fit of the three models discussed thus far.)

8.5 The Population-average (Marginal) Model

Marginal or population average models do not postulate a model for each subject but instead directly specify the marginal expectation and variance, $\boldsymbol{y}_i = \boldsymbol{X}_i\boldsymbol{\beta}+\boldsymbol{\delta}_i$ and $\boldsymbol{\delta}_i \sim \mathcal{N}(\boldsymbol{0}, \boldsymbol{\Sigma}_i(\boldsymbol{\alpha}))$. This is exactly the form of the marginal distribution of $\boldsymbol{y}_i$ in the random effects model except that in the random effects model $\boldsymbol{\Sigma}_i(\boldsymbol{\alpha})$ had a very specific form. Here we can specify any form we like. For example, we might try a 4×4 general covariance matrix for $\boldsymbol{\Sigma}_i$.

As in the random effects model we estimate $\boldsymbol{\beta}$ and $\boldsymbol{\alpha}$ by maximizing the log-likelihood which has the form

$$\sum_{i=1}^{M} -\log(|\boldsymbol{\Sigma}_i(\boldsymbol{\alpha})|) - \boldsymbol{r}_i(\boldsymbol{\beta})^T[\boldsymbol{\Sigma}_i(\boldsymbol{\alpha})]^{-1}\boldsymbol{r}_i(\boldsymbol{\beta})$$

where $\boldsymbol{r}_i(\boldsymbol{\beta}) = \boldsymbol{y}_i - \boldsymbol{X}_i\boldsymbol{\beta}$. Table 8.2 shows statistics evaluating the fit of six different models; the three random effects models discussed in Section 8.4 and three marginal models. The three marginal models differ in the choice of covariance matrices. Model 4 uses a general covariance matrix with a constant diagonal so that all observations have the same variance. Model 5 uses a completely general covariance matrix, allowing for a different variance at each time, while model 6 uses an AR(1) covariance structure.

We need criteria with which to choose from among these models. Since for nested models (see Section 8.8.1) the log-likelihood increases with the number

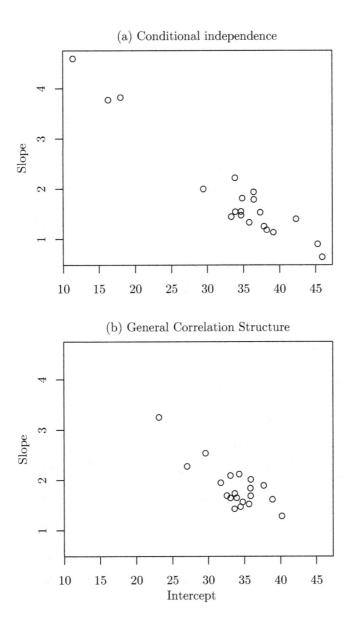

Figure 8.6 *Ramus height data, random effects fitted coefficients* $\hat{\beta} + \hat{b}_i$.

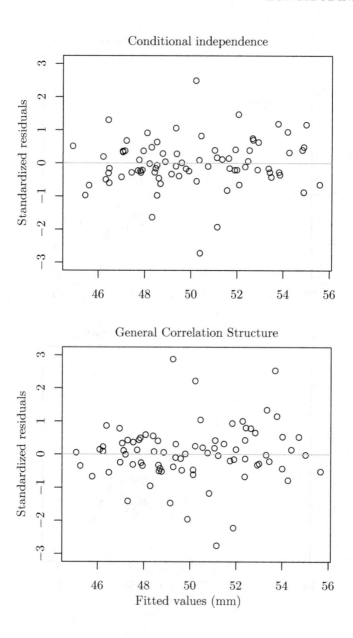

Figure 8.7 *Ramus height data, standardized conditional residuals.*

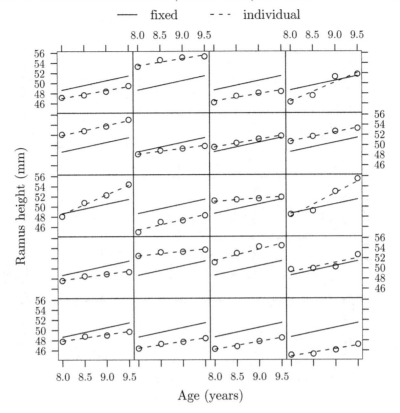

Figure 8.8 *Ramus height data and fitted curves for conditional independence model. Each panel contains data and fitted models for one subject. The solid line is the marginal fitted curve $X_i\hat{\beta}$ and does not vary by subject. The dashed lines are individual fitted curves $X_i\hat{\beta} + Z_i\hat{b}_i$.*

of parameters, and these models aren't nested, simply selecting the model with the largest log-likelihood is not satisfactory. Two other criteria are commonly used for selecting among non-nested models.

The *Akaike Information Criteria* (AIC) imposes a penalty equivalent to one log-likelihood unit for each additional parameter; AIC $= -2(\text{log-likelihood}-p)$ where p is the number of fixed parameters plus the number of variance parameters. The *Bayesian Information Criteria* (BIC) imposes a penalty equivalent to $\log(N)$ log-likelihood units for each additional parameter; i.e., BIC $= -2(\text{log-likelihood} - p\log(N^*))$. There appears to be some dispute regarding the definition of N^* for longitudinal data. Pinheiro and Bates (2000) define N^* to be the total number of observations while Fitzmaurice, Laird, and Ware (2004) define N^* to be the number of subjects, or alternatively, the "effective" number of subjects. Theoretically, the correct choice is related to the

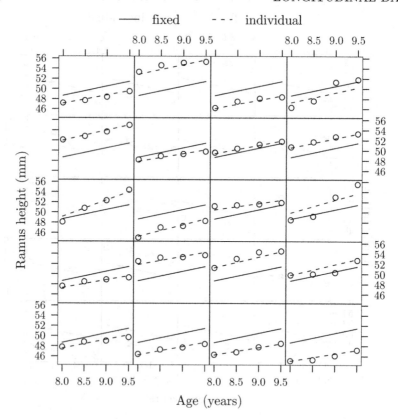

Figure 8.9 *Ramus height data and fitted curves for general conditional correlation model. Each panel contains data and fitted models for one subject. The solid line is the marginal fitted curve $X_i\hat{\beta}$ and does not vary by subject. The dashed lines are individual fitted curves $X_i\hat{\beta} + Z_i\hat{b}_i$.*

total information content. Note that while larger values of the log-likelihood are desirable, smaller values of AIC and BIC are desirable.

If we are interested only in the mean parameters we might pick marginal AR(1) since it has small AIC and BIC. If we need estimates of the subject-level parameters, a random effects model is required, and we would probably choose the random effects model with general conditional correlation and only the intercept random. The fitted fixed effects and standard errors do not differ substantially among the models (Table 8.3)

8.5.1 *Varying Design Matrices*

The subscript i on $\Lambda_i(\phi)$ indicates that the matrices depend on common parameter vectors, ϕ, but are subject specific—usually based on the timing of

Table 8.2 *Model comparison statistics for 6 models. (N = 80).*

Model	Marginal Var/Cov	p	AIC	BIC	Log-Like.
1) RE (I/S)	$\sigma^2 I + ZDZ^T$	6	245.97	260.27	-116.99
2) RE (I/S)	$\Lambda_{\text{general}} + ZDZ^T$	12	248.59	277.17	-112.29
3) RE (I)	$\Lambda_{\text{general}} + ZDZ^T$	11	244.98	268.80	-112.49
4) Marginal	General, equal Var.	9	242.97	264.41	-112.49
5) Marginal	General	12	248.46	277.04	-112.23
6) Marginal	AR(1) correlation	4	242.43	251.96	-117.22

Table 8.3 *Fixed effects estimates and standard errors for the models listed in Table 8.2.*

Model	Intercept	S.E.(Intercept)	Slope	S.E.(Slope)
1)	33.7475	2.2505	1.8660	0.2572
2)	33.7492	1.8022	1.8611	0.2039
3)	33.7447	1.8809	1.8615	0.2046
4)	33.7388	1.8811	1.8621	0.2045
5)	33.7604	1.8245	1.8616	0.2063
6)	33.7503	1.8455	1.8633	0.2010

the observations. For some of the variance-covariance structures that we have defined this generalization is natural. For example, independence, equal correlation (compound symmetric), general AR(1), and exponential correlation all generalize easily to varying observation times. For others, the generalization is not as obvious.

A general approach is to define the ordered vector of all unique values of the predictor variable, t_{complete}. We can think of this as the complete set of time points and think of each subject as having a potentially incomplete set of observed time points. We then use the t_{complete} vector to create a complete correlation matrix using any definitions we like; for example a general correlation matrix can be defined by

$$[\Lambda_{\text{complete}}(\phi)]_{hk} = [\Lambda_{\text{complete}}(\phi)]_{kh} = \begin{cases} v_{hk} & \text{for } h \neq k \\ 1 & \text{for } h = k. \end{cases}$$

To find Λ_i for a particular vector t_i we choose the relevant rows and columns of $\Lambda_{\text{complete}}$. For example, if wished to assume a general variance-covariance matrix and the time vectors for the first three subjects were

$$
\begin{aligned}
t_1 &= (1,2,4)^T \\
t_2 &= (1,3,4,5)^T \\
t_3 &= (2,3,4)^T
\end{aligned}
$$

then

$$t_{\text{complete}} = (1,2,3,4,5)^T$$

and

$$
\Lambda_{\text{complete}}(\boldsymbol{\phi}) =
\begin{bmatrix}
1 & \phi_1 & \phi_2 & \phi_3 & \phi_4 \\
\phi_1 & 1 & \phi_5 & \phi_6 & \phi_7 \\
\phi_2 & \phi_5 & 1 & \phi_8 & \phi_9 \\
\phi_3 & \phi_6 & \phi_8 & 1 & \phi_{10} \\
\phi_4 & \phi_7 & \phi_9 & \phi_{10} & 1
\end{bmatrix}
$$

and we would have

$$
\Lambda_1(\boldsymbol{\phi}) =
\begin{bmatrix}
1 & \phi_1 & \phi_3 \\
\phi_1 & 1 & \phi_6 \\
\phi_3 & \phi_6 & 1
\end{bmatrix}
$$

$$
\Lambda_2(\boldsymbol{\phi}) =
\begin{bmatrix}
1 & \phi_2 & \phi_3 & \phi_4 \\
\phi_2 & 1 & \phi_8 & \phi_9 \\
\phi_3 & \phi_8 & 1 & \phi_{10} \\
\phi_4 & \phi_9 & \phi_{10} & 1
\end{bmatrix}
$$

$$
\Lambda_3(\boldsymbol{\phi}) =
\begin{bmatrix}
1 & \phi_5 & \phi_6 \\
\phi_5 & 1 & \phi_8 \\
\phi_6 & \phi_8 & 1
\end{bmatrix} .
$$

Note that for this example, we would need more than these three subjects to estimate this correlation structure. A general correlation matrix can be estimated only when the vector $t_{complete}$ is not too large relative to the individual t_i vectors.

8.6 Restricted Maximum Likelihood Estimation (REML)

So far, our main tool for finding estimates has been maximum likelihood. Recall that the log-likelihood for the marginal model is

$$
\sum_{i=1}^{M} - \log(|\Sigma_i(\boldsymbol{\alpha})|) - r_i(\boldsymbol{\beta})^T [\Sigma_i(\boldsymbol{\alpha})]^{-1} r_i(\boldsymbol{\beta})
$$

where the $r_i(\boldsymbol{\beta}) = y_i - X_i \boldsymbol{\beta} Z$ are the marginal residuals. If we assume a random-effects subject-specific model, $\Sigma(\boldsymbol{\alpha})$ has the special form $\Sigma_i(\boldsymbol{\alpha}) = \sigma^2 \Lambda_i(\boldsymbol{\phi})_i + Z_i D Z_i^T$ and the parameter vector, $\boldsymbol{\alpha}$, includes σ, ϕ, and the entries in D. Unfortunately, the maximum likelihood (ML) estimates for the variance parameters, $\boldsymbol{\alpha}$, are biased. ML estimation does not take into account the fact that the number of degrees of freedom for estimating $\boldsymbol{\alpha}$ are reduced by the estimation of $\boldsymbol{\beta}$. In general, when using maximum likelihood we will tend to underestimate variances.

As an alternative, restricted maximum likelihood (REML) estimates have been proposed. There are a number of ways to derive the restricted likelihood but the most intuitive is as the likelihood for the data after a suitable linear transformation to remove the information about $\boldsymbol{\beta}$. For example, define

$$
N = \sum_{i=1}^{M} n_i \qquad \boldsymbol{X} = \begin{bmatrix} \boldsymbol{X}_1 \\ \boldsymbol{X}_2 \\ \vdots \\ \boldsymbol{X}_M \end{bmatrix} \qquad \boldsymbol{y} = \begin{bmatrix} \boldsymbol{y}_1 \\ \boldsymbol{y}_2 \\ \vdots \\ \boldsymbol{y}_M \end{bmatrix}
$$

and find an $(N-p) \times N$ matrix, $\boldsymbol{K}$, of maximal row rank such that $\boldsymbol{KX} = \boldsymbol{0}$. The log-likelihood for $\boldsymbol{Ky}$ is the restricted log-likelihood, $l_{\text{REML}}(\alpha)$, and has the form

$$
-\log(|\boldsymbol{X}^T[\boldsymbol{\Sigma}(\boldsymbol{\alpha})]^{-1}\boldsymbol{X}|) + \sum_{i=1}^{M} -\log(|\boldsymbol{\Sigma}_i(\boldsymbol{\alpha})|) - \boldsymbol{r}_i(\hat{\boldsymbol{\beta}}_i(\boldsymbol{\alpha}))^T[\boldsymbol{\Sigma}_i(\boldsymbol{\alpha})]^{-1}\boldsymbol{r}_i(\hat{\boldsymbol{\beta}}_i(\boldsymbol{\alpha}))
$$

where $\boldsymbol{\Sigma}(\boldsymbol{\alpha}) = \text{Diag}(\boldsymbol{\Sigma}_1(\boldsymbol{\alpha}), \boldsymbol{\Sigma}_2(\boldsymbol{\alpha}), \dots, \boldsymbol{\Sigma}_M(\boldsymbol{\alpha}))$ and $\hat{\boldsymbol{\beta}}(\boldsymbol{\alpha})$ is the generalized least squares (GLS) estimate of $\boldsymbol{\beta}$ given $\boldsymbol{\alpha}$. In other words,

$$
\hat{\boldsymbol{\beta}} = (\boldsymbol{X}^T[\boldsymbol{\Sigma}(\boldsymbol{\alpha})]^{-1}\boldsymbol{X})^{-1}\boldsymbol{X}^T[\boldsymbol{\Sigma}(\boldsymbol{\alpha})]^{-1}\boldsymbol{y}. \tag{8.6}
$$

For further details see Diggle, Liang, and Zeger (1994) Chapter 4, Section 5 and McCulloch and Searle (2001), Chapter 1, Section 7 and Chapter 6, Section 6. We note the following regarding REML estimation:

- The restricted log-likelihood is solely a function of $\boldsymbol{\alpha}$ and does not involve $\boldsymbol{\beta}$. Therefore the REML estimate of $\boldsymbol{\beta}$ is undefined. The GLS estimate of $\boldsymbol{\beta}$ (equation 8.6) and the BLUP estimate of $\boldsymbol{b}_i$ (equation 8.5), however, can be evaluated at the REML estimates of $\boldsymbol{\alpha}$ and should perform well.

- The maximum likelihood estimates of $\boldsymbol{\alpha}$ are invariant to any one-to-one transformation of the fixed effects. Since REML redefines the $\boldsymbol{X}_i$ matrices, however, the REML estimates are not.

- The REML estimates of the variance components are consistent whereas the maximum likelihood estimates will be too small. The size of this bias will depend on the particular data.

8.7 Standard Errors

Up to this point we have been discussing models and point estimates for the parameters in those models. In addition we are also interested in the variability of our estimators. Recall, the most general marginal model is $\boldsymbol{y}_i = \boldsymbol{X}_i\boldsymbol{\beta} + \boldsymbol{\delta}_i$ and $\boldsymbol{\delta}_i \sim \mathcal{N}(\boldsymbol{0}, \boldsymbol{\Sigma}_i(\boldsymbol{\alpha}))$. If we are using a random effects model we also have $\boldsymbol{\Sigma}_i(\boldsymbol{\alpha}) = \boldsymbol{Z}_i\boldsymbol{D}\boldsymbol{Z}_i^T + \sigma^2\boldsymbol{\Lambda}_i(\boldsymbol{\phi})$ and $\boldsymbol{\alpha} = (\sigma, \phi, \boldsymbol{D})$. In order to conduct inference regarding the parameters of interest, we may need standard errors for each of $\hat{\boldsymbol{\beta}}_{\mathrm{ML}}$, $\hat{\boldsymbol{\alpha}}_{\mathrm{ML}}$, $\hat{\boldsymbol{\alpha}}_{\mathrm{REML}}$, $\hat{\boldsymbol{\beta}}_{\mathrm{GLS}}(\hat{\boldsymbol{\alpha}}_{\mathrm{REML}})$, $\hat{\boldsymbol{b}}_i(\hat{\boldsymbol{\alpha}}_{\mathrm{ML}})$, and $\hat{\boldsymbol{b}}_i(\hat{\boldsymbol{\alpha}}_{\mathrm{REML}})$.

8.7.1 Maximum and Restricted Maximum Likelihood

Let $\boldsymbol{\theta} = [\boldsymbol{\beta}^T, \boldsymbol{\alpha}^T]^T$, then $\mathrm{Var}(\hat{\boldsymbol{\theta}}_{\mathrm{ML}}) = \mathcal{I}_{\mathrm{ML}}(\theta)^{-1}$ where $\mathcal{I}_{\mathrm{ML}}(\theta)$ is the Fisher information matrix

$$\mathcal{I}_{\mathrm{ML}}(\theta) = -E\left[\frac{\partial^2 \log l_{\mathrm{ML}}(\boldsymbol{\theta})}{\partial^2 \boldsymbol{\theta}}\right].$$

Also $\mathrm{Var}(\hat{\boldsymbol{\theta}}_{\mathrm{REML}}) = \mathcal{I}_{\mathrm{REML}}(\alpha)^{-1}$ where $\mathcal{I}_{\mathrm{REML}}(\alpha)$ is the information matrix

$$\mathcal{I}_{\mathrm{REML}}(\alpha) = -E\left[\frac{\partial^2 \log l_{\mathrm{REML}}(\boldsymbol{\alpha})}{\partial^2 \boldsymbol{\alpha}}\right].$$

In practice we use the observed information matrices, $\hat{\mathcal{I}}(\hat{\theta})$. Asymptotically, we also have that $\mathrm{Cor}(\hat{\boldsymbol{\beta}}_{\mathrm{ML}}, \hat{\boldsymbol{\alpha}}_{\mathrm{ML}}) = 0$.

If we assume $\boldsymbol{\Sigma}_i = \boldsymbol{\Sigma}_i(\hat{\boldsymbol{\alpha}})$, the variance of the estimates of the fixed effects has the simple form

$$\mathrm{Var}(\hat{\boldsymbol{\beta}}_{\mathrm{ML}}) = (\boldsymbol{X}^T[\boldsymbol{\Sigma}(\hat{\boldsymbol{\alpha}})]^{-1}\boldsymbol{X})^{-1}.$$

This estimate is biased downwards, however, because the variability in $\hat{\boldsymbol{\alpha}}$ is not taken into account.

8.7.2 Robust Estimation of Var($\boldsymbol{\beta}$)

As we have noted, estimates of the variance of $\hat{\boldsymbol{\beta}}$ that don't account for the estimation of $\boldsymbol{\alpha}$ are biased, so improved, robust estimates are required. We start by assuming the marginal model

$$\boldsymbol{y} = \boldsymbol{X}\boldsymbol{\beta} + \boldsymbol{\delta} \quad \boldsymbol{\delta} \sim \mathcal{N}(\boldsymbol{0}, \boldsymbol{\Sigma}). \tag{8.7}$$

If we knew $\boldsymbol{\Sigma}$, it would be possible to estimate $\boldsymbol{\beta}$ using the GLS estimator $\hat{\boldsymbol{\beta}}_{\boldsymbol{\Sigma}} = \left(\boldsymbol{X}^T\boldsymbol{\Sigma}^{-1}\boldsymbol{X}\right)^{-1}\boldsymbol{X}^T\boldsymbol{\Sigma}^{-1}\boldsymbol{y}$. Since we don't know $\boldsymbol{\Sigma}$, we can make an initial estimate, $\boldsymbol{W}$, called the *working* variance-covariance matrix. $\boldsymbol{W}$ is usually defined using a parsimonious structure, often AR(1). We then let

$$\hat{\boldsymbol{\beta}}_{\boldsymbol{W}} = \left(\boldsymbol{X}^T\boldsymbol{W}^{-1}\boldsymbol{X}\right)^{-1}\boldsymbol{X}^T\boldsymbol{W}^{-1}\boldsymbol{y}.$$

As we have seen $\hat{\boldsymbol{\beta}}_{\boldsymbol{W}}$ is not very sensitive to the specification of $\boldsymbol{W}$. On the other hand, the variance estimate of $\hat{\boldsymbol{\beta}}_{\boldsymbol{W}}$, calculated assuming that $\boldsymbol{W}$ is true, is $\left(\boldsymbol{X}^T\boldsymbol{W}^{-1}\boldsymbol{X}\right)^{-1}$ which can be seriously biased if $\boldsymbol{W}$ is incorrectly specified. Instead, we may compute the variance of $\hat{\boldsymbol{\beta}}_{\boldsymbol{W}}$ under the true model (Equation 8.7),

$$\mathrm{Var}(\hat{\boldsymbol{\beta}}_{\boldsymbol{W}}) = \left(\boldsymbol{X}^T\boldsymbol{W}^{-1}\boldsymbol{X}\right)^{-1}\boldsymbol{X}^T\boldsymbol{W}^{-1}\boldsymbol{\Sigma}\boldsymbol{W}^{-1}\boldsymbol{X}\left(\boldsymbol{X}^T\boldsymbol{W}^{-1}\boldsymbol{X}\right)^{-1}.$$

Note that if $\boldsymbol{W} = \boldsymbol{\Sigma}$ then this reduces to $\left(\boldsymbol{X}^T \boldsymbol{\Sigma}^{-1} \boldsymbol{X} \right)^{-1}$ as desired.

The so called *sandwich variance estimator* is this expression with $\boldsymbol{\Sigma}$ replaced by a consistent estimator. Usually we construct $\hat{\boldsymbol{\Sigma}}$ assuming as general a form as possible (completely general if the total number of time points is not too large). The sandwich estimator is consistent but can be inefficient compared to the standard estimate when the model is correct.

8.8 Testing

It is important in model building that we are able to assess whether particular model parameters, either fixed effects and variance components, are necessary or can be dropped. In many cases testing for the necessity of variance components is essential for finding a model for which reliable estimates of the parameters of interest can be found.

8.8.1 Nested Models

Two models are nested if they are identical except that some parameters are fixed at specified values (usually zero) in one of the models. Since we are using maximum likelihood estimates, a common approach to testing whether particular parameters are necessary is the likelihood ratio (LR) test (see Appendix A.3). If we have a model $\boldsymbol{y}_i = \boldsymbol{X}_i \boldsymbol{\beta} + \boldsymbol{\delta}_i$ and $\boldsymbol{\delta}_i \sim \mathcal{N}(\boldsymbol{0}, \boldsymbol{\Sigma}_i(\boldsymbol{\alpha}))$, and we want to test the null hypothesis, H_0, that some element of $\boldsymbol{\beta}$ or $\boldsymbol{\alpha}$ is zero (or any other value) we first fit the full model and calculate the likelihood, l_{FULL}.

Next, we fix some of the parameters at their values under the H_0, estimate the rest of the parameters using maximum likelihood, and compute the value of the likelihood, l_{REDUCED}. The LR test statistic is

$$2 \log \left(\frac{l_{\text{FULL}}}{l_{\text{REDUCED}}} \right).$$

Asymptotically (under certain conditions) this will have a χ^2 distribution with $p_{\text{FULL}} - p_{\text{REDUCED}}$ degrees of freedom under H_0, where p_{FULL} is the total number of parameters in the larger model and p_{REDUCED} is the total number of parameters in the smaller model.

Variance Components

Because variance components must be non-negative, $\boldsymbol{0}$ is on the edge of the corresponding parameter space and the LR tests for the variance components violate one of the required assumptions. In practice, however, the LR test works reasonably well (though it tends to be conservative) and no good alternatives exist so the LR test is still recommended for variance components. See Pinheiro and Bates (2000) Chapter 2, Section 4 for a detailed discussion. In summary, the LR test is conservative (overestimates p-values) for testing variance components.

Fixed Effects

The LR test can be quite anti-conservative (p-values are too small) for testing elements of $\boldsymbol{\beta}$. Instead, we recommend the conditional F- and t-tests (conditional on $\hat{\boldsymbol{\alpha}}$) (Pinheiro and Bates 2000).

If the null hypothesis is that $\boldsymbol{S\beta} = \boldsymbol{m}$ where $\boldsymbol{S}$ is $r \times p$ and if we let $\boldsymbol{\Sigma} = \sigma^2 \boldsymbol{V}$, where $\boldsymbol{V}$ is assumed known, and define

$$\hat{\sigma}^2 = \frac{\boldsymbol{y}^T(\boldsymbol{V}^{-1} - \boldsymbol{V}^{-1}\boldsymbol{X}(\boldsymbol{X}^T\boldsymbol{V}^{-1}\boldsymbol{X})^{-1}\boldsymbol{X}^T\boldsymbol{V}^{-1})\boldsymbol{y}}{N - p}$$

then

$$f = \frac{(\boldsymbol{S\hat{\beta}} - \boldsymbol{m})^T[\boldsymbol{S}(\boldsymbol{X}\boldsymbol{V}^{-1}\boldsymbol{X})^{-1}\boldsymbol{S}^T]^{-1}(\boldsymbol{S\hat{\beta}} - \boldsymbol{m})}{r\hat{\sigma}^2}$$

has an $F_{r,N-p}$ distribution under the null hypothesis. To calculate the test statistic in practice we must use an estimate for $\boldsymbol{V}$. We would typically use a maximum or restricted maximum likelihood estimator.

8.8.2 Non-nested Models

For choosing between non-nested models usually an information criterion such as AIC and BIC is used.

8.8.3 Example: Bone Density

Returning to the bone density example described in Section 8.1, Figure 8.10 shows bone density measurements over time for two treatment groups each containing 37 subjects. The trends for the subjects look relatively straight so we first fit a general, straight-line model assuming random intercept and slope and AR1 within-subject serial correlation. For the fixed effects, we consider the models defined in (8.1) and (8.2). The model for the variance components was chosen after comparison (using likelihood ratio tests) to other smaller models with various variance components removed.

The ANOVA tables for the fixed effects for both models are shown in Table 8.4. As indicated, the model with no intercept should be slightly more efficient, and the F-statistic is in fact larger, although differences in the F-statistics could be due to other factors. The fixed parameter estimates are shown in Table 8.5. In both models the interaction between day and treatment indicates a difference in the average slope of the two groups. The results are quite similar, suggesting that both models adequately fit the data. In each case the treatment group has a slightly less negative slope. In the model with no intercept, the standard error is slightly smaller, which might be attributed to improved efficiency. The estimates of the variance components for Model (8.1) are:

$$\hat{\boldsymbol{D}} = \begin{bmatrix} 4.99 \times 10^{-3} & -2.38 \times 10^{-7} \\ -2.38 \times 10^{-7} & 2.34 \times 10{-10} \end{bmatrix} \quad \hat{\sigma} = 2.03 \quad \hat{\phi} = 0.38$$

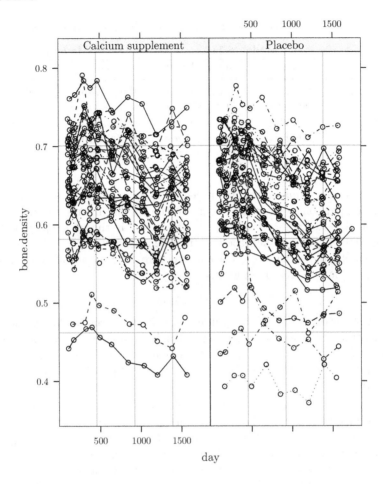

Figure 8.10 *Bone density measured at 10 or 11 times per subject. Observation days are not identical for each subject.*

Table 8.4 *ANOVA table for bone density example. The numerator and denominator degrees of freedom are the same for both models.*

			Model (8.1)		Model (8.2)	
	Num DF	Den DF	F-value	p-value	F-value	p-value
Intercept	1	725	5937.944	<.0001	5933.298	<.0001
trt	1	72	1.126	0.2921	–	–
day	1	725	158.270	<.0001	158.451	<.0001
trt:day	1	725	5.253	0.0222	6.223	0.0128

Table 8.5 *Fixed parameter estimates for bone density example.*

| | Model (8.1) | | Model (8.2) | |
	Value	Standard Error	Value	Standard Error
Intercept	0.6504759	0.011922357	0.6537246	0.008432233
trt	0.0064960	0.016858031	–	–
day	-0.0000392	0.000003727	-0.0000395	0.000003654
trt:day	0.0000121	0.000005269	0.0000126	0.000005064

where $\hat{\phi}$ is the estimated within-subject AR(1) correlation coefficient.

For comparison, we can also estimate the trt:day interaction using a two stage model. Let $\boldsymbol{\gamma}_{iz} = (\gamma_{i0z}, \gamma_{i1z})^T$ where γ_{i0z} is the intercept and γ_{i1z} is the slope of lines fit to subject i in treatment group z, $z = 0, 1$, assuming a conditional independence correlation structure. The mean difference between slopes for the two treatment groups,

$$\bar{\gamma}_{i01} - \bar{\gamma}_{i00}, \tag{8.8}$$

is a simple estimate of the trt:day interaction based on model (8.1) on page 232.

An estimate of the trt:day interaction can be computed under model (8.2) by making the assumption that $\hat{\boldsymbol{\gamma}}_{iz}$ is bivariate normal with mean $(\beta_0, \beta_1 + \beta_3 z)^T$. By applying standard results for bivariate normal data, conditional on $\hat{\gamma}_{i0z}$, we have

$$\hat{\gamma}_{i1z} = \beta_0' + \beta_1' \hat{\gamma}_{i0z} + \beta_3 z + e_{iz} \tag{8.9}$$

for parameters β_0' and β_1' that depend on β_0, β_1, and the correlation structure of $\hat{\boldsymbol{\gamma}}_{iz}$, and e_{iz} is a mean zero error term. Hence, one can estimate β_3 by fitting the regression model defined by equation (8.9) to the observed $\hat{\boldsymbol{\gamma}}_{iz}$. When $\hat{\gamma}_{i1z}$ and $\hat{\gamma}_{i0z}$ are correlated, the estimate from this model should be more efficient than the mean difference from equation (8.8). Estimates of β_0' and β_1' are not interpretable, and the estimate of β_3, the trt:day interaction, from this model is shown in Table 8.6.

Table 8.6 *Two-stage estimates of time-treatment interaction for bone density data.*

| | Equation (8.8) | | Equation (8.9) | |
	Value	Standard Error	Value	Standard Error
trt:day	0.0000122	0.0000056	0.0000130	0.0000054

8.9 Additional Levels of Clustering

By definition, longitudinal data are clustered within subjects. A linear mixed effects model with intercept terms only and with conditional independence is

Table 8.7 *Parameter definitions for a 2-level random effects model.*

Level	Parameter	Meaning
0	β	fixed mean
1	$b_k^{(1)} \sim \mathcal{N}(0, D_{1 \times 1}^{(1)})$	random effect for center k
2	$b_i^{(2)} \sim \mathcal{N}(0, D_{1 \times 1}^{(2)})$	random effect for subject i (in center k)
3	$e_{ij} \sim \mathcal{N}(0, \sigma^2)$	random effect (error) for observation j on subject i (in center k)

a simple mixed effects ANOVA model:

$$y_{ij} = \beta + b_i + e_{ij}$$

where

$$b_i \sim \mathcal{N}(0, D_{1 \times 1}) \qquad e_{ij} \sim \mathcal{N}(0, \sigma^2).$$

If we have an additional level of nesting (say subjects in a clinical trial are grouped into centers) we simply add an additional term to the model for center. In the following formulation, if we assume there are 15 subjects at each of 4 centers, index i runs from 1 to the total number of subjects $= 60$ rather than from 1 to 15. This method of numbering keeps the number of subscripts to a minimum. So we have, for subject i at center k,

$$y_{ij} = \beta + b_k^{(1)} + b_i^{(2)} + e_{ij}$$

where the parameters and their distributions are described in Table 8.7.

While having the advantage of simplicity, this is not a very interesting model for longitudinal data because there are no continuous predictors. We can generalize the model by adding back in the design matrices. The standard linear mixed effects model has the familiar form

$$\boldsymbol{y}_i = \boldsymbol{X}_i \boldsymbol{\beta} + \boldsymbol{Z}_i \boldsymbol{b}_i + \boldsymbol{e}_i$$

$$\boldsymbol{b}_i \sim \mathcal{N}(\boldsymbol{0}, \boldsymbol{D}) \qquad \boldsymbol{e}_i \sim \mathcal{N}(\boldsymbol{0}, \sigma^2 \boldsymbol{\Lambda}_i(\boldsymbol{\phi})).$$

We can extend it as above to include an additional level of nesting. For subject i in center k we have

$$\boldsymbol{y}_i = \boldsymbol{X}_i \boldsymbol{\beta} + \boldsymbol{Z}_i^{(1)} \boldsymbol{b}_k^{(1)} + \boldsymbol{Z}_i^{(2)} \boldsymbol{b}_i^{(2)} + \boldsymbol{e}_i \qquad (8.10)$$

where the definitions of the parameters are given in Table 8.8.

To continue the multi-center clinical trial example, assume we observe a straight line response at times $1, \ldots, 6$ for each subject. If we wish to include random effects for intercept and slope at both the center and subject level we

Table 8.8 *Definitions and distributions for fixed and random effects in a 2 level clustered model with more than one random effect at each level.*

Level	Parameter	Meaning
0	$\boldsymbol{\beta}$	fixed effects
1	$\boldsymbol{b}_k^{(1)} \sim \mathcal{N}(\boldsymbol{0}, \boldsymbol{D}^{(1)})$	random effect vector for center k
2	$\boldsymbol{b}_i^{(2)} \sim \mathcal{N}(\boldsymbol{0}, \boldsymbol{D}^{(2)})$	random effect vector for subject i (in center k)
3	$\boldsymbol{e}_i \sim \mathcal{N}(0, \sigma^2 \boldsymbol{\Lambda}_i(\boldsymbol{\phi}))$	random effect (error) vector for subject i (in center k)

would have

$$\boldsymbol{X}_i = \boldsymbol{Z}_i^{(1)} = \boldsymbol{Z}_i^{(2)} = \begin{bmatrix} 1 & 1 \\ 1 & 2 \\ 1 & 3 \\ 1 & 4 \\ 1 & 5 \\ 1 & 6 \end{bmatrix}.$$

Under these assumptions, $\boldsymbol{\beta}$ (in Equation 8.10) is the overall mean intercept and slope, $\boldsymbol{b}_k^{(1)}$ for $k = 1, \ldots, 10$ are random intercept and slope effects for center, and $\boldsymbol{b}_i^{(2)}$ for $i = 1, \ldots, 60$ are random intercept and slope effects for subject i.

8.10 Generalized Estimating Equations for Non-normal Data

Thus far we have restricted attention to continuous responses that we have assumed to be normally distributed. Often, the response that is measured over time is not a continuous measure, but is the occurrence of a particular event, or the number of such events occurring in a particular interval, for example, the number of asthma exacerbations or epileptic seizures during each month of follow-up. Whenever we have a parametric form for the distribution of the data and can write down the probability of the data given the parameters we can use maximum likelihood estimation. It is often the case, however, that we do not know the exact distribution. If we are willing to specify a functional form for the expectation and the marginal variance, generalized estimating equation (GEE) methods can be used.

8.10.1 Examples

We motivate the GEE methods by first considering simple examples for non-normal data without repeated measures.

Example 8.1. Suppose that $y_1, y_2, \ldots, y_n$ have a binomial distribution with probability p_i and size m_i. Then the log-likelihood has the form

$$
\begin{aligned}
\log L_{\boldsymbol{p}}(Y) &= \sum_{i=1}^{n} y_i \log \frac{p_i}{1 - p_i} + m_i \log(1 - p_i) + \log \binom{m_i}{y_i} \\
&= \sum_{i=1}^{n} y_i \theta_i - m_i \log(1 + e^{\theta}) + C(Y) \qquad (8.11)
\end{aligned}
$$

where $\theta_i = \log p_i/(1 - p_i)$. If we let $\theta_i = x_i^T \beta$, where x_i is a covariate vector for subject i and β is a parameter vector, then equation (8.11) has a form similar to the likelihood for Gaussian data, equation (A.2) in Appendix A.2.
□

Example 8.2. Suppose that $y_1, y_2, \ldots, y_n$ have a Poisson distribution with mean λ_i. The log-likelihood has the form

$$
\begin{aligned}
\log L_{\boldsymbol{p}}(Y) &= \sum_{i=1}^{n} y_i \log \lambda_i - \lambda_i - \log y_i! \\
&= \sum_{i=1}^{n} y_i \theta_i - e^{\theta} + C(Y) \qquad (8.12)
\end{aligned}
$$

where $\theta_i = \log \lambda_i$. Again, if we let $\theta_i = x_i^T \beta$, we have a form similar to equation (A.2).
□

8.10.2 The Model for Longitudinal Data

Typically we specify the model by first specifying the connection between the mean curve and the predictors. Letting $\boldsymbol{\mu}_i(\boldsymbol{\beta}) = E(\boldsymbol{y}_i)$, we model the mean structure by

$$
h(\boldsymbol{\mu}_i(\boldsymbol{\beta})) = \boldsymbol{X}_i \boldsymbol{\beta}
$$

where h is a known one-to-one *link* function and $\boldsymbol{\beta}$ is a vector of unknown parameters. Since the range of $E(y_{ij})$ may be restricted, between zero and one for Bernoulli data, or positive for Poisson data for example, one purpose of the link function is to transform the range of the expected values of $\boldsymbol{y}_i$ to the real line, ensuring that $\boldsymbol{X}_i \boldsymbol{\beta}$ always corresponds to valid values of $h(\cdot)$.

For example, if we have Bernoulli data $E(\boldsymbol{y}_i) = \boldsymbol{p}_i$ and if we wish to model $h(\boldsymbol{p}_i) = \boldsymbol{X}_i \boldsymbol{\beta}$ the most commonly used link function is the logit transformation,

$$
h(p_{ij}) = \log(p_{ij}/(1 - p_{ij}))
$$

which transforms the interval (0,1) to the entire real line. Also, from the Bernoulli distribution we might assume

$$
\text{Var}(y_{ij}) = p_{ij}(1 - p_{ij}).
$$

For Poisson data, we would typically choose the log link, and the variance equal to the mean.

In general, the variance matrix is $A = \mathrm{Diag}(A_1, A_2, \ldots, A_M)$, where $A_i = \mathrm{Diag}(\mathrm{Var}(y_{i1}), \mathrm{Var}(y_{i2}), \ldots, \mathrm{Var}(y_{in_i}))$ is the diagonal variance matrix for subject i.

As in the normal case we can specify a working correlation matrix $R = \mathrm{Diag}(R_1, R_2, \ldots, R_M)$, where R_i is the working correlation matrix for subject i.

Then the working covariance matrix is

$$W = R^{1/2} A R^{1/2}$$

where $R^{1/2}$ is a symmetric matrix such that $R^{1/2} R^{1/2} = R$.

The estimate of β is found by solving the "working score equations",

$$\sum_{i=1}^{M} \tilde{X}(\beta)^T W^{-1} (y_i - \mu_i(\beta)) = 0,$$

where $\tilde{X}_i(\beta) = \frac{\partial \mu_i(\beta)}{\partial \beta}$. Once again, the variance of $\hat{\beta}_W$ calculated assuming that W is true has the form $\left(\tilde{X}^T W^{-1} \tilde{X} \right)^{-1}$ and can be seriously biased if W is incorrectly specified. Instead we compute the variance of $\hat{\beta}$ under the true model,

$$\mathrm{Var}(\hat{\beta}_W) = \left(\tilde{X}^T W^{-1} \tilde{X} \right)^{-1} \tilde{X}^T W^{-1} \Sigma W^{-1} \tilde{X} \left(\tilde{X}^T W^{-1} \tilde{X} \right)^{-1}.$$

The so called "sandwich variance estimator" is this expression with a consistent estimator for Σ. This is a marginal approach because it directly models the marginal variance of the data. It is possible to use GEE to fit models to non-normal data which are derived from a conditional specification based on random effects. We do not provide details here.

8.10.3 Example: Epilepsy Data

Thall and Vail (1990) present data on epileptic seizures for 59 individuals. We will use this data to demonstrate the generalized estimating equation (GEE) approach. The data have the format shown in Table 8.9 where seizures is the number of seizures in the two weeks preceding the visit, tmt is the treatment: progabide (1) or placebo (0), base is the number of seizures in the 8 weeks before randomization to treatment group, age is age in years, id is a subject id, and
textttvisit is the visit number (1 to 4).

We fit a GEE model without a main effect for treatment and using a link and variance function derived from the Poisson distribution, that is

$$E(y_i) = \exp(X_i \beta) = \mu_i(\beta)$$

Table 8.9 *First 19 observations in the epilepsy data example.*

seizures	treatment	base	age	id	visit
5	0	11	31	1	1
3	0	11	31	1	2
3	0	11	31	1	3
3	0	11	31	1	4
3	0	11	30	2	1
5	0	11	30	2	2
3	0	11	30	2	3
3	0	11	30	2	4
2	0	6	25	3	1
4	0	6	25	3	2
0	0	6	25	3	3
5	0	6	25	3	4
4	0	8	36	4	1
4	0	8	36	4	2
1	0	8	36	4	3
4	0	8	36	4	4
7	0	66	22	5	1
18	0	66	22	5	2
9	0	66	22	5	3

and

$$\mathrm{Var}(y_{ij}) = E(y_{ij}).$$

We also used a conditional independence correlation matrix. The parameter of interest in this model is the time-treatment interaction, visit:tmt.

The estimated coefficients and naive (based on independence correlation structure) and robust standard errors are shown in Table 8.10. Treatment does not appear to have a significant effect on the number of seizures. The estimate of the time-treatment interaction coefficient is -0.0119 with a standard error of 0.0650 (a significant negative coefficient would suggest that treatment reduces the seizure rate).

8.11 Missing Data

Missing data are discussed in more detail in Chapter 11, so here we only briefly discuss the effect of missing data on longitudinal data analysis. We first note that we consider data to be *missing* if a well defined response is unobserved. This definition excludes, for example, responses that cannot be observed because the subject has died, in which case the responses cannot be coherently defined. Frangakis and Rubin (2002) consider such responses to be *truncated* by death, and these require a different kind of analysis.

Table 8.10 *Estimated coefficients for epilepsy data.*

	Estimate	Naive S.E.	Robust S.E.	Robust z	p-value
Intercept	-3.94	0.91	1.05	-3.75	0.0002
log(base)	1.22	0.07	0.15	8.05	< 0.0001
log(age)	0.579	0.237	0.286	2.02	0.043
visit	-0.0527	0.0484	0.0573	-0.92	0.358
visit:tmt	-0.0119	0.0390	0.0650	-0.18	0.857

Second, unobserved responses are considered *missing completely at random* (MCAR) (Little and Rubin 2002) if the probability that an observation is missing is independent of both the observed and unobserved responses, and considered *missing at random* (MAR) (Little and Rubin 2002) if the probability that an observation is missing depends only on the observed data. If neither of these holds, the observations are considered *missing not at random*. Unfortunately, it is not possible to determine directly from the data which of these is the case. In some special cases, such as when responses are missing solely because they occur after some prespecified data cutoff date, it can be known that the missingness is MAR. Otherwise, we can rarely be confident that we know the nature of the missingness.

In the first case, all the modeling results discussed in this chapter are directly applicable. In the second case, unbiased estimates of model parameters are obtainable if the model is properly fit. For example, suppose that subjects with a greater rate of decline are more likely to withdraw from the study and therefore have more missing observations, especially at later follow-up times. If the mixed or marginal models of sections 8.4 and 8.4.4 are naively applied, the rate of decline is likely to be underestimated. This happens because the subjects with fewer observations both are given less weight in the model fitting process and are more likely to have greater rates of decline. The two stage model is not likely to suffer from this bias because (assuming the model is correct) the observed slope for each subject is an unbiased estimate of the true slope for the given subject, and, therefore, the (unweighted) average observed slope is an unbiased estimate of the population average slope.

8.12 Summary

Longitudinal data analysis is an important tool for the clinical trial statistician. Nonetheless, it is important to keep in mind that clinical trial results may be less compelling when based on complicated analyses requiring strong assumptions. Since the primary outcome analysis is prespecified, it must be as robust as possible to departures from assumptions. It is also important to be aware of the effect that missing data might have on the analysis, and select an analysis that is as robust as possible to the effect of missing data. In clinical trials, a two stage analysis in which all subjects receive equal weight may often be preferred, both because of its simplicity and its robustness.

CHAPTER 9

Quality of Life

Outcome measures in clinical trials traditionally have been objective evaluations such as assessments of physical function (e.g., survival, lung capacity) or biological markers of response to treatment (e.g., blood cell counts, tumor size, etc.). For example, in a clinical trial examining the effectiveness of a new asthma medication, key outcomes might include measures of an individual's respiratory capacity. Similarly, a study evaluating the efficacy of a new heart disease treatment might use outcomes such as myocardial infarction or long-term survival, depending on the goal of the treatment. While these measures of an individual's biological status are important, they do not give an indication of the individual's perception of treatment-associated benefits such as emotional well-being, physical function, or performance of daily activities. A group of instruments called "patient-reported outcomes" (PROs) has emerged during recent decades to fill this gap in the comprehensive assessment of treatment effectiveness.

An outcome is considered a PRO if it is obtained from patient reports such as diet diaries, symptoms checklists, or questionnaires (Willke, Burke, and Erickson 2004). The use of PROs as outcomes in clinical trials has become so pervasive that the Food and Drug Administration (FDA) sponsored a task force in 2001 to explore key issues related to the use of PROs in clinical trials (Acquadro et al. 2003). This chapter provides a brief overview of statistical considerations related to the use of a broad class of PROs called quality of life (QoL) measurements. Those interested in broader exploration of QoL may refer to recent texts such as those by Fairclough (2002); Fayers and Hays (2005); Fayers and Machin (2000); and Mesbah, Cole, and Lee (2002).

As we illustrate in this chapter, analysis of QoL outcomes often involves the estimation of model parameters and some QoL models are quite complex, requiring strong model assumptions. As such, analyses of QoL data can be subject to bias or difficulties in interpretation when the assumptions (generally untestable) fail to hold. Furthermore, because the assessments can be highly subjective, QoL results may lack credibility with some investigators. Consequently, unless QoL results are extremely compelling, additional evidence of efficacy based on clinical outcomes may be required before a new intervention gains acceptance.

9.1 Defining QoL

Although there is no single definition of QoL, most definitions are rooted in the World Health Organization's 1948 definition of health as a "state of complete physical, mental, and social well-being."[1] Thus, it is generally agreed that QoL is multi-dimensional, encompassing an individual's self-report of functional status over a range of health-related domains that include social, emotional, psychological, and physical well being (Speith and Harris 1996; Quittner 1998). Another key feature of QoL outcomes is that they reflect the individual's subjective and objective evaluation of how an illness and its therapy affect the individual functionally across these multiple domains.

9.2 Types of QoL Assessments

There are two basic forms of QoL assessments: those assessing individual preferences and those assessing health status and function (Fairclough 2002; Yabroff, Linas, and Shulman 1996). One or both types may be used as outcomes for any given study, depending on the goal of the assessment.

9.2.1 Subject Preference Measures

Subject preference measures are most often used to examine a subject's preference for quantity versus quality of life. For example, a clinical trial may be designed to compare the effects of a palliative treatment versus a more invasive or side-effect ridden treatment that could prolong life 6-9 months in a population with advanced cancer. A preference-oriented QoL measure would evaluate whether a subject would be willing to tolerate the side effects of the more invasive treatment in return for the additional few months of life. QoL measures that assess preferences are called utility measures and yield data that can be summarized in units of well year equivalents or *Quality Adjusted Life Years* (QALYs). These measures are derived by weighting time spent in a compromised state by a number between zero and one where the former represents death and the latter represents "asymptomatic full function" (Kaplan et al. 1998). Utility measures are often used in health policy decision making and are useful in that they allow treatment comparisons both within and across disease states.

The *Quality of Well-Being Scale* (QWB) (Kaplan et al. 1998) and the *Medical Study Outcomes Short-Form 36* (SF–36) (Ware 2000) are examples of widely used utility QoL measures. The QWB is composed of the following five scales: Mobility, physical activity, social activity, physical symptom status, and mental health. Preferences on questions across all these domains are combined to yield a single health index that ranges from zero to one. The

---

[1] Preamble to the Constitution of the World Health Organization as adopted by the International Health Conference, New York, 19-22 June, 1946; signed on 22 July 1946 by the representatives of 61 States (Official Records of the World Health Organization, no. 2, p. 100) and entered into force on 7 April 1948.

SF-36 consists of 36 questions and is composed of eight scales (Ware 2000) which are listed in Table 9.1. Summary scores are obtained for each of the eight scales as well as for summary measures of physical health (scales 1-4) and mental health (scales 5-8).

Table 9.1 *Quality of well-being scales for SF-36.*

Scale	Description
1)	Physical Function: Limitations in physical activities because of health problems
2)	Role-Physical: Limitations in usual role activities because of physical health problems
3)	Bodily pain
4)	General health perceptions
5)	Vitality: Energy and fatigue
6)	Social Function: Limitations in social activities because of physical or emotional problems
7)	Role-Emotional: Limitations in usual role activities because of emotional problems
8)	General mental health perceptions

9.2.2 Health Status and Functional Measures

Instruments that assess health status and function fall into two categories, *general health profiles* and *disease-specific measures* (Fairclough 2002; Quittner 1998; Koscik et al. 2005). General health profiles are also referred to as generic health profiles and, as such, give the subject an opportunity to rate function in multiple areas that are relevant to QoL for a variety of diseases and illness conditions (Speith and Harris 1996). For example, the *Child Health Questionnaire* (CHQ) (Landgraf, Abetz, and Ware 1996) is a general health profile that has questions representing 12 QoL dimensions, including physical function, role/social limitations, family activities, self-esteem, and others. Each dimension is summarized using a scale score that ranges from zero (worst) to 100 (best possible QoL). The items on these instruments tend to be very general and broad and while they are often not sensitive enough to use for efficacy studies, they may be useful for comparing groups with differing diseases or health states.

In contrast to generic health instruments, disease-specific measures consist predominantly of items that are directly associated with disease symptoms and characteristics. For example, Figure 9.1 shows the items on the *Minnesota Living with Heart Failure* (MLHF) questionnaire (Rector, Kubo, and Cohn 1993). The MLHF questionnaire is a self-administered, 21-question tool assessing emotional and physical parameters that measure how an individual

with heart failure lives compared to how they would like to live. All answers
to the 21 questions can be combined to yield a global summary score of "how
heart failure and treatments impact an individual's quality of life" (Rector,
Kubo, and Cohn 1993). Other disease-specific measures yield summary scores
for multiple functional domains. For example, the *Cystic Fibrosis Questionnaire* (CFQ) uses disease symptom and characteristic-oriented items to yield
scale scores from zero (worst QoL) to 100 (best QoL) for "typical" dimensions of QoL (e.g., physical function, vitality, health perceptions) as well as
for dimensions quite specific to CF that include treatment burden, respiratory function, and digestive function (Quittner et al. 2005). Disease-specific
measures tend to be more useful than generic measures in treatment efficacy
studies, but disease-specific measures are not available for all diseases.

Did your heart failure prevent you from living as you wanted during the past month (4 weeks) by −	No	Very Little				Very Much
1. causing swelling in your ankles or legs	0	1	2	3	4	5
2. making you sit or lie down to rest during the day?	0	1	2	3	4	5
3. making your walking about or climbing stairs difficult?	0	1	2	3	4	5
4. making your working around the house or yard difficult?	0	1	2	3	4	5
5. making your going places away from home difficult?	0	1	2	3	4	5
6. making your sleeping well at night difficult?	0	1	2	3	4	5
7. making your relating to or doing things with your friends or family difficult?	0	1	2	3	4	5
8. making your working to earn a living difficult?	0	1	2	3	4	5
9. making your recreational pastimes, sports, or hobbies difficult?	0	1	2	3	4	5
10. making your sexual activities difficult?	0	1	2	3	4	5
11. making you eat less of the foods you like?	0	1	2	3	4	5
12. making you short of breath?	0	1	2	3	4	5
13. making you tired, fatigued, or low on energy?	0	1	2	3	4	5
14. making you stay in a hospital?	0	1	2	3	4	5
15. costing you money for medical care?	0	1	2	3	4	5
16. giving you side effects from medications?	0	1	2	3	4	5
17. making you feel you are a burden to your family or friends?	0	1	2	3	4	5
18. making you feel a loss of self-control in your life?	0	1	2	3	4	5
19. making you worry?	0	1	2	3	4	5
20. making it difficult for you to concentrate or remember things?	0	1	2	3	4	5
21. making you feel depressed?	0	1	2	3	4	5

Figure 9.1 *Minnesota Living with Heart Failure Questionnaire (MLHF).*

9.3 Selecting a QoL Instrument

There are numerous QoL instruments available to researchers. Valid QoL assessments require that the instruments used be suitable for the intended task. In practice, researchers often choose validated, off-the-shelf instruments to evaluate QoL (Sloan and Dueck 2004). For example, in oncology clinical trials, an off-the-shelf instrument frequently used to identify general problems and symptoms is FACT-G (Cella et al. 1993). It comprises 27 questions that assess four primary dimensions of QoL: physical, social and family, emotional, and functional well-being. A drawback to off-the-shelf instruments is that they may not be sensitive to the differences in the QoL domains targeted by the treatment in a given trial and they may not be validated in the population being tested. Moreover, these instruments tend to be lengthy and may include irrelevant questions that might negatively affect compliance. Customized instruments, on the other hand, can be simple and targeted to a particular disease. These instruments, however, must be first validated to the trial population. It is also important that the instrument selected is sensitive to either between-group differences in function or within-subject changes or both as required. Each of these areas is explored briefly in the following paragraphs.

9.3.1 Purpose of the Assessment

QoL assessments are included as primary or secondary outcomes in clinical trials in order to accomplish a number of purposes. Fayers and Hays (2005) outline several general purposes including: determining the effectiveness of treatments with curative intent as well as those with palliative intent; evaluating the extent to which treatments provide symptom relief or rehabilitation; facilitating communication with future patients, for example, about the range of problems that are likely to affect patients who receive a particular intervention; identifying patient preferences about various health conditions, for example, exploring the degree to which patients are willing to experience unpleasant side effects in return for prolonged life expectancy; identifying problems of psychosocial adaptation that occur late in treatment or even after treatment is completed; and assisting in medical decision-making.

9.3.2 Validity

Validity is a term that refers to the degree to which an instrument "does what it is intended to do" (Carmines and Zeller 1979). A good instrument will possess adequate *construct, criterion,* and *content* validity. *Construct validity* refers to the relationship among items and between items and scales. *Criterion validity,* in contrast, concerns whether the instrument (or scale) shows an empirical relationship to one or more established measures of that domain. Finally, *content validity* refers to the overall degree to which the items reflect the domain(s) of interest. Comprehensive assessment of any given domain is key to ensuring adequate content validity. Statistical methods used in establishing the validity of an instrument include, but are not limited to, item response theory, factor analysis, and multitrait-multimethod analysis (Fayers and Machin 2000).

9.3.3 Reliability

Reliability refers to the degree to which an assessment tool will yield consistent results if given multiple times under similar conditions. Reliability can be assessed empirically several ways, including test-retest, split-half, alternative form, and Cronbach's α coefficient (Carmines and Zeller 1979). The first three describe a measure's stability over time while the latter is used to describe an instrument or scale's internal reliability (or consistency). The formula for computing the Cronbach's α coefficient is given by

$$\alpha = \frac{k}{k-1} \left(1 - \frac{\sum_{i=1}^{k} s_i^2}{s_T^2} \right),$$

where k is the number of items, s_i^2 the variance of the ith item, and s_T^2 the variance of the total score that is formed by summing up all the items. If all items are identical, then all the s_i^2 will be equal and $s_T^2 = k^2 s_i^2$, so that $\alpha = 1$. If, on the other hand, the items are all independent, then $s_T^2 = \sum_{i=1}^{k} s_i^2$ so that $\alpha = 0$.

Regardless of the method used, the higher the reliability, the less measurement error there is, so a high degree of reliability is desired. A scale or whole questionnaire may be revised based on the reliability data obtained during the validation process.

9.3.4 Sensitivity and Responsiveness

Sensitivity and *responsiveness* are related, though distinct, characteristics of QoL instruments that must be considered when selecting a QoL instrument and estimating the required sample size. First, *sensitivity* refers to an instrument's ability to measure clinically meaningful differences in function between treatment groups. Sensitivity is typically assessed using cross-sectional data and comparing QoL scores between groups where QoL is expected to differ. Second, *responsiveness* refers to an instrument's ability to measure a clinically meaningful change within a subject over time for any given state of function and is evaluated using longitudinal assessment of subjects (Fayers and Machin 2000). Although the terms are presented as distinct concepts, be aware that they are often used interchangeably in the QoL literature.

Interestingly, an instrument can have adequate reliability, but lack sensitivity or responsiveness (or both). For example, the Child Health Questionnaire described earlier has well-established reliability and validity of its 12 scales. When the instrument was used with a pediatric sample of subjects with cystic fibrosis, however, the scores were at or near the maximum score of 100 for a substantial percentage of the subjects across most of the instrument's dimensions (Koscik et al. 2005). This phenomenon is referred to as a *ceiling effect*. When ceiling effects are present, an instrument will not be able to detect differences between groups, and will therefore lack sensitivity.

9.3.5 Determining Clinically Meaningful Differences

When designing any study, power, and sample size calculations are based on the specification of a desired effect size Δ (see Chapter 4). QoL data are no exception to this rule and this Δ is often referred to as the "minimally important difference" (MID) (Crosby, Kolotkin, and Williams 2003). Determining exactly what constitutes the MID in QoL scores is a difficult task, and there are two general approaches that are typically taken to defining clinical significance, anchor-based and distribution-based. Anchor-based methods identify clinically meaningful change in QoL scores by comparing QoL scores with other measures of a subject's status. For example, if QoL is being measured in a disease with levels of disease severity that can be objectively determined (e.g., mild, moderate, severe), differences in QoL scores between adjacent severity categories can be used to estimate what constitutes a clinically meaningful difference in QoL scores. Distribution-based methods, on the other hand, rely on the statistical properties of the responses to estimate clinically meaningful differences. For example, many researchers have used a change of one half of one standard deviation as the MID while others (see, for example, Samsa et al. (1999)) have argued that differences as small as 0.2 standard deviation units constitute the MID. Those interested in expanded descriptions of anchor- and distribution-based methods and their limitations should refer to Crosby, Kolotkin, and Williams (2003).

9.4 Developing a QoL Instrument

A research team may find that after a thorough search of the literature and/or piloting of available QoL instruments with their study population, no measure QoL suitable for their purposes exists. The team may then decide to develop a new questionnaire and the statistician can play an integral role in ensuring that the new instrument meets all of the needs outlined in Section 9.3. It is beyond the scope of this text to provide detail on the many steps that are needed to develop a valid, reliable, and sensitive instrument and interested readers should refer to Fayers and Machin (2000), Fowler (1995, 2002), or Rea and Parker (1997) for comprehensive guidance in instrument development.

9.5 Quality of Life Data

9.5.1 General Issues

Because responses are multidimensional, QoL analyses may require statistical methods that differ from those used for the more traditional, univariate, outcomes. Before describing the details of statistical methods typically used to analyze QoL data, we briefly summarize the main characteristics of QoL data in clinical trials. First, we note that QoL assessments typically consist of multiple outcomes measuring different aspects of a subject's emotional and physical well-being. The presence of multiple outcomes may present difficulties, including adjustments for multiple comparisons and problems presenting and interpreting the results. Second, QoL assessments are obtained at several, possibly unequally spaced times, and it is often of interest to evaluate changes in QoL over a time period. One of the major challenges in the analysis of longitudinal data is the handling of missing data that is an inherent feature in QoL evaluations (Fairclough, Peterson, and Chang 1998). In advanced diseases, non-compliance with QoL assessments is often a result of death or other medical reasons. For example, Hürny et al. (1992) reported that the compliance rate in some oncology trials was less than 30%. The concern with missing data in QoL evaluations is that it may lead to bias, due either to incomplete evaluations or evaluations that are missing entirely because subjects have discontinued their participation in the trial (Olschewski and Schumacher 1990). Consequently, QoL data should be analyzed with care and missing data problems should be properly considered. A number of statistical methods have been proposed to handle the missing data problem. As we discuss in more detail in Chapter 11 (see also Little and Rubin (2002)), missing data are often categorized as either *Missing Completely at Random* (MCAR), *Missing at Random* (MAR), or *Missing Not at Random* (MNAR). These categories are useful for describing the assumptions required for a particular analytic technique to provide valid inference. MCAR is the least restrictive, but generally also the least plausible. MNAR is the most difficult to account for, but in many cases is the most plausible.

In QoL assessments, there are two forms of missing data. First, there could be single item non-responses that might occur when a response has not been provided for at least one question from a questionnaire. Single item non-responses may cause problems when calculating global QoL scores and many standard questionnaire manuals suggest methods of dealing with single missing items, usually by using extrapolation (Stephens 2004). Second, multiple item non-responses might arise, for example, if an entire questionnaire is missing. This may result from a single missed visit or the withdrawal of a subject from the trial altogether. Since in each case the missingness is likely to be related to the health status of the subject, this form of missingness is generally considered to be MNAR.

9.5.2 Data Collection Considerations

A comprehensive discussion of general issues related to data collection is provided in Chapter 6. In this section, we summarize some of the data collection issues that are specific to QoL assessments. Measurement of QoL in a clinical trial can be based on self-administered questionnaires or interviews. Data collected using self-administered questionnaires are more vulnerable to non-compliance, but might be less costly and the only feasible option in many clinical trials. Interview-based data collection requires training of interviewers and can be done either during clinic visits or using a phone interview. Some subjects may feel uncomfortable being interviewed before or directly after receiving treatment and self-administered questionnaires may be preferred from a subject's perspective as they can be filled out in a safe and comfortable environment. Regardless of whether the data collection is based on self-administered questionnaires or interviews, practical steps should be taken to ensure that the QoL evaluations are incorporated successfully into the clinical trial. First, in order to maximize the compliance rate, the QoL evaluation should be mandatory. Second, it is important to identify instruments that are appropriate to the study, are not too lengthy, and do not include irrelevant questions. Moreover, it should be ensured that questionnaires are available in the appropriate language. Finally, the schedule of QoL assessments should be convenient to the subject while including sufficiently many assessments to capture changes in QoL profiles.

9.6 Analysis of QoL Data

Statistical methods frequently applied to QoL data range from simple descriptive methods to complex multivariate models. The choice of the appropriate method is influenced by study objectives and the type of QoL outcomes. An overview of statistical methods commonly used to analyze QoL data in clinical trials will be given in this section.

9.6.1 Longitudinal Data Analysis

In a clinical trial, QoL data are typically collected over an extended time period. The analysis and interpretation of longitudinal data can be complex, particularly when data are missing.

Graphical Summaries

As an initial step, a simple exploratory analysis can provide important insights. Graphical procedures are useful exploratory tools that can reveal trends, outliers, and patterns of non-compliance (Billingham, Abrams, and Jones 1999). Graphical summaries of longitudinal QoL data include profile plots of individual subjects and group profile plots. Profile plots of individual QoL responses help to identify general trends over time and may provide information about inter-individual variability. For example, Machin and Weeden (1998) recommend plotting QoL scores from individual subjects versus the time from randomization. Profile plots of individual subject's QoL scores can be displayed as a set of small graphs or overlaid in one graph. Figure 9.2 shows the profile plots of the global QoL score of the MLHF questionnaire (see Section 9.2) for a subgroup of subjects from the Vesnarinone Trial (VesT) (Cohn et al. 1998). The global MLHF score is computed as a sum of all 21 individual item scores and ranges from 0 (best QoL) to 105 (worst QoL). The VesT study was a double-blind, placebo controlled, randomized phase III trial that assessed mortality, morbidity, and quality of life of subjects with severe heart failure. A total number of 3833 subjects at 189 study centers were randomized to receive either 30 *mg* daily dose of vesnarinone, 60 *mg* daily dose of vesnarinone, or placebo. The MLHF questionnaire was filled out by the subject in the VesT study at baseline, and at weeks 8, 16, and 26.

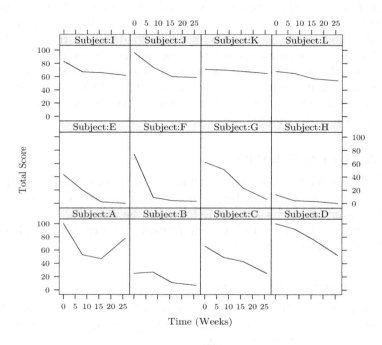

Figure 9.2 *Profile plots of individual subjects' global MLHF scores from the VesT trial. Lower scores indicate better quality of life.*

Figure 9.2 suggests that there is considerable variability both between and within subjects and that there is an overall decrease in the total QoL score over time. Of course for large trials, examining individual profile plots of all subjects becomes impractical. In these situations, group summary measures should be used. For example, if the data are on a continuous scale, the means with the corresponding confidence intervals can be plotted. If the data are on a categorical scale, the proportions of responses that fall into particular categories can be plotted over time. Profile plots of summary measures should be interpreted with caution when informative drop-out occurs (Billingham, Abrams, and Jones 1999). Figure 9.3 shows the profile plots of means of the global MLHF scores of the VesT trial along with the corresponding 95% confidence intervals for the three treatment groups. Ignoring the potential effects of missing data, Figure 9.3 suggests that all three treatment groups saw an improvement in QoL during follow-up. At the 8 and 16 week assessments, the means of the QoL total scores for the 60 *mg* vesnarinone treated group were significantly lower than those in the placebo group.

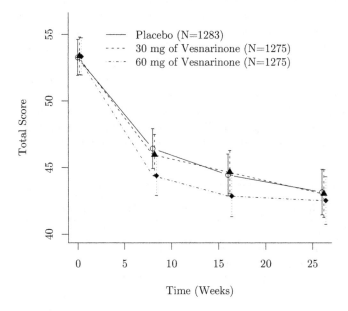

Figure 9.3 *Profile plots of means of the global MLHF scores in the VesT trial along with the corresponding 95% confidence intervals.*

Summary Measures

Summary measures can reduce the repeated measures of an individual subject's assessment into a single measure. Longitudinal data can be summarized using a variety of standard summary measures that can be easily computed. The disadvantage of summarizing repeated QoL assessments into a single measure is that information about patterns of change over time may be lost. Furthermore, if subjects drop out, the analysis of these measures might lead to biased results.

The most commonly used summary measure of longitudinal QoL outcomes is the area under the curve (AUC). Letting T_{ij} denote the jth time ($j = 1, \cdots, K$) for subject i and x_{ij} the QoL score of the ith subject at the jth time, the AUC can be computed using the trapezoidal rule by

$$\text{AUC}_i = \frac{1}{2} \sum_{j=2}^{K} \left(x_{ij} + x_{i(j-1)} \right) \left(T_{ij} - T_{i(j-1)} \right).$$

QoL scores missing at individual times can be imputed by interpolation. For example, if an intermediate observation is missing, the corresponding QoL score could be computed using only the non-missing observations. This is equivalent to imputation using linear interpolation. If a subject drops out and follow-up QoL assessments are missing, the corresponding missing QoL scores could be imputed by extrapolating from the last observations. Alternatively, the AUC can be considered as censored at the last available QoL assessment. Censoring, however, can be informative and standard survival analysis techniques can lead to biased estimation (Billingham, Abrams, and Jones 1999). A bias adjustment procedure has been proposed by Korn (1993) using estimates of the cumulative distribution function of an interpolated AUC. Other standard summary measures include the mean, median, or the lowest or highest values reported. All these summary measures are straightforward to compute and can be easily interpreted. The summary measure should be chosen to most directly address the primary questions of the trial.

Table 9.2 *Mean and standard deviation AUC of MLHF global score of VesT study.*

Group	Mean	Standard Deviation
Placebo	1882.79	908.07
30 *mg* vesnarinone	1871.44	921.40
60 *mg* vesnarinone	1863.64	917.13

Table 9.2 shows the means and standard deviations for the AUCs of the MLHF global scores for the three treatment arms of the VesT study (Cohn et al. 1998). The AUCs were computed from the baseline to the 26 week assessment. For subjects who died or underwent heart transplantation before the 26 weeks assessment, the worst possible MLHF score was imputed for the missing assessments. The mean AUC in the placebo arm is 11.35 units higher than the mean AUC in the 30 *mg* vesnarinone arm and 19.15 units higher than the mean AUC in the 60 *mg* vesnarinone arm.

Analysis at each Time Separately

If the QoL assessments are made at fixed times, an analysis can be conducted separately at each time. The analysis is then reduced to independent observations at each time for which standard parametric or nonparametric statistical procedures are available (e.g., t-tests, ANOVA, or Wilcoxon rank sum tests). QoL scores are often summarized using means and standard deviations for each time. Percentage changes between baseline and follow-up assessments are typically reported. Changes between baseline and follow-up assessments can be evaluated using paired comparisons. While this analysis is intuitive and the results easily interpretable by the researcher, there are several drawbacks to this approach. First, if the assessments are made over more than two times, information about the profile across time is lost. Second, biased results might be obtained when some values are missing. Finally, since multiple analyses are involved, multiple testing issues arise.

Statistical Modeling for Repeated QoL Measurements

There are a number of modeling approaches to analyze longitudinal data. A comprehensive description of longitudinal data analysis models is given in Chapter 8. The choice of an appropriate model depends on several factors, including the type of outcome, distribution assumptions, and the types of missing values.

Repeated Measures ANOVA If QoL outcomes are on a continuous scale, a repeated measurements analysis of variance (RMANOVA) can be used. RMANOVA have the advantage that many clinicians are familiar with it and that it can be easily implemented using most statistical software packages. The main feature of the analysis of variance approach is that it can model the mean change over time. On the other hand, the RMANOVA may not be appropriate for the QoL analysis in clinical trials because of restrictive model assumptions. First, this approach does not allow for a flexible covariance structure among repeated measurements, i.e., it is assumed that the correlations among repeated QoL assessments over all times within a subject are the same (*sphericity* or *compound symmetry*), although approximate adjustments are available that attempt to account for departures from sphericity. Furthermore, analysis of variance requires observations at the same times for all subjects. This is rarely the case in QoL evaluations in clinical trials because of irregular visit schedules and missing visits.

When data are missing, a complete case analysis or data imputation is required. A complete case analysis is valid only if the missing data are MCAR. One commonly used imputation technique, usually referred to as *last observation carried forward* (LOCF), imputes the last observed value for each subsequent missing value. This imputation technique has serious drawbacks, however, and is not recommended (see Section 11.3.3 on page 361 for additional discussion). A preferred alternative is *multiple imputation* which can be used when data are MAR. Multiple imputation is complex and will not be described in detail in this book; a brief discussion appears in Section 11.3.3.

Mixed Effects Models The mixed effects model is a flexible tool for the analysis of QoL data with less restrictive assumptions than the traditional linear model. (See Chapter 8 for detailed discussion of mixed effects models.) Specifically, mixed effects models allow flexible dependence structures to accommodate within-subject correlations. This is particularly useful in the clinical trial setting where measurements are often obtained at unequally spaced times. Moreover, mixed effects models can accommodate hierarchical data structures (e.g., multicenter studies) or situations where the data are clustered. Parameters can be estimated using either maximum likelihood (ML) or restricted maximum likelihood (REML).

Since QoL scores are usually treated as continuous measurements, linear mixed effects models are frequently used for the primary QoL analysis. Several standard software packages can be used to fit linear mixed effects models, for example, `PROC MIXED` in SAS/STAT or the `lme` function in S-Plus or R.

In some situations, however, QoL outcomes are on a categorical scale so that linear mixed effects models cannot be used. In these situations, the method of generalized estimating equations (GEE), as described in Chapter 8, can be utilized. Parameters are estimated using iterative procedures. `PROC NLMIXED` in SAS/STAT or the `glme` function in S-Plus can also be used to fit generalized linear mixed effects models.

The major limitation of the mixed effects modeling approach for the analysis of QoL data is the MAR assumption. In practice, a subject may drop-out for a variety of reasons, including excessive toxicity, disease progression, and death. Therefore, the MAR assumption is often violated. When data are MNAR, the standard linear or generalized mixed effects model could give biased parameter estimates (Little and Raghunathan 1999). Longitudinal data analysis with MNAR data requires more complex models. Several different parametric and semiparametric approaches to analyze longitudinal with MNAR data or informative drop-outs have been proposed. For example, Schluechter (1992) proposed a joint mixed-effects and survival model that accounts for informative drop-outs. Let T_i denote the time to drop-out the ith subject. In the joint mixed-effects and survival model it is assumed that the joint distribution of the random components b_i in the standard mixed effects model and a function $f(T_i)$, for example, $f(T_i) = \log(T_i)$, have a multivariate normal distribution

$$\begin{pmatrix} b_i \\ f(T_i) \end{pmatrix} \sim N \left(\begin{pmatrix} 0 \\ \mu_T \end{pmatrix}, \begin{pmatrix} G & \sigma_{bt} \\ \sigma_{bt} & \tau^2 \end{pmatrix} \right).$$

Maximum likelihood estimates of the model parameters can be obtained using the EM algorithm (Dempster, Laird, and Rubin 1977).

Wu and Carroll (1988) use a probit model to model the relationship between the probability of drop-out and the trajectory of the response variable. Diggle and Kennward (1994) propose an outcome-dependent logistic drop-out selection model. Software to fit these models is not readily available, however.

9.6.2 Multivariate Analysis

A Global Test Statistic

Most QoL instruments consist of many items that may be grouped into categories measuring various aspects of a subject's quality of life. While this grouping reduces the number of outcome variables, it does not eliminate the problem multiple comparisons and there is no consensus regarding the approach that best accounts for the multiplicity in QoL outcomes (Fayers and Machin 2000). It is common practice in clinical trials to analyze each outcome separately and use an adjustment for multiple comparisons in order to control the overall type I error rate. (See Section 11.5 for a more detailed discussion of multiple comparisons.) For example, the simplest adjustment method is the Bonferroni adjustment in which the adjusted p-value is computed by multiplying the nominal p-value by the number of outcomes to be compared. Since the individual instrument items are likely correlated, however, the Bonferroni adjustment can be too extreme and separate analysis of each item may be inefficient when evaluating the overall treatment effect. The test of O'Brien (1984) described in Chapter 2, equation (2.19), can be applied in this situation. A drawback of this method is that it does not give an estimate of the treatment difference.

For example, scores on the MLHF questionnaire can be subdivided into "emotional well-being" and "physical well-being" scores. Table 9.3 shows t-statistic values for comparing "emotional well-being" and "physical well-being" (change from baseline) scores between the placebo and 60 *mg* vesnarinone arm of the VesT study (Cohn et al. 1998) at weeks 8, 16, and 26.

Table 9.3 *T-statistic values for comparing "emotional well-being" and "physical well-being" MLHF scores between placebo and 60 mg vesnarinone arm in the VesT study*

Time	"emotional well-being"	"physical well-being"
week 8	3.38	2.69
week 16	2.86	2.65
week 26	1.45	0.84

The empirical pooled correlations between the "emotional well-being" and "physical well-being" scores (change from baseline) for the 8, 16, and 26 week assessments are 0.53, 0.57, and 0.59, respectively. Therefore, the Z test statistic value for the comparison of multiple outcomes at the 8 week assessment is 3.47 so that $P < 0.001$. Analogously, the Z test statistic values for the comparisons at the 16 and 26 week assessments are 3.11 ($P = 0.002$) and 1.28 ($P = 0.200$), respectively.

Latent Variable Models

QoL states can be treated as *latent* (not directly observable) variables. Therefore, latent variable models can be useful tools for the analysis of QoL data (Fayers and Hand 1997). Latent variable modeling is a multivariate technique commonly used in social and behavioral sciences to describe an underlying structure that cannot be observed directly. The models used for these analyses relate all observed outcomes to latent common factors. The simplest form of a latent variable model is the linear measurement model (Bollen 1989) that assumes that a $k \times 1$ vector $y_i = (y_{1i}, \cdots, y_{ki})'$ of observed items and a $q \times 1$ ($q < k$) unobserved vector of latent variables ξ_i for the ith subject satisfies

$$y_i = \mu + \Lambda \xi_i + \epsilon_i. \tag{9.1}$$

In the linear measurement model, (9.1), ϵ_i is a vector of unobserved measurement errors and the parameters μ and Λ denote the matrix of overall intercept and the slope parameters. The standard assumption is that the latent variables have a multivariate normal distribution with unknown mean μ_ξ and covariance matrix Σ_ξ. The measurement errors ϵ_i are assumed to be independently and identically distributed with $E(\epsilon_i) = \mathbf{0}$ and covariance matrix Ψ. Furthermore, it is assumed that the latent variables ξ_i and the measurement errors ϵ_i are independent. Even with these assumptions, model (9.1) is not identifiable (overparameterized) without further restrictions. A standard identifiable form of model (9.1) is given by

$$y_i = \begin{pmatrix} 0 \\ \mu_0 \end{pmatrix} + \begin{pmatrix} I_q \\ \Lambda_0 \end{pmatrix} \xi_i + \epsilon_i, \tag{9.2}$$

where I_q denotes the q-dimensional identity matrix. The elements of the $k-q$ dimensional vector μ_0 and of the $(k-q) \times q$ dimensional matrix Λ_0 may contain unrestricted parameters.

The elements of the latent variable ξ_i may represent individual QoL subscales. For a clinical trial with G study arms, model (9.2) can be written for the gth $(g = 1, \cdots, G)$ study arm as

$$y_i^{(g)} = \begin{pmatrix} 0 \\ \mu_0^{(g)} \end{pmatrix} + \begin{pmatrix} I_q \\ \Lambda_0^{(g)} \end{pmatrix} \xi_i^{(g)} + \epsilon_i^{(g)}. \tag{9.3}$$

Since in clinical trials the same QoL instrument is administered to all study arms simultaneously, it is reasonable to assume that the measurement properties are invariant across study arms, i.e., $\mu_0^{(1)} = \cdots = \mu_0^{(G)}$ and $\Lambda_0^{(1)} = \cdots = \Lambda_0^{(G)}$. The distribution parameters of the latent variables remain unrestricted so that differences in QoL between study arms can be directly assessed by comparing latent variable means and covariances between arms. Since in validated QoL instruments the subscale structure is known, certain elements of Λ_0 are fixed at zero. For example, the MLHF questionnaire consists of an "emotional well-being" and a "physical well-being" component. The "physical well-being" component consists of eight items $j = 1, \cdots, 8$, with (index, j, in parentheses) "rest during day" (1), "walking and climbing stairs" (2), "working around the house" (3), "going away from home" (4), "sleeping" (5), "doing things with others" (6), "dyspnea" (7), and "fatigue" (8). The "emotional well-being" component consists of five items $j = 9, \cdots, 13$, with "feeling burdensome" (9), "feeling a loss of self-control" (10), "worry" (11), "difficulty concentrating and remembering" (12), and "feeling depressed" (13). Therefore, the measurement model (9.2) for QoL data obtained from the MLHF instrument can be written as

$$
\begin{pmatrix} y_{1i}^{(g)} \\ y_{2i}^{(g)} \\ \vdots \\ y_{8i}^{(g)} \\ y_{9i}^{(g)} \\ y_{10i}^{(g)} \\ \vdots \\ y_{13i}^{(g)} \end{pmatrix} = \begin{pmatrix} 0 \\ \mu_2 \\ \vdots \\ \mu_8 \\ 0 \\ \mu_{10} \\ \vdots \\ \mu_{13} \end{pmatrix} + \begin{pmatrix} 1 & 0 \\ \lambda_2 & 0 \\ \vdots \\ \lambda_8 & 0 \\ 0 & 1 \\ 0 & \lambda_{10} \\ \vdots \\ 0 & \lambda_{13} \end{pmatrix} \begin{pmatrix} \xi_{1i}^{(g)} \\ \xi_{2i}^{(g)} \end{pmatrix} + \begin{pmatrix} \epsilon_{1i}^{(g)} \\ \epsilon_{2i}^{(g)} \\ \vdots \\ \epsilon_{8i}^{(g)} \\ \epsilon_{9i}^{(g)} \\ \epsilon_{10i}^{(g)} \\ \vdots \\ \epsilon_{13i}^{(g)} \end{pmatrix}. \quad (9.4)
$$

The λ's are unknown slope parameters, the latent variable $\xi_{1i}^{(g)}$ represents the "physical well-being" component and the latent variable $\xi_{2i}^{(g)}$ represents the "emotional well-being" component of the gth study arm. Larger values of $\xi_{1i}^{(g)}$ and $\xi_{2i}^{(g)}$ indicate a worse health state. The slope parameters λ's represent the direct effects of the latent variables ("physical well-being" or "emotional well-being") on the observed responses of the MLHF questions. Model (9.4) is illustrated in the path diagram in Figure 9.4. Table 9.4 shows the maximum likelihood estimates of the latent variables means for the 8 weeks post-treatment assessment of the VesT study.

Table 9.4 *Maximum likelihood estimates (standard errors) of the latent variable means for the 8 weeks post-treatment assessment of the VesT study.*

Group	"physical well-being" (ξ_1)	"emotional well-being" (ξ_2)
Placebo	2.37 (0.036)	1.63 (0.010)
3mg vesnarinone	2.31 (0.035)	1.63 (0.009)
60mg vesnarinone	2.26 (0.036)	1.62 (0.010)

The basic measurement model, (9.1), can be extended to a structural equation model (Bollen 1989). A structural equation model allows us to specify relations between unobserved and observed variables while controlling for measurement errors and correlations among both the measurement errors and the latent variables. Parameter estimation is typically performed using maximum likelihood estimation based on iterative procedures. Latent variable models can be fit using specialized software packages, including LISREL (Jöreskog and Sörbom 1996) and Mplus (Muthén and Muthén 1998).

Quality-Adjusted Survival Analysis

Survival time is the most important outcome in the evaluation of the treatment of a life threatening disease such as cancer. There is often a trade-off,

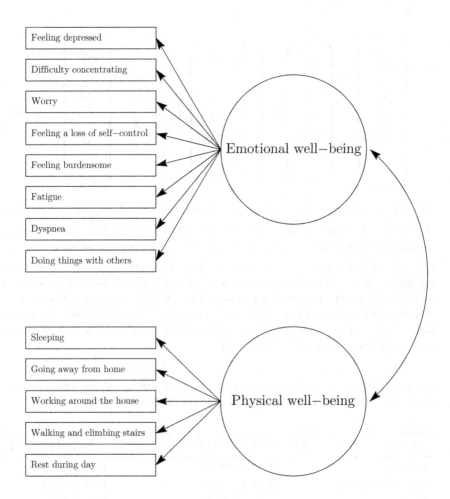

Figure 9.4 *Path diagram for measurement model for MLHF instrument.*

however, between clinical benefit measured by prolonged survival and side effects that might reduce the quality of life. Quality-adjusted survival analysis is a method for combining survival and quality of life into a single measure. Q-TWiST, "Quality-adjusted Time Without Symptoms of disease and Toxicity of treatment", was introduced by Goldhirsch et al. (1989) as a means to combine quality of life information and survival analysis. The Q-TWiST analysis consists of three steps. In the first step, several clinical health states are defined. In the original application for which Q-TWiST was developed, three health states were defined (Goldhirsch et al. 1989): time with toxicity (TOX), time without symptoms and toxicity (TWiST), and time after progression or relapse (REL). In the second step, Kaplan-Meier curves for the clinical health transition times are used to partition the area under the overall survival curves (see Zhao and Tsiatis (1997, 1999)). The average time spent in each health state in calculated separately for each treatment as illustrated in Figure 9.5.

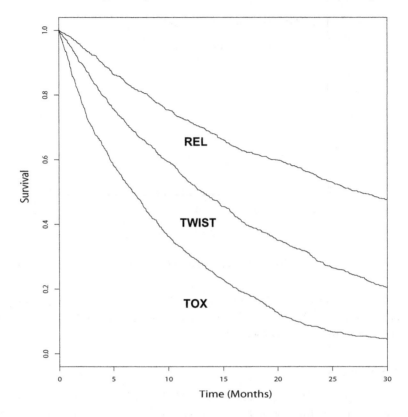

Figure 9.5 *Partitioned survival curve for Q-TWiST.*

In the third step, utility weights between 0 and 1 are assigned to each health state by considering how valuable a time period with toxicity or relapse is to each subject. The treatment regimens are then compared using the weighted sum of the mean durations of each clinical health status calculated in step 2. For example, in the original application (Goldhirsch et al. 1989), Q-TWiST was calculated as

$$\text{Q-TWiST} = u_t \text{TOX} + \text{TWiST} + u_R \text{REL},$$

where u_t and u_R are the utility weights for estimated time with toxicity and estimated time after progression or relapse, respectively. In most situations, the utility weights u_t and u_R are unknown. One approach in these situations is to perform a threshold utility analysis as illustrated in Figure 9.6. In a threshold utility analysis, the Q-TWiST treatment effect is evaluated for all possible combinations of utility weight values.

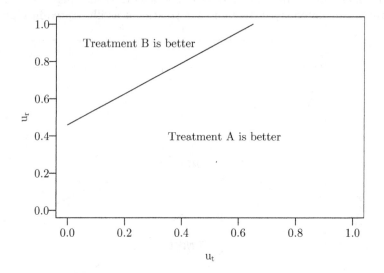

Figure 9.6 *Threshold utility analysis.*

Some more recent work regarding the joint modeling of QoL scores and survival is due to Wang, Douglas, and Anderson (2002) and Chi and Ibrahim (2006, 2007) but is not presented here.

9.7 Summary

In this chapter we have presented some of the basic issues encountered when using Quality of Life measures as either a primary or a secondary outcome measure. In either case, the best choice of a QoL instrument is one that is specific to the needs of the trial. That is, the instrument should be targeted to a specific disease and its direct consequences, or targeted to specific QoL dimensions. General, non-specific QoL instruments tend not to be sensitive to the concerns most relevant in a particular trial and subject population. Inappropriate instruments may not only be insensitive to the intervention effect but may be so irrelevant or awkward for the subject that it may even discourage them from continuing to participate.

In addition to selecting a targeted QoL instrument, the analysis for that instrument is generally more complex than for other outcome measures. Plans for analysis must be laid out in advance, especially if this is the primary outcome measure. Design aspects including sample size are more complicated than for continuous, binomial, longitudinal, or survival analysis and may require simulation methods. Missing data in an instrument can be a common problem that must be addressed in any analysis plan.

Nonetheless, QoL is an important measure of the effects of an intervention in a subject population, and should be included as an outcome measure when appropriate. With proper design and planning, many trials have successfully utilized QoL instruments.

CHAPTER 10

Data Monitoring and Interim Analysis

The term *interim analysis* refers to statistical analysis conducted during the course of a clinical trial for the purpose of monitoring efficacy and safety. While interim analyses serve a variety of purposes, a primary goal of interim analyses is to determine if the trial should stop before its planned termination time if the superiority of the intervention under study is clearly established, if the ultimate demonstration of a relevant intervention difference has become unlikely (futility), or if unacceptable adverse effects are apparent. Also, as a result of interim analyses, the intervention may be modified or elements of the experimental design, such as subject eligibility criteria, changed. Since all interventions have the potential for causing harm, there is an ethical obligation to the study participants that a trial not continue beyond the point at which the potential risks to the study participants outweigh the potential benefits. On the other hand, if one intervention is conclusively demonstrated to be substantially superior to another intervention, there is an ethical obligation not to continue to expose subjects to an inferior therapy. Finally, if it is clear that the study is unlikely to provide definitive answers to the study question, continued participation in the trial may expose subjects to potential risk with minimal scientific justification. The statistical issues related to early stopping because of unexpected adverse side effects are more complex and sound decision making generally requires a combination of careful statistical analysis and informed clinical judgment. It is difficult, if not impossible, to prespecify stopping criteria that address all possible safety issues that might arise. Consequently, formal stopping rules for safety monitoring are typically specified for a small number of safety outcomes such as all-cause mortality or adverse events of particular concern such as liver abnormalities that may be suspected of being associated with the treatment.

These are complex issues and in order to ensure ethical conduct of clinical trials, the National Institutes of Health (NIH), the Food and Drug Administration (FDA), and the International Conference on Harmonization of Technical Requirements for Registration of Pharmaceuticals for Human Use (ICH) have issued principles governing data and safety monitoring and guidelines for data and safety monitoring procedures. We will review general issues in monitoring of data and safety in Section 10.1. To illustrate the issues in data and safety monitoring, two examples are introduced in Section 10.2 and will be used in subsequent sections to illustrate various issues in interim analysis. A typical interim analysis will use one of three general approaches: group sequential tests, triangular tests, and stochastic curtailment tests. These three approaches will

be described in Sections 10.4, 10.5, and 10.6, respectively. Sequential methods
for interim analysis have implications for statistical inference such as point
and confidence intervals and the observed significance. Methods for statistical
inference following sequential tests will be described in Section 10.7.

10.1 Data and Safety Monitoring

All clinical trials require some degree of data and safety monitoring to minimize risks to participants and reassess the risk/benefit ratio throughout the
study period. The extent of monitoring should depend on the nature of the
disease and the therapy under investigation, and the method of monitoring
should be appropriate to the size, scope, and complexity of clinical trials.

The need for ongoing monitoring of data and safety in clinical trials was
perhaps first recognized formally in late 1960s for large-scale randomized, controlled trials sponsored by the National Heart Institute (subsequently renamed
the National Heart, Lung, and Blood Institute) and was documented in what
has come to be known as the *Greenberg Report*, issued in 1967 and later published in 1998 (Heart Special Project Committee 1998). The first NIH policy
on data and safety monitoring developed by the NIH Clinical Trials Committee was issued in June 1979 based largely on the recommendations given in
the Greenberg Report. In 1994, the Office of Extramural Research established
the Committee on Clinical Trial Monitoring to review the oversight and management practices for phase III clinical trials. The committee's findings and
recommendations formed a basis of the NIH notice issued in June of 1998.[1]
This policy announcement requires "a system for the appropriate oversight
and monitoring of the conduct of clinical trials to ensure the safety of participants and the validity and integrity of the data for all NIH-supported or
conducted clinical trials." It also requires "the establishment of the data and
safety monitoring boards (DSMBs) or data monitoring committees (DMCs)
for multi-site clinical trials involving interventions that entail potential risk
to the participants." In addition, it emphasizes that "the data and safety
monitoring functions and oversight of such activities are distinct from the requirement for study review and approval by an Institutional Review Board
(IRB)."

The ICH Harmonized Tripartite Guideline E6[2] defines Good Clinical Practice (GCP) as "an international ethical and scientific quality standard for
designing, conducting, recording, and reporting of trials that involve participation of human subjects." The monitoring of clinical trials for safety of
participants, integrity of data leading to valid conclusions from clinical trials,
and considerations for early termination of clinical trials to avoid unnecessary
experimentation on human subjects can be thought of as direct responses to
the GCP requirements. A recent draft guidance document [3] from the FDA

also describes guidelines on establishment and operation of clinical trial data monitoring committees.

Data and safety monitoring activities should be conducted by a body of experts from various scientific disciplines and recommendations regarding study conduct provided to the sponsor. These recommendations are reviewed and addressed by the study team. Institutional Review Boards or Ethics Committees are usually kept abreast of findings from adverse event reports and recommendations from the DMC. The reporting relationship between the DMC for NIH-supported multicenter clinical trials and the local IRBs was established in a 1999 NIH notice[4] that, in particular, provides guidelines on reporting of adverse events to IRBs.

The specific individuals involved in monitoring activities and their associated responsibilities will depend on the design and phase of the trial. The monitoring of multicenter phase III clinical trials is typically performed by an independent DMC, consisting of clinical trial experts, biostatisticians, bioethicists, and clinicians knowledgeable about the disease under investigation and the protocol intervention. In order to maintain independence, DMC members monitoring outcomes of a trial should have no other involvement in the trial. The composition of the DMC, its responsibilities, policy, and procedures including confidentiality and conflict of interest should be clearly delineated in its charter. Practical guidelines for data and safety monitoring boards have been documented in Ellenberg, Fleming, and DeMets (2002).

The monitoring of early phase I and phase II clinical trials does not require an independent DMC. In a separate NIH notice[5] issued in 2000, the NIH provides further guidance on data and safety monitoring for early phase clinical trials. This guidance recognizes that clinical investigators conducting clinical trials and their support staff such as clinical research associates or research nurses are the vanguard of subject safety, with clearly specified mechanisms for the reporting of adverse events.

The primary responsibilities of a DMC include review of the study protocol and data and safety monitoring plan; evaluation of the progress of the study, including participant recruitment, periodic assessments of data quality and completeness of follow-up, compliance with the protocol, performance of clinical sites, and other factors that can affect study outcome; assessments of risks versus benefits; and finally making recommendations to the sponsor, local IRBs, and investigators concerning continuation, modification, or termination of the trial(s); and protection of the confidentiality of the trial data and the results of monitoring.

In the remainder of the chapter, we will address statistical issues regarding data and safety monitoring in phase III randomized, controlled trials. Monitoring of data and safety in randomized, controlled clinical trials is usually conducted via a series of interim analyses. Because the number, methods, and

---

[4] http://grants.nih.gov/grants/guide/notice-files/not99-107.html
[5] http://grants.nih.gov/grants/guide/notice-files/NOT-OD-00-038.html

consequences of these analyses affect the interpretation of the trial results, interim analyses should be carefully planned in advance and described explicitly in the protocol. When an interim analysis is planned with the intention of deciding whether or not to terminate a trial early, this is usually accomplished by the use of a procedure from one of three general classes known as *group sequential procedures*, *triangular tests*, and *stochastic curtailment*.

10.2 Examples

Two examples of randomized, control trials will be introduced here and will be used throughout the chapter to illustrate different interim analysis procedures and issues to consider in early termination of clinical trials.

10.2.1 Beta-Blocker Heart Attack Trial

By the middle of the 1970s, a class of drugs known as beta-blockers were commonly used to treat subjects with coronary heart disease for symptomatic relief of angina pectoris. In experimental animal models these agents were demonstrated to decrease myocardial ischemia and to limit infarct size. A number of small clinical trials using beta-blockers had been carried out in the long-term treatment of survivors of myocardial infarction (MI) because of preliminary evidence that they would be beneficial. Several of these trials showed trends favoring the use of beta-blockers. Because of small sample size or other limitations in design and analysis, however, the results were inconclusive. Based on these results, a trial of sufficient size was initiated to address the question of benefit of beta-blockade in subjects experiencing an MI.

The Beta-blocker Heart Attack Trial (BHAT) was a randomized, double-blind, placebo-controlled, multicenter trial designed to test the effect of a beta-blocker, propranolol hydrochloride, on total mortality in subjects who had at least one documented MI (Beta-Blocker Heart Attack Trial Research Group 1982). The primary objective was to determine whether the daily administration of propranolol hydrochloride in subjects who had at least one documented MI would result in a significant reduction in mortality from all causes during a 2–4 year follow-up period. Secondary objectives were to study the effect of chronic administration of propranolol on congestive heart disease (CHD) mortality, sudden cardiac death, and CHD mortality plus definite nonfatal MI. The protocol treatment was either 180mg/day or 240mg/day of propranolol or a matched placebo. Subjects were to be 30–69 years of age and 5–21 days post MI. Subject accrual began in June 1978 and continued until October 1981 with a total of 3837 subjects. Follow-up was to be terminated in June 1982 with an average follow-up of approximately 3 years. An independent Policy and Data Monitoring Board (PDMB) received the reports on interim analyses of accumulating data semi-annually.

10.2.2 Multicenter Automatic Defibrillator Implantation Trial

Each year approximately 450,000 people suffer sudden cardiac death, and a large majority of deaths (80%–90%) are caused by ventricular fibrillation. Approximately 100,000 lives are saved by prompt cardiopulmonary resuscitation. When the Cardiac Arrhythmia Suppression Trial (The Cardiac Arrhythmia Suppression Trial (CAST) Investigators 1989), in which encainide and flecainide were compared to placebo, was abruptly terminated due to excessive deaths on active treatments, there was a sense of urgency to evaluate the competing therapy with amiodarone and automatic implantable cardioverter defibrillator (AICD). The hypothesis was that the implantation of AICD would reduce death or prolong survival when compared to conventional pharmacological therapy.

The Multicenter Automatic Defibrillator Implantation Trial (MADIT) was a phase III trial designed to compare the effects of prophylactic therapy using an automatic implantable cardioverter defibrillator to conventional medical therapy with amiodarone on overall survival in subjects with previous MI and left ventricular dysfunction (MADIT Executive Committee 1991). The primary objective of the study was to determine whether implantation of AICD would reduce death when compared to conventional pharmacological treatment. Secondary outcomes included cardiac death, aborted sudden cardiac death, sustained life-threatening ventricular tachycardia, and operative morbidity and mortality in subjects with AICD. Eligible subjects were randomized between AICD and amiodarone stratified by clinical centers and whether a prior MI was within the previous 6 months or not. The primary analysis was based on the log-rank test stratified by the type of implant, but not by center and by time since prior MI, according to the intention-to-treat principle.

10.3 The Repeated Testing Problem

While ethical demands for interim data monitoring often require the repeated examination of evolving data, this process, when applied naively, causes a repeated testing problem aptly termed "sampling to a foregone conclusion" by Anscombe (1954), and described in detail in the following subsection.

10.3.1 Sampling to a Foregone Conclusion

Let $X_1, X_2, \ldots$ be independent and identically distributed (iid) Gaussian random variables with mean μ and variance 1, i.e., $N(\mu, 1)$, and consider test of $H_0: \mu = 0$ against $H_1: \mu \neq 0$. With a fixed sample of size k, one would reject H_0 at a significance level α if and only if

$$|S_k| > Z_{1-\alpha/2}\sqrt{k} \tag{10.1}$$

or equivalently

$$|Z_k| > Z_{1-\alpha/2}$$

where $S_k = \sum_{i=1}^{k} X_i$ denotes the partial sum of $X_1, \ldots, X_k$ and $Z_k = S_k/\sqrt{k}$ is a standardized test statistic.

Now, suppose that k is not fixed in advance, and data become available one observation at a time. If S_k is computed for each $k \geq 1$, then by the law of the iterated logarithm, $|S_k|$ is certain to exceed $Z_{1-\alpha/2}\sqrt{k}$ for some $k < \infty$, even when H_0 is true.

Thus a naive experimenter might be tempted to take a sample of size

$$k^* = \inf\{k \geq 1 \colon |S_k| > Z_{1-\alpha/2}\sqrt{k}\},$$

i.e., the smallest sample size for which the fixed sample test significance is reached, and report it as a fixed sample size and claim rejection of H_0 at a significance level α. On the other hand, he could be waiting quite a while since $E(k^*) = \infty$. Inference based solely on the likelihood principle or Bayesian methods, without regard to type I and type II errors, is formally unaffected by stopping rules, whereas the frequentist inference, based on sampling distributions, is extremely sensitive to the stopping rules. Nonetheless, whatever statistical approach is used, ultimately a decision must be made to either accept or reject an intervention and this leads to the opportunity to make one of two types of errors: a false positive, or type I error, or a false negative, or type II error. The goal of the data monitoring procedures we discuss is to conduct inference that controls these error rates.

Armitage, McPherson, and Rowe (1969) and McPherson and Armitage (1971) studied the effect of optional stopping on statistical inference in the frequentist setting. Their work considered the probability of obtaining a "significant" result at a particular nominal significance level as a function of the maximum number of tests, i.e., the *overall type I error rate*. Table 10.1 shows the probability of rejection of H_0 as a function of the number of observations and the size of the test when (10.1) is applied sequentially. Clearly, unless repeated testing is accounted for, type I error rates can be severely inflated. Most of the remainder of this chapter is devoted to methods for performing interim analyses without an accompanying increase in the overall type I error rate.

10.3.2 The General Setup

The simple repeated testing problem described in the previous section is a simplification of that encountered in randomized controlled trials. Generally we have two or more treatment groups, although typically monitoring plans are based on comparisons of only two groups and a single primary outcome. In trials with more than two groups or multiple primary outcomes, the monitoring plan may involve only one pairwise comparison (say high dose versus placebo), have separate monitoring plans for each pairwise comparison, or use the comparison of all active groups combined with control. Thus in this chapter we will focus on monitoring plans that involve the comparison of two groups and a single primary outcome.

Table 10.1 *Probabilty of rejection of the null hypothesis as a function of the number of observations and nominal significance level. (See Armitage et al. (1969).)*

K	Nominal Significance Level		
	0.05	.02	.01
1	0.0500	0.0200	0.0100
2	0.0831	0.0345	0.0177
3	0.1072	0.0456	0.0237
4	0.1262	0.0545	0.0286
5	0.1417	0.0620	0.0327
10	0.1933	0.0877	0.0474
20	0.2479	0.1163	0.0640
30	0.2801	0.1338	0.0744
40	0.3029	0.1464	0.0820
50	0.3204	0.1563	0.0880

The first sequential trials frequently enrolled pairs of subjects, one on each treatment, and evaluated the effectiveness of treatment after each pair. For example, in the 6-Mercaptopurine in Acute Leukemia trial (Freireich et al. 1963) described in Chapter 7 (Example 7.5), pairs of subjects were enrolled and one given 6-MP and the other placebo. The *preferred* treatment from each pair was the treatment with the longest remission time. The test statistic was the difference between the number of preferences for 6-MP and the number of preferences for placebo. The trial stopped after 21 pairs (18 preferring 6-MP and 3 preferring placebo) when the difference became sufficiently large. Sequential designs based on pairing of individual subjects has not been widely adopted in more recent years for a variety of reasons. First, subjects are typically paired solely because they are enrolled at the same time. Since paired subjects may differ widely with respect to underlying risk or prognosis, there is likely to be a loss of efficiency. Second, especially in large, multicenter trials, pairing is more difficult, and the logistical difficulties make the continual reassessment of the status of enrolled subjects required to implement these kinds of procedures difficult. Alternative approaches are necessary to improve efficiency and enable data monitoring to be conducted in a wide range of situations.

Before describing the details of data monitoring procedures, we note that rarely are the statistical tests used in clinical trials based simply on sums of i.i.d. random normal random variables, so interim monitoring procedures are required that can accommodate a variety of statistical tests. In the general setting we will consider, we have a sequence of analysis "times", $t_1, t_2, \ldots, t_K$ and a sequence of test statistics $S(t_1), S(t_2), \ldots, S(t_K)$ so that for S_k defined in the previous section, $S_k = S(t_k)$. In the cases we have considered thus far, the "times" represent the number of observations or pairs. While the

t_k can be the actual calendar times at which the analyses are performed, it is usually more mathematically convenient to consider "time" to be on the *information* scale (see Appendix A.5 for a more detailed discussion of information). In the simple case in the previous section, we could simply let $t_k = k$, the number of observations at the kth analysis. Alternatively, the t_k could represent the *information fraction*, relative the complete information at the planned conclusion of the trial, $t_k = k/K$ where K is the maximum sample size (or information). In this case we have $t_k \in (0, 1]$.

The test statistics, $S(t_k)$, can arise from a number of different settings, but for the most part we will focus on those arising from *score tests* (see Appendix A.3). For simplicity, first suppose that the data are iid observations from a single parameter family of distributions, where μ is the parameter of interest and the null hypothesis is H_0: $\mu = 0$. Let the score function be $U_k(\mu)$ at analysis k and $S_k = -U_k(0)$. The Fisher information is

$$\mathcal{I}(\mu) = -E[U_\mu(\mu)]$$

where the subscript μ indicates differentiation with respect to μ. Note that by expanding $U(\mu)$ in a Taylor series about $\mu = 0$, and using the fact that $E[U(\mu)] = 0$ (see Appendix A.2), we have

$$E[S_k] = -E[U_k(0)] \approx \mathcal{I}_k(0)\mu.$$

If μ is sufficiently small, then $\mathcal{I}_k(\mu) = \mathcal{I}_k(0)$, so we have that

$$S_k \overset{a}{\sim} N(\mu \mathcal{I}_k, \mathcal{I}_k), \tag{10.2}$$

where we suppress dependence on μ and write $\mathcal{I}_k$ in place of $\mathcal{I}_k(0)$. The case in which we have a multi-parameter family with density $f(x_1; \mu, \phi)$, where ϕ is a *nuisance* parameter, is more complicated, but the result in (10.2) still holds (see Whitehead (1997) or Whitehead (1978)).

These test statistics often have the form $S(t_k) = \sum_i (y_i(t_k) - E\{y_i(t_k)\})/\phi$ where the sum is over observations, $y_i(t_k)$, in, say, the experimental group available at time t_k, the expectation $E\{y_i(t_k)\}$ is computed under the null hypothesis of no difference between groups, and ϕ is a scale parameter (and may be known or estimated). Many commonly used tests can be written in this form (Scharfstein et al. 1997) and the methods described in this chapter will apply. Examples include:

- Normal observations: For normal observations, $S(t_k) = \sum(y_i - \hat{\mu}_k)/\hat{\sigma}^2$, where $\hat{\mu}_k = (\sum_j x_j + \sum_i y_i)/(n_x + n_y)$ is the overall mean of the observations at time t_k. The Fisher information is $\mathcal{I}_k = \sigma^2 n_x n_y/(n_x + n_y)$ which does not depend on μ and, assuming that the proportion n_x/n_y remains constant, is proportional to the total number of observations at t_k. $S(t_k)/\sqrt{\mathcal{I}_k}$ is the t-statistic.

- Binary observations: $S(t_k) = y_k - n_{yk}\hat{p}_k$, where y_k is the number of events in the experimental group, n_{yk} is the total number of observations in the experimental group, and $\hat{p}_k$ is the aggregate event rate over the two groups, ignoring treatment. $\mathcal{I}_k$ is $p(1 - p)n_{xk}n_{yk}/(n_{xk} + n_{yk})$. $S(t_k)^2/\mathcal{I}_k$ is the

Pearson chi-square test statistic, and alternatively, $S(t_k)/\sqrt{\mathcal{I}_k}$ has, approximately, a standard normal distribution.

- Failure time observations: $S(t_k) = \sum_j d_{jyk} - (d_{jxk} + d_{jyk})n_{jyk}/(n_{jxk} + n_{jyk})$ (equation (7.3) on page 217) is the log-rank statistic (Mantel 1966), where the sum is over distinct failure times, d_{jxk} and d_{jyk} are the number of failures, and n_{jxk} and n_{jyk} are the number of subjects at risk in the control and experimental groups, respectively, at the jth failure time. $\mathcal{I}_k$ is given by $\sum_j d_{j \cdot k}(n_{j \cdot k} - d_{j \cdot k})n_{jxk}n_{jyk}/n_{j \cdot k}^2(n_{j \cdot k} - 1)$, where $d_{j \cdot k} = d_{jxk} + d_{jyk}$ and $n_{j \cdot k} = n_{jxk} + n_{jyk}$. (See Tsiatis (1982, 1981) for a proof that the log-rank statistic has the desired structure.)

Because the Wilcoxon rank-sum test can be considered the score test for a proportional odds model (Section 2.3.1), it can also be placed into this framework. In each case, we can define t_k to satisfy either $t_k = \mathcal{I}_k$ or $t_k = \mathcal{I}_k/\mathcal{I}_K$. Lee and DeMets (1991) discuss monitoring in the longitudinal data setting for normal data and Gange and DeMets (1996) in the longitudinal data setting for non-normal data.

We note that each of the above test statistics can be shown to (asymptotically) satisfy 3 properties:

1. $S(t_1), S(t_2), \ldots, S(t_K)$ have a multivariate normal distribution,

2. $E\{S_k\} = t_k \mu$, for some μ, and

3. for $k_1 < k_2$, $\mathrm{Cov}(S(t_{k_1}), S(t_{k_2})) = \mathcal{I}_k(0)$.

Because processes satisfying these three properties behave like sums of iid random variables, Proschan et al. (2006) refer to a process satisfying these properties as an *S-process* (this definition differs slightly from that of Lan and Zucker (1993)). Specifically, if a process satisfies these properties, for $t_{k_1} < t_{k_2}$, $E\{S(t_{k_2}) - S(t_{k_1})\} = \mu(t_{k_2} - t_{k_1})$ and $S(t_{k_2}) - S(t_{k_1})$ is independent of $S(t)$ for $t \leq t_{k_1}$. The latter property is sometimes referred to as the *independent increments* property.

Another process of interest is the so called *B*-value (Lan and Wittes 1988),

$$B(t_k) = S_k/\mathcal{I}_k, \qquad (10.3)$$

where $t_k = \mathcal{I}_k/\mathcal{I}_K$. In this case, the process $B(t)$ satisfies

B1 $B(t_1), B(t_2), \ldots, B(t_K)$ have a multivariate normal distribution,

B2 $E\{B_k\} = t_k\theta$, for some θ, sometimes referred to as the *standardized treatment difference*, and

B3 for $t_{k_1} < t_{k_2}$, $\mathrm{Cov}(B(t_{k_1}), B(t_{k_2})) = t_{k_1}$.

These properties imply that for $t_{k_1} < t_{k_2}$, $B(t_{k_1})$ and $B(t_{k_2}) - B(t_{k_1})$ are independent and $\mathrm{Var}(B(t_{k_2}) - B(t_{k_1})) = t_{k_2} - t_{k_1}$.

For simplicity, the discussion that follows will generally be framed in terms of sums of i.i.d. normal random variables. While this makes the formulation easier, keep in mind the results generally apply to any test statistic satisfying properties 1, 2, and 3 above.

10.3.3 Repeated Significance Tests

Again letting $S_k = \sum_{i=1}^{k} X_i$, where the X_i are iid $N(\mu, 1)$, a *repeated significance test* is a procedure in which observations accrue until, for some constant $c > 0$,

$$|S_k| > c\sqrt{k},$$

where S_k is defined in the previous section, or until a maximum sample size, K, is reached. Define k^* by

$$k^* = \inf\{k \colon 1 \le k \le K \text{ and } |S_k| > c\sqrt{k}\}$$

and reject H_0 if and only if $|S_{k^*}| > c\sqrt{k^*}$. The probability of rejecting H_0 is then

$$\alpha^* = \Pr(|S_k| > c\sqrt{k}, \text{ for some } k \le K),$$

which may be controlled by choice of c.

Letting $c_k = c\sqrt{k}$ the probability distribution of k^* can be found as follows (see Armitage et al. (1969)). First, note that S_k is observed only if $k^* \ge k$, and, therefore, for $k > 1$, S_k doesn't have a sampling distribution in the usual sense. We can, however, define a *sub-density* function $f_k(\cdot; \mu)$, with the property that

$$\int_{-\infty}^{\infty} f_k(u; \mu)du = \Pr\{k^* \ge k\}.$$

That is, the density function of S_k, given that $k^* \ge k$, is $f_k(s; \mu)/\Pr\{k^* \ge k\}$.

Because $S_1 = X_1$, we have

$$f_1(s; \mu) = \phi(s - \mu) \qquad (10.4)$$

where $\phi(\cdot)$ is the standard normal density function. If we write $S_k = S_{k-1} + X_k$, then, because S_{k-1} and X_k are independent, for $k > 1$, $f_k(\cdot; \mu)$ is the convolution of the (sub)-densities of S_{k-1} and X_k,

$$f_k(s; \mu) = \int_{-c_{k-1}}^{c_{k-1}} f_{k-1}(u; \mu)\phi(s - u - \mu)du. \qquad (10.5)$$

The probability of stopping at or before k is given by

$$P_k(\mu) = \Pr\{k^* \le k | \mu\} = 1 - \int_{-c_k}^{c_k} f_k(u; \mu)du. \qquad (10.6)$$

(The integral on the right hand side of (10.6) is the probability of not rejecting H_0 through stage k.) The overall type I error rate is the probability of rejecting H_0 when it is true, $P_K(0)$, and the power for $H_1 \colon \mu = \mu_1$ is $P_K(\mu_1)$. Iterative numerical integration can be used to determine c and the maximum sample size K so that the overall type I error is α and the power to detect a specified alternative $\mu = \mu_1$ is $1 - \beta$. (See Reboussin et al. (2000) for a discussion of computational issues.) Software for performing these calculations is available at http://www.biostat.wisc.edu/landemets.

10.4 Group Sequential Tests

Repeated significance tests and other early sequential designs described earlier are formulated assuming that accumulating data are assessed continuously. A *group sequential* procedure (GSP) allows monitoring to occur periodically, after possibly unequal sized groups of observations have accrued. In this section we describe the most commonly used group sequential approaches.

10.4.1 Classical Group Sequential Methods

Suppose that the response is a normal random variable with known variance σ^2 and means μ_A and μ_B for groups A and B, respectively, and that we enroll equal numbers of subjects in each group. Letting the treatment difference be $\delta = \mu_B - \mu_A$, consider tests of $H_0 \colon \delta = 0$ against $H_1 \colon \delta \neq 0$. For the purpose of this discussion we will consider two-sided tests.

A fixed sample size test at significance level α with n subjects in each group will reject H_0 when

$$Z = \left| \frac{\overline{X}_A - \overline{X}_B}{\sqrt{2\sigma^2/n}} \right| \geq Z_{1-\alpha/2}$$

where $\overline{X}_A$ and $\overline{X}_B$ denote the sample means for groups A and B, respectively.

Now suppose that we assess the accumulating data after every $2n$ observations (n from each treatment arm) up to a maximum of K interim analyses, or *looks*, and a maximum of $2nK$ observations. Let $S_k = \sqrt{2/n\sigma^2} \sum_{j=1}^{k} \overline{X}_{Aj} - \overline{X}_{Bj}$, where $\overline{X}_{Aj}$ and $\overline{X}_{Bj}$ are the means of the observations in the jth groups for treatments A and B, respectively. S_k has mean $k\delta\sqrt{n/2\sigma^2} = k\delta^*$ and variance k. Using the repeated significance test of Section 10.3.3, we would stop and reject H_0 if $|S_k| \geq c\sqrt{k}$.

The constant c can be found using the formula (10.5). Using this procedure, the nominal significance level required to reject H_0 is the same at each k. In general, however, we may want a procedure in which the nominal significance level varies over the course of the trial. A more general group sequential procedure can be defined by the number, K, of interim looks and the corresponding critical values, c_k, defined so that we would stop and reject H_0 if $|S_k| \geq c_k$ for some $k = 1, 2, \ldots, K$. We require that the overall type I error rate for the procedure be controlled at level α, and that the procedure have power $1 - \beta$ for a particular alternative, $\delta = \delta_1$.

We now describe two classical group sequential tests, one discussed by Pocock (1977a)[6] and the other by O'Brien and Fleming (1979). The Pocock (P) group sequential test rejects the null hypothesis the first time that

$$|S_k| \geq c_k = c_P\sqrt{k}$$

---

[6] Note that Pocock does not advocate the use of the Pocock boundary (Pocock and White 1999).

or equivalently

$$\left|\frac{S_k}{\sqrt{k}}\right| \geq c_P,$$

i.e., when the standardized partial sum of accumulating data exceeds a constant critical value c_P. The O'Brien-Fleming (OBF) group sequential test rejects H_0 the first time that

$$|S_k| \geq c_k = c_{OBF}\sqrt{K},$$

i.e., when the partial sum of accumulating data exceeds a fixed boundary that is a constant c_{OBF} multiplied by $\sqrt{K}$. Equivalently,

$$\left|\frac{S_k}{\sqrt{k}}\right| \geq c_{OBF}\sqrt{K/k}.$$

When $\alpha = 0.05$ and $K = 5$, $c_P = 2.41$ for the Pocock group sequential test and $c_{OBF} = 2.04$ for the O'Brien-Fleming group sequential test (see Figure 10.1). Therefore, when $\alpha = 0.05$ and $K = 5$, the Pocock group sequential test rejects the null hypothesis the first time that

$$|Z_k| = \left|\frac{S_k}{\sqrt{k}}\right| \geq 2.41,$$

which corresponds to a constant nominal p-value of 0.0158 at each look. In comparison, the O'Brien-Fleming group sequential test rejects the null hypothesis the first time that

$$|Z_k| = \left|\frac{S_k}{\sqrt{k}}\right| \geq 2.04\sqrt{5/k}, \tag{10.7}$$

which corresponds to a nominal p-value of 0.00000504 at the first look, 0.00125 at the second look, 0.00843 at the third look, 0.0225 at the fourth look, and 0.0413 at the last look. Note, however, that both group sequential tests yield the type I error probability of 0.05.

An alternative to these tests, proposed by Haybittle (1971) and Peto et al. (1976), uses a fixed critical value of 3.0 for interim analysis and a fixed sample critical value of 1.96 for the final analysis for an overall signficance level of approximately 0.05. The use of a large critical value for the interim analysis ensures that the resulting group sequential test will have overall significance level close to, but not exactly, the desired level with no additional adjustment. Precise control of the overall type I error rate can be achieved by adjusting the final critical value once the trial is completed. For example, if 4 equally spaced interim analyses are conducted using a critical value of 3.0, a final critical of 1.99 will ensure an overall type I error rate of 0.05.

With group sequential designs which allow early termination solely for statistical significance in the observed treatment differences, there is a reduction in power relative to the fixed sample test of the same size. Maintenance of power requires that the maximum sample size be increased by an amount that depends on the choice of boundary. For given δ_1 under the alternative

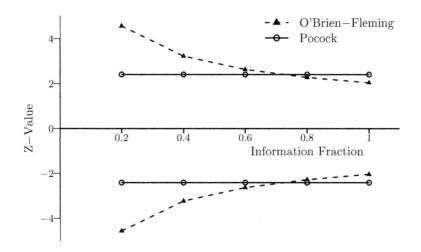

Figure 10.1 *Pocock and O'Brien-Fleming boundaries with $\alpha = 0.05$ and $K = 5$.*

hypothesis, one can compute the power of the group sequential test as

$$1 - \beta = 1 - \Pr(|S_1| < c_1, \ldots, |S_K| < c_K; \delta_1^*),$$

where $\delta_1^* = \delta_1 \sqrt{n/2\sigma^2}$.

Conversely, given the desired power $1 - \beta$ of the group sequential test, one can determine the value of $\delta_1^* = \tilde{\delta}$ that satisfies the above equation. The value of $\tilde{\delta}$ depends on α, K, $1 - \beta$, and $\mathbf{c} = (c_1, c_2, \ldots, c_K)$, i.e., $\tilde{\delta} = \tilde{\delta}(\alpha, K, \mathbf{c}, 1 - \beta)$. The required group size, $\tilde{n}$, satisfies

$$\tilde{\delta} = \delta_1 \sqrt{\frac{\tilde{n}}{2}}$$

so one can solve for $\tilde{n}$ to determine the necessary group size, i.e.,

$$\tilde{n} = 2 \left(\frac{\tilde{\delta}}{\delta_1} \right)^2.$$

Hence the maximum sample size for the group sequential design becomes

$$2\tilde{n}K = 4 \left(\frac{\tilde{\delta}\sqrt{K}}{\delta_1} \right)^2.$$

For example, with $\alpha = 0.05$, $K = 5$, and $1 - \beta = 0.8$, $\tilde{\delta} = 1.387$ for the Pocock group sequential test, and $\tilde{\delta} = 1.270$ for the O'Brien-Fleming group sequential test. Therefore, if we take $\delta_1 = 1$, for the Pocock test we have

$$\tilde{n} = 2(1.387)^2 = 3.86 \text{ and } 2\tilde{n}K = 38.6$$

and for the O'Brien-Fleming test

$$\tilde{n} = 2(1.270)^2 = 3.23 \text{ and } 2\tilde{n}K = 32.3.$$

This is in contrast to a fixed sample design with the sample size of 31.4. We see that for the O'Brien-Fleming boundary, the sample size increase is quite small.

In general, for a fixed sample design with $K = 1$, the necessary sample size to detect a difference δ_1 with power $1 - \beta$ at a two-sided level α test is

$$2\tilde{n} = 4^2 \left(\frac{Z_{\alpha/2} + Z_\beta}{\delta_1} \right)^2.$$

For a group sequential design with $K > 1$, the maximum sample size as derived above is

$$2\tilde{n}K = 4 \left(\frac{\tilde{\delta}\sqrt{K}}{\delta_1} \right)^2$$

$$= 4 \left(\frac{Z_{\alpha/2} + Z_\beta}{\delta_1} \right)^2 \times \left(\frac{\tilde{\delta}\sqrt{K}}{Z_{\alpha/2} + Z_\beta} \right)^2,$$

thus a constant multiple of the corresponding sample size for the fixed sample design. This constant multiple

$$\mathcal{F} = \left(\frac{\tilde{\delta}\sqrt{K}}{Z_{\alpha/2} + Z_\beta} \right)^2$$

is referred to as the *inflation factor*.

As noted above, with $\alpha = 0.05$, $K = 5$, and 80% power, the inflation factor is $\mathcal{F} = 38.58/31.40 = 1.23$ for the Pocock procedure and $\mathcal{F} = 32.29/31.40 = 1.03$ for the O'Brien-Fleming procedure. We note that the inflation factor is determined in large part by the final critical value, c_K. Because, for the Pocock boundary with $\alpha = .05$ and $K = 5$, $c_K = 2.41$ is substantially larger than the nominal 1.96 for the fixed sample test, the inflation factor is large. Conversely, for the O'Brien-Fleming boundary, the corresponding value of c_K is 2.04, and the inflation factor is near one.

Table 10.2 gives the inflation factors for the group sequential design with the maximum number of interim analyses including the final analysis, $K = 2, 3, 4, 5$, for both Pocock and O'Brien-Fleming designs with power, $1 - \beta = 0.8, 0.90, 0.95$, at a two-sided test with significance level, $\alpha = 0.05, 0.01$. A simple, conservative, approximation to this formal adjustment uses the final critical value in place of $Z_{1-\alpha}$ in the sample size formulas described in Chapter 4.

The increase in the *maximum* sample size required to maintain the power of a group sequential trial relative to a fixed size trial may seem to be a disadvantage of group sequential procedures. If an experimental treatment is in fact beneficial, however, the result may be obtained much sooner in a group sequential procedure, resulting in a smaller trial.

Table 10.2 *Inflation factors for Pocock (P) and O'Brien-Fleming (OBF) group sequential designs.*

		\multicolumn{8}{c}{K}							
		\multicolumn{2}{c}{2}	\multicolumn{2}{c}{3}	\multicolumn{2}{c}{4}	\multicolumn{2}{c}{5}
α	$1-\beta$	P	OBF	P	OBF	P	OBF	P	OBF
0.05	.80	1.11	1.01	1.17	1.02	1.20	1.02	1.23	1.03
	.90	1.10	1.01	1.15	1.02	1.18	1.02	1.21	1.03
	.95	1.09	1.01	1.14	1.02	1.17	1.02	1.19	1.02
0.01	.80	1.09	1.00	1.14	1.01	1.17	1.01	1.19	1.02
	.90	1.08	1.00	1.12	1.01	1.15	1.01	1.17	1.01
	.95	1.08	1.00	1.12	1.01	1.14	1.01	1.16	1.01

To quantify this observation, if $2n$ subjects are added at each look, let k^* denote the number of looks at the time of stopping. The expected sample size for the group sequential design, known as the average sample number (ASN), is given by

$$\text{ASN} = 2n\text{E}(k^*).$$

Since k^* is a discrete random variable,

$$
\begin{aligned}
\text{E}(k^*) &= 1\Pr(k^*=1) + 2\Pr(k^*=2) + \cdots + K\Pr(k^*=K) \\
&= 1 + \Pr(k^*>1) + \Pr(k^*>2) + \cdots + \Pr(k^*>K-1) \\
&= 1 + \sum_{k=1}^{K-1} \int_{-c_k}^{c_k} f_k(u;\delta^*)du
\end{aligned}
$$

where $f_k(\cdot)$ is defined in (10.4) and (10.5), and $\delta^* = \delta\sqrt{n/2\sigma^2}$. For GSPs with $K=5$, $\alpha = 0.05$, and that maintain $1-\beta = .80$,

$$
\text{E}(k^*) = \begin{cases} 3.25 & \text{for the Pocock boundary} \\ 3.98 & \text{for the O'Brien-Fleming boundary.} \end{cases}
$$

Hence,

$$
\text{ASN} = \begin{cases} 2(3.86)(3.25) = 25.1 & \text{for the Pocock boundary} \\ 2(3.23)(3.98) = 25.7 & \text{for the O'Brien-Fleming boundary.} \end{cases}
$$

For the fixed sample size design, it remains at 31.4, so the GSP results in an average reduction in sample size. For designs with higher power, the relative reduction in sample size for the GSP is greater.

10.4.2 Early Stopping in Favor of the Null Hypothesis: One-Sided Tests

In the two-sided tests of the previous section, early stopping is allowed solely to reject H_0, either in favor of the experimental arm or the control arm. If the responses to both treatments are similar, H_0 will not be rejected, and the trial will continue to its planned conclusion. This procedure treats the experimental and control arms symmetrically. In practice, however, the question is rarely symmetrical. If a treatment is widely accepted, for example the use of certain anti-arrhythmic drugs as in the CAST example (see Section 2.4.2), compelling evidence of harm may be required to change clinical practice and symmetric boundaries may be desirable. On the other hand, development of a novel therapy may be discontinued based on evidence suggesting that there is little likelihood that the therapy is beneficial, especially in the face of potential adverse effects. In this setting the question is asymmetric and early stopping may be desirable if the treatment is shown to be beneficial or if there is either a low probability of showing benefit were the trial to continue, or one has sufficient evidence to rule out clinically meaningful benefit. See DeMets, Pocock, and Julian (1999) for a discussion of this and related issues.

DeMets and Ware (1980, 1982) proposed asymmetric boundaries to account for the fundamental asymmetry in the clinical question. Emerson and Fleming (1989) subsequently proposed a group sequential test for a one-sided test of $H_0 : \delta \leq 0$ against $H_1 : \delta \geq \delta_1$ for $\delta_1 > 0$, in which early stopping is allowed if either H_0 or H_1 is rejected. Specifically we stop and reject H_0 the first time that

$$S_k \geq c_k^U$$

and stop and reject H_1 the first time that

$$S_k \leq k\delta_1^* - c_k^L,$$

where $\delta_1^* = \delta_1 \sqrt{n/2\sigma^2}$. The boundary is constructed to provide power for H_1 of $1 - \beta$ at an overall significance level α.

If we require that the boundaries meet at the last look, then

$$\delta_1^* = (c_K^U + c_K^L)/K,$$

which will in turn determine the necessary group size n on each intervention. The values of the group sequential boundaries, $c_1^L, \ldots, c_K^L$ and $c_1^U, \ldots c_K^U$, can be determined using a variation of equations (10.4) and (10.5) in which asymmetric limits are used. Emerson and Fleming suggest that H_0 and H_1 be treated symmetrically so that $c_k^U = c_k^L = c_k$.

An example of Emerson and Fleming boundaries is shown in Figure 10.2. Here $K = 5$ and $c_k = 4.502/\sqrt{k}$, so the upper boundary is similar to the O'Brien-Fleming boundary in equation (10.7). We note that for this boundary, the final critical value is 2.01 which is smaller than the corresponding value from the O'Brien-Fleming boundary of 2.04. This happens because the possibility of early stopping to accept H_0 reduces the overall type I error rate, effectively "buying back" type I error probability that can then be used to lower the upper efficacy boundary. This may be considered an undesirable feature since, because the decision to stop a trial is complex, involving both statistical and non-statistical considerations, a data monitoring committee may choose to allow a trial to continue even though the lower boundary

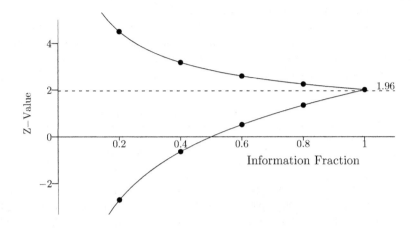

Figure 10.2 *Emerson and Fleming boundary with early stopping in favor of* H_0. *Here* $\alpha = 0.025$ *(one-sided),* $K = 5$, *and* $c_k = 4.502/\sqrt{k}$ *(from Emerson and Fleming (1989)) so that the upper boundary is similar to an OBF boundary.*

was crossed. If the upper and lower boundaries were constructed as one-sided $(\alpha/2$ level) tests without regard to the other boundary, the resulting proce- dure would be conservative (after accounting for the probability of crossing the lower boundary, the (one-sided) type I error rate would be less than $\alpha/2$), but would not suffer from these difficulties.

The group sequential method for early stopping for the null hypothesis can be extended to two-sided tests, the so called *inner wedge* tests, similar to what one might obtain by reflecting the top half of Figure 10.2 about the x-axis.

10.4.3 Early Termination in BHAT

The BHAT trial was one of the first large, randomized trials to employ a group sequential monitoring plan. BHAT was designed to begin in June 1978 and last 4 years, ending in June 1982, with a mean follow-up of 3 years. An O'Brien-Fleming monitoring boundary with $K = 7$ and $\alpha = .05$, so that $c_{OBF} = 2.063$, was chosen with the expectation that analyses would be con- ducted every six months after the first year, with approximately equal incre- ments of information between analyses. In October 1981 the data showed a 9.5% mortality rate in the placebo group (183 deaths) and a 7% rate in the propranolol group (135 deaths) corresponding to a log-rank Z-score of 2.82, well above the critical value for the sixth analysis of $2.063/\sqrt{6/7} = 2.23$. The details of the statistical aspects of early stopping in this trial are given by DeMets et al. (1984). The independent Policy and Data Monitoring Board

(PDMB) recommended that the BHAT be terminated in October 1981. The interim analyses are summarized in Table 10.3.

The target number of deaths (total information) was not prespecified, so for our purpose, we will assume that an additional 90 deaths, for a total of 408 deaths, would have occurred between the point that the trial was stopped and the planned conclusion in June 1982.

Table 10.3 *Interim analyses in BHAT.*

Interim Date	Propranolol	Placebo	Information Fraction (%)	c_k	Z
May 1979	22/860	34/848	13.7	5.46	1.68
October 1979	29/1080	48/1080	18.9	3.86	2.24
March 1980	50/1490	76/1486	30.9	3.15	2.37
October 1980	74/1846	103/1841	43.4	2.73	2.30
April 1981	106/1916	141/1921	60.5	2.44	2.34
October 1981	135/1916	183/1921	77.9	2.23	2.82*

* PDMB terminated BHAT

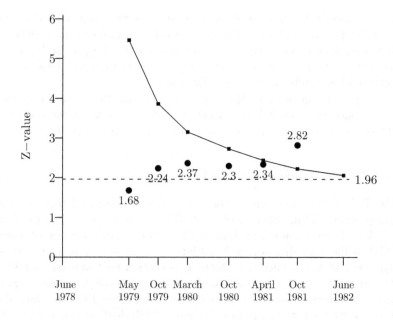

Figure 10.3 *Group sequential monitoring in BHAT. (Adapted from DeMets et al. (1984).)*

BHAT is typical in that, while the boundary was computed under the assumption of equally spaced analyses, it is difficult in practice to enforce a prespecified monitoring schedule. The boundary values that were used were based on type I error probabilities computed using equations (10.4) and (10.5), which assume equal increments of information. The actual overall type I error, assuming an additional final analysis with 408 total deaths and accounting for the timing of the interim analyses, is 0.055, so, in this example, the unequal spacing results in slightly inflated type I error. We further note that the accumulated boundary crossing probability at the time of the October 1981 analysis was 0.034. Therefore, in spite of the deviation of the actual timing of the interim analyses from the planned schedule, the overall type I error could still have been strictly controlled by adjusting the critical value at the final analyses slightly upward. That is, while the planned final critical value was 2.06327, by using a generalization of equation (10.5) that accommodates unequal increments (equation (10.11) in the next section), we can compute a new critical value of 2.06329, ensuring that the overall type I error will be exactly 0.05. Clearly the difference between these critical values is negligible, and in this case, the unequal spacing does not pose a serious problem.

In addition, note that the recalculated value does not depend on the observed test statistics, but only on the timing of the interim analyses. This idea can be applied, not only to the final analysis, but can, in principle, be applied to each interim analysis in turn so that the cumulative type I error rate is controlled at each stage, regardless of the actual timing of the analyses. This reasoning led to the development of the *alpha spending* approach that is the subject of the next section.

10.4.4 Alpha Spending Approach

In the group sequential procedures discussed so far, interim looks were equally spaced and the maximum number was prespecified. In practice, as illustrated by the BHAT example, it is generally not feasible to know when and how many times the study will be monitored. Lan and DeMets (1983) proposed the use of a prespecified *alpha spending function* that dictates the rate at which the total type I error probability accumulates as data accrue. Specifically, let $\alpha(t) = \Pr\{|S_k| > c_k$ for some $t_k \leq t\}$.

First, consider the group sequential procedures from Section 10.4.1. For $K = 5$ and $\alpha = 0.05$, the cumulative probabilities of rejecting H_0 at or before the kth analysis for $k = 1, \ldots, 5$ are given in Table 10.4 and plotted in Figure 10.4 for the Pocock and O'Brien-Fleming boundaries. (Note that as it is defined, $\alpha(t)$ is constant between t_k and t_{k+1}; however, in Figure 10.4 we have used linear interpolation to suggest that $\alpha(t)$ is a continuous function.) Note that there is a one-to-one correspondence between $\alpha(t_k)$, $k = 1, 2, \ldots, K$ and the critical values, c_k. Therefore, rather than defining the stopping boundary in terms of the critical values, one could choose an increasing function, $\alpha(t)$,

Table 10.4 *Nominal and cumulative probabilities of rejecting H_0 when H_0 is true.*

	Pocock		O'Brien-Fleming	
	Nominal	Cumulative	Nominal	Cumulative
1	0.0158	0.0158	0.00000504	0.00000504
2	0.0158	0.0275	0.00125	0.00126
3	0.0158	0.0365	0.00843	0.00891
4	0.0158	0.0439	0.0225	0.0256
5	0.0158	0.0500	0.0413	0.0500

and define $c_1, c_2, \ldots, c_K$ to satisfy

$$\Pr\{|S_1| > c_1\} = \alpha(t_1) \tag{10.8}$$

and

$$\Pr\{|S_k| > c_k, |S_l| < c_l, l = 1, \ldots, k - 1\} = \alpha(t_k) - \alpha(t_{k-1}). \tag{10.9}$$

Lan and DeMets (1983) noted that if $\alpha(t)$ is specified for $t \in [0, 1]$, then

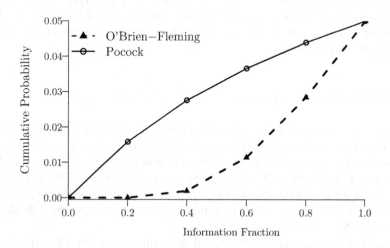

Figure 10.4 *Cumulative probabilities of rejecting H_0 for Pocock (solid line) and O'Brien-Fleming (dotted line) tests with $\alpha = 0.05$ and $K = 5$. (Note that linear interpolation is used to suggest that the cumulative probability is a continuous function.)*

neither $K, t_1, t_2, \ldots$ nor $c_1, c_2, \ldots$ need to be prespecified. Therefore, the timing and number of the interim analyses are flexible, and once $t_1, t_2, \ldots t_k$ have been determined, $c_1, c_2, \ldots, c_k$ can be determined sequentially using (10.8) and (10.9). The function $\alpha(t)$ is known as the *alpha spending function* or *error spending function*.

Recall that equations (10.4) and (10.5) require the increments in the test statistic to have variance one. To compute the probabilities in equations (10.8) and (10.9), we need a slight modification of (10.4) and (10.5). For convenience we formulate the testing procedure in terms of the B-value defined in Section 10.3.2. Given a sequence $t_1, t_2, \ldots$, if we stop the first time that $|B(t_k)| > b_k$, letting $f_k(\cdot)$ be the sub-density function of its argument and $\theta = E[B(1)]$, we have that

$$f_1(b; \theta) = \phi(b/t_1 - \theta)/t_1 \qquad (10.10)$$

and

$$f_k(b; \theta) = \int_{-b_{k-1}}^{b_{k-1}} f_{k-1}(u; \theta)\phi\left(\frac{b - u}{t_k - t_{k-1}} - \theta\right)\frac{1}{t_k - t_{k-1}}du, \text{ for } k > 1.$$
$$(10.11)$$

Equations (10.10) and (10.11) provide a computational algorithm for nearly any group sequential procedure.

Lan and DeMets (1983) determined that a boundary approximating the Pocock boundary can be generated using the alpha spending function

$$\alpha(t) = \alpha \log\{1 + (e - 1)t\}$$

which is known as the "Pocock type alpha spending function."

An alpha spending function that generates O'Brien-Fleming-like boundaries can be constructed as follows. Letting $K \to \infty$, and the maximum of $|t_k - t_{k-1}| \to 0$ then the process $B(t_1), B(t_2), \ldots$, approaches a Brownian motion process (see Appendix A.6). If observation stops the first time that $|B(t_k)| > b$ for a fixed b, then by property 2 on page 403, the probability that we stop prior to time t is approximately

$$\alpha(t) = 2\{1 - \Phi(Z_{1-\alpha/2}/\sqrt{t})\} \qquad (10.12)$$

where Φ is the standard normal distribution. Thus, the function defined by (10.12) is known as the "O'Brien-Fleming type alpha spending function." Two other proposed spending functions that are intermediate between α_P and α_{OBF} are

- $\alpha_3(t) = \alpha t$ (see Lan and DeMets (1983))
- $\alpha_4(t) = \alpha t^{3/2}$ (see Kim and DeMets (1987b)),

  or more generally

- $\alpha_5(t) = \alpha t^\rho$ for $\rho > 0$.

Examples of these spending functions are shown in Figure 10.5.

While the boundaries we have constructed from alpha spending functions have generated symmetric tests, as indicated in Section 10.4.2, the clinical questions are rarely symmetrical and these ideas can be easily extended to asymmetric tests as suggested by Kim and DeMets (1987b). The simplest way

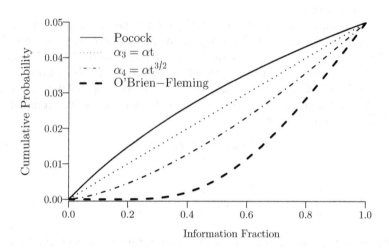

Figure 10.5 *Pocock and O'Brien-Fleming type alpha spending functions with $\alpha = 0.05$.*

is to independently construct upper and lower one-sided boundaries, each with overall type I error probability $\alpha/2$. This is technically a slightly conservative approach because the two stopping regions are not disjoint in the space of sample paths. The probability of a path lying in the intersection is negligible, however (approximately 5×10^{-7} for the Pocock boundary and 5×10^{-11} for the O'Brien-Fleming boundary). Thus, one could, for example, select an O'Brien-Fleming spending function for the upper boundary, and a Pocock spending function for the lower boundary. This monitoring plan would require substantial evidence of benefit to stop early, but allow earlier stopping with moderate evidence of harm. Since the boundary for harm is to be used only to terminate the trial in the event of an adverse effect, the fact that it has a more conservative final critical value would not be of concern. The alpha spending function approach has also been extended to accommodate early stopping in favor of the null hypothesis in a manner similar to that in Section 10.4.2 for both one-sided and two-sided tests by Pampallona and Tsiatis (1994).

The power associated with a given alpha spending function, $\alpha(t)$, depends relatively little on the number of looks and when the looks are made. Therefore, when deciding how large the terminal or maximum sample size is needed to achieve certain power, we can use the same technique based on the inflation factor we described earlier. That is, inflate the fixed sample by 25–30% for the Pocock procedure and by 3–5% for the O'Brien-Fleming procedure. Alternatively, a conservative sample size estimate can be obtained by treating the trial as if it were of fixed size, using the final expected critical value. Conversely, Lakatos (2002) proposed techniques for designing trials with survival outcomes that account for interim monitoring and allow for time dependent hazard rates, including non-proportional hazard alternatives for which condition 2 on page 297 does not hold. Software necessary to compute boundary values is available on the world wide web[7] or commercially in several software packages including EaSt (Cytel Software Corporation 2000).

10.5 Triangular Test

For a sequence of i.i.d. observations, $x_1, x_2, \ldots$, Wald's sequential probability ratio test (SPRT) (Wald 1947) of $H_0 \colon \mu = \mu_0$ versus $H_1 \colon \mu = \mu_1$ has a continuation region defined by $a < \sum_{i=1}^{n} \log(f(x_i; \mu_1)/f(x_i; \mu_0)) < b$, where $f(\cdot; \mu)$ is the density function for x_i given μ and a and b are predetermined constants that can be chosen provide the desired type I and type II error rates. The error probabilities for this test are based on large sample approximations for which it is assumed that the data are monitored continuously. This procedure has been shown to be optimal in the sense that among all tests with type I and II error probabilities α and β, it minimizes $\mathrm{E}(k^*|\mu_0)$ and $\mathrm{E}(k^*|\mu_1)$ (Wald 1947). Furthermore, the procedure is *open* in the sense that there is no fixed maximum sample size. Specifically, at $\mu = (\mu_0 + \mu_1)/2$, $\mathrm{E}(k^*|\mu)$ may be unacceptably large. Moreover, for this value of μ, $\Pr(k^* \geq n) > 0$ for any given $n > 0$ so the sample size is unbounded. To avoid this problem, Anderson (1960) developed a *closed* procedure, known as the *triangular test*, that minimizes $\mathrm{E}(k^*|\mu)$ at $\mu = (\mu_0 + \mu_1)/2$. This idea was further developed by Whitehead and Stratton (1983) and Whitehead (1997).

10.5.1 *Triangular Test for Normal Data*

Let $X_1, X_2, \ldots$ be i.i.d. from $N(\mu, 1)$, let $S_n = \sum_{i=1}^{n} X_i$ and consider tests of $H_0 \colon \mu = 0$ *vs* $H_1 \colon \mu = \mu_1 > 0$. The general form of the continuation region of the triangular test is

$$S_n \in (-a + b_L n, a + b_U n).$$

The calculations are mathematically complicated, but it can be shown (see Whitehead (1997)) that for type I error probability α and type II error probability $\beta = \alpha$

$$b_L = \frac{3}{4}\mu_1 \text{ and } b_U = \frac{1}{4}\mu_1$$

and

$$a = \frac{2}{\mu_1} \log \frac{1}{2\alpha}.$$

The maximum sample size is

$$m = \frac{4a}{\mu_1}.$$

---

[7] http://www.biostat.wisc.edu/landemets/

10.5.2 General Form of the Triangular Test for Continuous Monitoring

In the general case, we will assume that at each interim analysis we observe the pair[8] (S, V) where $V = \text{Var}[S] = \mathcal{I}(\mu)$ and $S \sim N(\mu V, V)$.

Given the statistics S and V, the general form of the triangular test is defined by a continuation region of the form

$$S \in (-a + 3cV, a + cV),$$

with the apex of the triangle at $V = a/c$ and $S = 2a$ (see Figure 10.6). If $\alpha/2$ is the probability of crossing the upper boundary when H_0 is true, and $1 - \beta$ is the probability of crossing the lower boundary when H_1 is true, in the special case where $\alpha/2 = \beta$, it can be shown that

$$a = -2(\log \alpha)/\mu_1 \text{ and } c = \mu_1/4.$$

The case in which $\alpha/2 \neq \beta$ is more complex, and we do not present the computations here. See Whitehead (1997) for details.

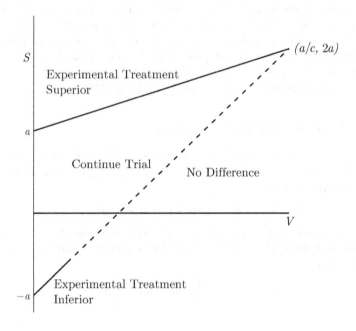

Figure 10.6 *Stopping boundaries for continuous monitoring based on the triangular test (Adapted from Whitehead (1997)).*

---

[8] Whitehead uses "Z" to denote the score statistic, $-U(0)$. For consistency with notation used elsewhere in this text, we use "S" to denote the score statistic used in the triangular test.

10.5.3 Triangular Test with Discrete Monitoring

The type I and type II error rates for the triangular test as defined above are computed under the assumption that data are monitored continuously. In practice interim analyses take place at discrete times, so an adjustment is required to maintain the desired error rates. When data are monitored continuously, because the S is a continuous function of V, the point at which the upper boundary is crossed, (V^*, S^*), satisfies $S^* = a + cV^*$. On the other hand, when data are monitored periodically, we have that $S^* \geq a + cV^*$. The overshoot R is the vertical distance between the final point of the sample path and the continuous boundary defined as

$$R = S^* - (a + cV^*).$$

A reliable correction to the boundary can be made using the expected amount of overshoot. Specifically, the continuous stopping criterion

$$S \geq a + cV$$

is replaced by

$$S \geq a + cV - A$$

where

$$A = E(R; \mu),$$

the expected value of the overshoot at the time of boundary crossing, leading to what is sometimes referred to as the "Christmas tree adjustment" (see Figure 10.7). Whitehead (1997) claims that the $A = 0.583\sqrt{V_i - V_{i-1}}$ where V_i is the value of V at analysis i (see also Siegmund (1985)). Because a greater information difference, $V_i - V_{i-1}$, between consecutive assessments leads to larger values of A, larger adjustments are required when monitoring is less frequent.

10.5.4 Triangular Test in MADIT Study

The accrual goal for the MADIT study was 280 subjects from 24 centers over 18 months at an enrollment rate of 0.65 subjects per month with an additional 6 months of follow-up after the last subject is enrolled, for a total study duration of 2 years. The sample size was based on a two-sided level $\alpha = 0.05$ triangular test and power $1 - \beta = 0.85$ to detect a 46% reduction in 2-year mortality from 30% on conventional therapy to 16.3% on AICD. It also accounted for a drop-in/drop-out rate of $< 5\%$. The corresponding fixed sample size was 300 subjects. Note that the triangular boundary is truncated at $V = 37$ with little loss both because there is a low probability that a sample path would find its way into the narrowest part of the triangle, and the correction for discrete monitoring effectively introduces truncation as suggested by Figure 10.7.

The results from the MADIT study were reported by Moss et al. (1996). The design of the study was modified on three occasions. First, on August 27, 1993,

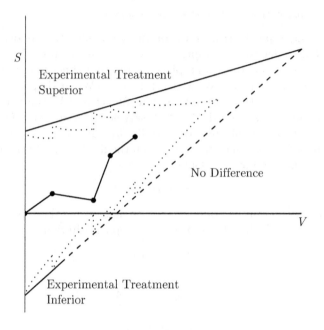

Figure 10.7 *Triangular test with "Christmas tree" adjustment.*

a new stratification factor was introduced in the randomization, transthoracic *vs* transvenous. This was necessitated by the approval of non-thoracotomy transvenous leads. Second, on September 1, 1993, the power requirement was increased from 85% to 90%, but with no apparent change in sample size requirements to account for a potential change in referral pattern due to transvenous leads. More important, from a statistical point of view, it was decided on November 12, 1995 that follow-up times would be censored at 5 years to compensate for the slow rate of enrollment.

After the first 10 deaths were reported, interim analyses were performed weekly. The upper triangular boundary was crossed on March 18, 1996 (see Figure 10.8) leading to early termination of the study due to statistically significant reduction in all cause mortality in subjects given AICD. At study termination there were 196 randomized in the study with 101 on conventional therapy and 95 on AICD enrolled between December 27, 1990 and March 18, 1996. The first subject had 61 months of follow-up, while the last subject had less than 1 month of follow-up, for an average follow-up of 27 months. There were 98 subjects in the transthoracic stratum and 98 in the transvenous stratum.

At the time that the study was terminated, there were a total of 51 deaths. By the time of study close-out on April 19, 1996, an additional 3 deaths had been discovered, making a total of 39 deaths on conventional therapy and

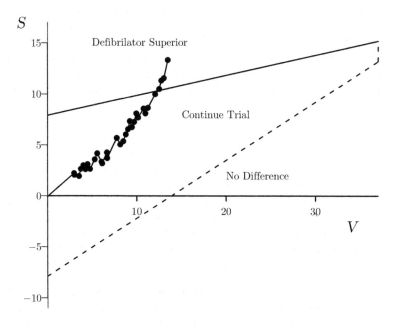

Figure 10.8 *Triangular test in MADIT. Once interim monitoring had begun, the monitoring frequency is high enough that the adjustment for discrete monitoring is quite small and does not meaningfully change the result. (Figure adapted from Moss et al. (1996).)*

15 deaths on AICD with a nominal p-value of 0.009. The maximum information was approximately $V = 37$ corresponding to $148 \approx 37 \times 4$ deaths. At early termination with 54 deaths (36% information), $V \approx 54/4 = 13.5$.

10.6 Curtailment Procedures

Curtailment, whether stochastic or deterministic, refers to early termination on the grounds that there is either no chance (deterministic) or a very small chance (stochastic) that the result observed at an interim analysis will change were the study to continue to its planned termination. Stopping a trial for *futility*—the probability that a trial will be "successful" if allowed to continue is too small to justify continuation—is a form of curtailment. We begin with a discussion of *deterministic curtailment*.

10.6.1 Deterministic Curtailment

We illustrate deterministic curtailment with the following simple numerical example based on an illustration from Alling (1963). (See also Halperin and Ware (1974).)

Example 10.1. Suppose that 20 subjects, 10 in each of two treatment groups, are simultaneously enrolled. The primary outcome is time to failure (assumed to be eventually observed on all subjects) and treatment comparisons made using the Wilcoxon rank-sum test. When all failure times are known, the sum of ranks over both treatment groups will be 210, and the experimental treatment will be considered to be superior if the rank sum for this group is at least 131, or, equivalently, if the rank sum for the control group is at most 79. Because there is a common start time, the rank for a given subject is determined at the time of failure (e.g., the first failure has rank one, the second, rank two, and so on). Now suppose that at the time of the eighth failure in the control group the rank sum is at most 40. (If there were no failures in the experimental group by this time, the rank sum would be 36.) Because the ranks for the final two subjects will be at most 19 and 20, it is known at this point that regardless of the order of the remaining failures, the rank sum for the control group cannot exceed 79, so the outcome is not in doubt. Unless additional information beyond the hypothesis test is of interest, there is no reason to continue the trial.   □

To make this concept concrete statistically, let S denote a test statistic that measures the intervention difference and let the sample space, Ω, of S consist of disjoint regions, an acceptance region, A, and a rejection region, R, such that at the end of the study

$$\Pr(S \in R|H_0) = \alpha \text{ and } \Pr(S \in A|H_1) = \beta$$

where α and β are the type I and II error probabilities. Let t denote the time of an interim analysis, and let $D(t)$ denote the accumulated data up to time t. A deterministic curtailment test rejects or accepts the null hypothesis H_0 if

$$\Pr(S \in R|D(t)) = 1 \text{ or } \Pr(S \in A|D(t)) = 1,$$

respectively, regardless of whether H_0 or H_1 is true. Note that this procedure does not affect the type I and II error probabilities. For test statistics of the form $S_n = \sum_{i=1}^{n} x_i$, where the $x_1, x_2, \ldots$ are i.i.d., deterministic curtailment is possible only when the range of the x_i is finite (see DeMets and Halperin (1982)). In Example 10.1, had the analysis used a t-test for difference in *mean* failure time, deterministic curtailment would not have been possible, because the mean failure time for the control group could be arbitrarily large depending on timing of the two remaining failures. The use of ranks constrains the influence of the remaining observations.

10.6.2 Stochastic Curtailment

In general, deterministic curtailment is conservative, requiring that the eventual decision is known with certainty. A more practical procedure might require that the eventual decision is known only to a sufficient degree of certainty. To motivate the idea of stochastic curtailment, consider the following simple example.

Example 10.2. Suppose we conduct a single arm phase II trial involving 40 subjects in which the treatment will be of interest if the response rate is greater than $\pi = 0.3$, and will only pursue further investigation if we reject $H_0 \colon \pi \leq 0.3$. Thus, we require at least 19 responses out of 40 subjects, or the compound will be dropped. In addition, we believe that the largest value that π might reasonably be expected to take is 0.6. If, after 30 subjects we have observed only 11 responses, we will require 8 of the remaining 10 subjects to respond. Under the assumption that the true response rate is 0.6, the probability of at least 8 responses is $\binom{10}{8} 0.6^8 0.4^2 + \binom{10}{9} 0.6^9 0.4^1 + \binom{10}{10} 0.6^{10} 0.4^0 = 0.167$. Under the assumption that the true response rate is 0.5, this probability drops to 0.05. Since the data suggest that a true response rate as high as 0.6 may be unlikely, an investigator may conclude that these probabilities are too small to justify continuing the trial. □

The concept of stochastic curtailment and the consequence of its use were first proposed by Halperin et al. (1982) and further investigated by Lan et al. (1982). Consider a fixed sample size test of $H_0 \colon \mu = 0$ at a significance level α with power $1 - \beta$ to detect the intervention difference $\mu = \mu_A$. The conditional probability of rejection of H_0, i.e., *conditional power*, at μ is defined as

$$P_C(\mu) = \Pr(S \in R | D(t); \mu).$$

For some $\gamma_0, \gamma_1 > 1/2$, using a stochastic curtailment test we reject the null hypothesis if

$$P_C(\mu_A) \approx 1 \text{ and } P_C(0) > \gamma_0$$

and accept the null hypothesis (reject the alternative hypothesis) if

$$P_C(0) \approx 0 \text{ and } P_C(\mu_A) < 1 - \gamma_1.$$

Lan et al. (1982) established that the type I and II error probabilities are inflated but remain bounded from above by

$$\alpha' = \alpha/\gamma_0 \text{ and } \beta' = \beta/\gamma_1.$$

Generally stochastic curtailment tests of this type are quite conservative, and if $\gamma_0 = 1 = \gamma_1$, they become deterministic curtailment.

10.6.3 B-value and Conditional Power

The stochastic curtailment procedure described in the preceding section involved formal rejection of acceptance of H_0 based on conditional power at an interim analysis. In practice, conditional power is likely to be used in conjunction with other accumulating information such as adverse effect profiles to stop a trial for futility—the trial is not likely to demonstrate benefit and to continue would unnecessarily expose subjects to additional risk and waste time and resources. Here we describe a procedure that can be used to assess conditional power in a variety of settings.

Recall that the sequential test can be defined in terms of the B-value, $B(t)$, defined in equation (10.3). Suppose that we have observed $B(t_0)$, $t_0 < 1$, and that at the end of the study, $t = 1$, we will reject H_0: $\theta = 0$ in favor of H_1: $\theta = \theta_0$ if $B(1) \geq b(1)$. (Note that if an alpha spending function is in use, the final critical value will depend on the number and timing of interim analyses between time t and time 1, so $b(1)$ may not be known exactly.) We wish to calculate the probability, $P_C(\theta)$, that we will reject H_0 at $t = 1$. First, we can write $B(1) = B(t_0) + B(1) - B(t_0)$ and exploit the following three properties of $B(t)$ to compute conditional power:

1. $B(t_0)$ and $B(1) - B(t_0)$ are independent,

2. $\mathrm{Var}\{B(1) - B(t_0)\} = 1 - t_0$, and

3. $E(B(1) - B(t_0)) = (1 - t_0)\theta$.

We have that

$$
\begin{aligned}
P_C(\theta) &= \Pr\{B(1) > b(1)|B(t_0), \theta\} \\
&= \Pr\left\{\frac{B(1) - B(t_0) - (1 - t_0)\theta}{\sqrt{1 - t_0}} > \right. \\
&\qquad\qquad \left.\frac{b(1) - B(t_0) - (1 - t_0)\theta}{\sqrt{1 - t_0}}\middle| B(t_0), \theta\right\} \\
&= 1 - \Phi\left(\frac{b(1) - B(t_0) - (1 - t_0)\theta}{\sqrt{1 - t_0}}\right). \qquad (10.13)
\end{aligned}
$$

The last equality holds because the random variable on the left hand side of the inequality in the previous line has mean zero and variance one. Equation (10.13) can also be written

$$
P_C(\theta) = 1 - \Phi\left(\frac{b(1) - Z(t_0)\sqrt{t_0} - (1 - t_0)\theta}{\sqrt{1 - t_0}}\right).
$$

Example 10.3. Suppose that we conduct 3 interim analyses at information fractions 0.2, 0.4, and 0.6. Using the O'Brien-Fleming boundary defined by equation (10.7). This boundary is equivalent to $|B(t)| \geq 2.04$. The corresponding Z statistics are 0.5, -0.6, and 0.3, with B-values $.5\sqrt{.2} = .223$, $-.6\sqrt{.4} = -.379$, and $.3\sqrt{.6} = .232$. (See Figure 10.9.) Suppose that the trial is powered for a standardized difference of $\theta = 3.24$ (for fixed sample power of 90% at two-sided $\alpha = 0.05$). Conditional power assuming that this is the true value of θ is

$$
1 - \Phi\left(\frac{2.041 - 0.232 - (1 - 0.6) \times 3.24}{\sqrt{1 - 0.6}}\right) = .209.
$$

Thus under the original sample size assumption, the probability of showing benefit is just over 20%. On the other hand, the current estimate of the treatment difference is $\hat{\theta} = 0.3/.6 = 0.5$, with a 95% (unadjusted) confidence interval of (-2.14, 2.92), so the assumed value of θ may be considered incon-

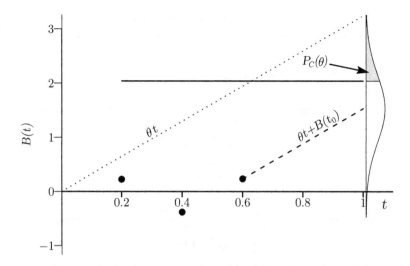

Figure 10.9 *Conditional power computed using B-value in Example 10.3. The dotted line represents the unconditional expected value of $B(t)$ (prior to the collection of any study data). The dashed line represents the expected value of $B(t)$ given $B(t_0)$, for $t_0 = 0.6$.*

sistent with the observed data and we may want to consider a range of values for θ, creating the following table:

θ:	0	0.5	1	2	2.92	3	3.24
$P_C(\theta)$ (%):	0.2	0.5	1.3	5.5	15.6	16.8	20.9

We see that under both $H_0\colon \theta = 0$ and the observed difference $\theta = \hat{\theta} = .5$, the probability of showing benefit is less than 1%. Under values of θ within the 95% confidence interval, we have $P_C(\theta) < 16\%$. We might consider that these probabilities are too small to justify continuation, although other factors should be considered.   □

The interpretation of the parameter, θ, depends on the nature of the data being analyzed. Table 10.5 provides the interpretation of θ for several commonly used data types.

If desired, one can formalize futility monitoring by creating a boundary with fixed conditional power for a given value of θ. Figure 10.10 shows possible futility boundaries for $\theta = 3.24$ (required for 90% fixed sample power) and intermediate value of $\theta = 1$. The boundaries based on $\theta = 1$ would probably be considered too aggressive—signaling early termination before most monitoring committees would seriously consider it. Because the upper efficacy boundary is computed independent of the futility boundary, the overall type I error is reduced slightly depending on the specific lower boundary selected, and the procedure is slightly conservative. Similarly, when $\theta > 0$, power is reduced

Table 10.5 *Parameter for conditional power* $(\theta = E[Z_N^*])$.

1. Survival $\theta = \sqrt{D/4}\log(\lambda_C/\lambda_T)$ $D = \text{total events}$

2. Binomial $\theta = \dfrac{P_C - P_T}{\sqrt{2\bar{p}\bar{q}/(N/2)}}$ $N = \text{total sample size}$

   $\qquad\qquad = \dfrac{(P_C - P_T)\sqrt{N/4}}{\sqrt{\bar{p}\bar{q}}}$

   $\qquad\qquad = \dfrac{(P_C - P_T)\sqrt{N}}{2\sqrt{\bar{p}\bar{q}}}$

3. Means $\theta = \left(\dfrac{\mu_C - \mu_T}{\sigma}\right)\sqrt{N/4}$ $N = \text{total sample size}$

   $\qquad\qquad = \left(\dfrac{\mu_C - \mu_T}{2\sigma}\right)\sqrt{N}$

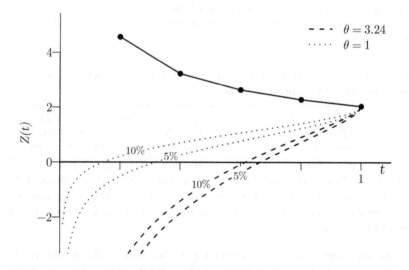

Figure 10.10 *Conditional power boundaries for O'Brien-Fleming boundary with* $K = 5$ *and (one-sided)* $\alpha = 0.025$ *for true* $\theta = 3.24, 1$, *and conditional power 5% and 10%.*

slightly. For the boundaries based on $\theta = 3.24$, however, the power loss is well below 1%.

Note that a key assumption in the calculation of conditional power is assumption B2 on page 297. If this condition fails, then $E[B(t)]$ will not follow a straight line as shown in Figure 10.9. This might happen, for example, in a survival trial in which there is a delay in the effect of treatment. Analyses conducted early in the trial, when all or most subjects have yet to receive the benefit of treatment, may show little or no systematic difference between groups. As more subjects have sufficient follow-up, the difference between groups should emerge and strengthen throughout the remainder of the trial. Thus, caution is advised in settings where such an effect is a possibility.

10.6.4 Predictive Power

Note that the conditional power given by (10.13) depends on both the current data through $B(t_0)$, and the presumed value of θ. If $B(t_0)$ is small, rejection of H_0 requires that the increment, $B(1) - B(t_0)$, be large, which may be unlikely unless θ is large. On the other hand, small values of $B(t_0)$ suggest that large values of θ are implausible. Therefore, if t_0 is large enough, small values of $B(t_0)$ are detrimental in two ways: large increments in $B(t)$ are required to show benefit, and the large values of θ required to make large increments likely are inconsistent with the evidence regarding θ obtained thus far.

In Example 10.3, we computed conditional power for a range of values of θ. The decision to stop for futility requires, among other considerations, that one assess which of these values are credible in the light of both the observed data and current scientific understanding. For example, the value upon which the trial was designed, $\theta = 3.24$, seems unlikely given the current estimate of $\hat{\theta} = 0.5$, and hence one may discount conditional power computed under this assumption. On the other hand, if the data are inconsistent with prior experience, one might wish to discount the current evidence and be more cautious. One quantity that can make use of both prior scientific knowledge and data from the current trial into an estimate of the likelihood of success is known as *predictive power*.

Predictive power was proposed by Spiegelhalter et al. (1986) and is computed by averaging the conditional power $P_c(\theta)$ over *likely* values of θ. Since the usual frequentist viewpoint does not allow for the notion of *likely values*, one is required to assume a Bayesian point of view, considering the posterior distribution of θ, $\pi(\theta|B(t))$. We define predictive power to be

$$P_P = \int P_C(\theta)\pi(\theta|B(t))d\theta$$

where $B(t)$ denotes the accumulated data by time t of the interim analysis, and $\pi(\theta|B(t)) = M(B(t))f(B(t);\theta)\pi(\theta)$ where $f(B(t);\theta)$ is the likelihood function for $B(t)$, $\pi(\theta)$ is a given *prior* distribution, and $M(B(t))$ is chosen so that $\pi(\theta|B(t))$ is a proper probability distribution. The primary difficulty with this approach is that the choice of $\pi(\theta)$ is somewhat subjective.

To illustrate, suppose that *a priori* θ is distributed $N(\eta, 1/\nu)$, so that η is the prior mean and ν is the prior *precision* of θ. Given $B(t_0)$ and using Bayes' theorem, the posterior distribution of θ is

$$\pi(\theta|B(t_0)) \sim N\left(\frac{B(t_0) + \eta\nu}{\nu + t_0}, \frac{1}{\nu + t_0}\right).$$

Since $B(1) - B(t_0) \sim N(\theta(1 - t_0), 1 - t_0)$, and integrating out the unknown

θ, we have that

$$\pi(B(1)|B(t_0)) \sim N\left(\frac{B(t_0)(\nu+1)+\eta\nu(1-t_0)}{\nu+t_0}, \frac{(\nu+1)(1-t_0)}{\nu+t_0}\right),$$

so clearly the predictive power, $P_P(\eta,\nu)$, depends on the prior parameters, η and ν.

We note two special cases. If $\nu \to \infty$, so that the prior precision is large, we have $\pi(B(1)|B(t_0)) \sim N(B(t_0)+\eta(1-t_0), 1-t_0)$ and predictive power is identical to conditional power when $\theta = \eta$. Conversely, if $\nu \to 0$, the prior variance of θ is large, so the prior distribution is diffuse and uninformative; we have $\pi(B(1)|B(t_0)) \sim N(B(t_0)/t_0, (1-t_0)/t_0)$, so predictive power is similar to conditional power using the current estimate $\hat{\theta}$, except that the variance is larger by a factor of $1/t_0$, reflecting the uncertainty in $\hat{\theta}$.

Example 10.4. Continuing Example 10.3, using the diffuse prior ($\nu = 0$), then predictive power is 2.1%, larger than the conditional power assuming $\theta = \hat{\theta}$ (0.5%), but suggesting that a successful trial is unlikely given the current data. If we take $\eta = 3.24$ and $\nu = 1$, so that we have a strong belief that the treatment is beneficial, but with uncertainty regarding the size of the effect, the $P_P(3.24,1) = 9.2\%$. In spite of our strong belief, the evidence against $\theta = 3.24$ is sufficiently strong that the predictive power is relatively small.   □

Predictive power was part of the rationale for early termination of a trial in traumatic hemorrhagic shock (Lewis et al. 2001). In this trial, a diffuse (uninformative) prior distribution was used and at the time that the trial was stopped, the predictive probability of showing a benefit was extremely small (0.045%).

10.7 Inference Following Sequential Tests

Clinical trials using sequential tests such as those discussed in the chapter are designed explicitly to test hypotheses; they allow stopping at the point that a decision to accept or reject particular hypotheses can be made. In a fixed sample trial, in addition to a formal hypothesis test, one will generally compute a p-value that quantifies the strength of evidence against the null hypothesis, a point estimate of the treatment difference and a corresponding confidence interval. In each case, inference is based on the sampling distribution of the summary statistics. When data are sampled sequentially, however, the sampling distributions of the summary statistics depend on the sequential procedure and inference that ignores the procedure will be incorrect. Specifically, when interim analyses are conducted at unequally spaced intervals, the sampling distribution of the cumulative sums, S_k, are defined by equations (10.10) and (10.11).

An idea central to inference in this setting is that of the ordering of the sample space. This idea is especially crucial in the construction of a p-value.

In the fixed sample case, the usual definition of a p-value is that it is the *probability of observing a result at least as extreme as the one observed when the null hypothesis is true*. For fixed sample tests this definition is generally straightforward to implement. For example, for a (two-sided) two sample t-test, the $p = \Pr\{|T| > |t^*|\}$ where t^* is the observed t-statistic and T is a random variable with a t-distribution with the same number of degrees of freedom. In this case "at least as extreme" means that the t-statistic is at least as large in absolute value.

In sequential trials, the definition of "at least as extreme" is not as clear. Specifically, the observed result may be represented by a pair (k^*, S^*) where k^* indicates the analysis at which the boundary was crossed or $k = K$ if the trial was not stopped early and S^* is the corresponding test statistic at the terminal analysis. We also let I_k be the Fisher information at analysis k. For the triangular test the idea is similar, with (k^*, S^*) replaced by (V^*, S^*). Hence, the observed response is two dimensional and there are many possible orderings. In the remainder of this section, we discuss the construction of p-values, confidence intervals, and point estimates that are consistent with the sequential procedure. The choice of ordering of the observations (k, S) will play a key role in such inference.

10.7.1 Observed Significance

Following sequential procedure, one may want to report the observed significance (p-value) of the observed intervention effect as is done with a fixed sample study. Recall that, by definition, a p-value is the probability of observing a result at least as extreme as the one observed when the null hypothesis is true. Since, as discussed earlier, there are many possible definitions of "at least as extreme" we begin with a discussion of possible orderings of the sample space. For simplicity, we consider only procedures in which stopping is allowed solely for benefit. This excludes, for example, procedures that allow early stopping to accept H_0. We will also consider only one-sided tests and one-sided p-values. A two-sided p-value can be most easily obtained by doubling the one-sided p-value.

When, for a particular ordering, an observation (k', S') is more extreme than (k, S), we write $(k', S') \succ (k, S)$. Jennison and Turnbull (2000) discuss four possible orderings:

1. *Stage-wise ordering (SW)*. Using the SW ordering, $(k', S') \succ (k, S)$ if one of the following holds:

   (a) $k' = k$ and $S' > S$,

   (b) $k' < k$.

2. *MLE ordering*. We consider $(k', S') \succ (k, S)$ if the $\hat{\mu}' = S'/I_{k'} > \hat{\mu} = S/I_k$.

3. *Likelihood Ratio (LR) ordering*. $Z = S/I_k^{1/2}$ is a monotone function of the likelihood ratio so we consider $(k', S') \succ (k, S)$ if $S'/I_{k'}^{1/2} > S/I_k^{1/2}$.

4. *Score ordering.* In this ordering $(k', S') \succ (k, S)$ if $S' > S$.

For a given ordering, O, the (one-sided) p-value for an observation, (k^*, S^*), is

$$p_O = \Pr\{(k, S) \succ (k^*, S^*) | \mu = 0\}.$$

First consider the **SW ordering**. This ordering was proposed by Siegmund (1978) and Fairbanks and Madsen (1982). Using the SW ordering, for a given pair (k, S), any realization of the trial data in which the boundary is crossed earlier is considered more extreme. Also, any realization for which the boundary is crossed at the same analysis time, k, but with a larger value of S is considered more extreme.

With that in mind, define $\alpha_1, \ldots, \alpha_K$ such that

$$\alpha_1 = \Pr(S_1 \geq c_1),$$

and

$$\alpha_k = \Pr(S_1 < c_1, \ldots, S_{k-1} < c_{k-1}, S_k \geq c_k)$$

for $k = 2, \ldots, K$. Then $\sum_{k=1}^{K} \alpha_k = \alpha$, the overall significance level of the test.

If the test terminates at the k^*th interim analysis with a terminal observed value of the test statistic S^*, the SW p-value for the test is defined as

$$p_{SW} = \sum_{j=1}^{k-1} \alpha_j + p^* \tag{10.14}$$

where

$$p^* = \Pr(S_1 < c_1, \ldots, S_{k-1} < c_{k-1}, S_k \geq S^*).$$

Clearly, if $k^* = 1$, p_{SW} is identical to the corresponding fixed sample p-value. Furthermore, the p-value will be smaller if the test terminates at interim analysis $k - 1$ than if it terminates at interim analysis k regardless of the value of S^*. The SW ordering is the only ordering for which more extreme observations cannot occur at future analysis times. Thus the SW ordering has the desirable property that the p-value can be computed solely from the analyses conducted up to the point at which the trial is stopped without regard for the timing or critical values for planned future analyses.

The **MLE ordering** orders observations based on the point estimate $\hat{\mu}$. Unlike the SW ordering, a more extreme observation can occur at an analysis time beyond the one at which the trial is stopped. Thus, to compute the p-value exactly, one needs to know both the timing and critical values for all planned future analyses. Since these analyses will never be conducted, when flexible procedures are used, their timing—possibly even their number—can only be hypothesized at study termination. The p-value is computed as

$$p_{MLE} = \Pr\{S_1 \geq I_1 \hat{\mu} \vee c_1\} + \sum_{k=2}^{K} \Pr\{S_j < c_j, j = 1, \ldots, k-1, S_k \geq I_1 \hat{\mu} \vee c_k\}$$

where "$\vee$" denotes that maximum of its arguments. Under this ordering, there can exist realizations of the trial data for which the boundary is crossed at an earlier time, but that are not considered "more extreme." This phenomenon is less likely to occur with the MLE ordering than with the LR and score orderings because boundaries usually cannot be crossed at the earliest analyses times unless the point estimates, $\hat{\mu}$, are quite large.

The **LR ordering** is similar to the MLE ordering in that the p-value depends on the timing and critical values at future analyses. The p-value is computed in a similar fashion to that for the MLE ordering,

$$p_{LR} = \Pr\{S_1 \geq (I_1/I_{k^*})^{1/2}S^* \vee c_1\} + $$
$$\sum_{k=2}^{K}\Pr\{S_j < c_j, j = 1, \ldots, k-1, S_k \geq (I_k/I_{k^*})^{1/2}S^* \vee c_k\}.$$

The appeal of the LR ordering is that it is a direct generalization of the ordering from the fixed sample case—to the extent that $S/I^{1/2}$ captures the strength of evidence against H_0, only those realizations with stronger evidence are considered more extreme. As with the MLE ordering, the difficulty with the LR ordering is its dependence on the timing and critical values of planned future analyses.

Finally, the **score ordering** is based directly on the cumulative sums, S_k, and the p-value is computed using

$$p_{score} = \Pr\{S_1 \geq S^* \vee c_1\} + \sum_{k=2}^{K}\Pr\{S_j < c_j, j = 1, \ldots, k-1, S_k \geq S^* \vee c_k\}.$$

Given that variance of S_k, I_k, is an increasing function of k, under the score ordering it is unlikely for a extreme observation to occur early in a trial. This gives the p-value from the score ordering undesirable properties as noted by Chang et al. (1995) and Cook (2002a).

Jennison and Turnbull (2000) and Proschan et al. (2006) recommend that the SW ordering be used, principally because the p-value does not depend on the timing and critical values of future analyses. Other authors recommend the LR ordering, arguing that it is less conservative than the SW ordering. Chang et al. (1995) and Gillen and Emerson (2005) recommend the LR ordering because it demonstrates increased "power" in the sense that under alternative hypotheses, the probability of small p-values is greater. Cook (2002a) recommends the LR ordering because it produces p-values that are more consistent with evidence in the data against the null hypothesis, while noting that the dependence on future analyses is small, and one can maximize with respect to likely future analysis times and produce bounds on the p-value that are much less conservative than those produced by the SW ordering. For example, the MERIT-HF study (MERIT-HF Study Group 1999) stopped with approximately 50% information and a nominal p=value of 0.00009 for mortality. The p-value obtained using the SW ordering is 0.0062, which is 68 times larger than the nominal p-value. The p-value obtained using the LR ordering is 0.00015 which is much more consistent with the evidence against H_0 in the data. Similarly, the COPERNICUS study (Packer et al. 2001) was stopped at approximately 35% information and the final value of Z was 3.82. The nominal p-value was 0.00013, the SW p-value was 0.0014, and the LR p-value, assuming two additional interim analyses, was 0.00056. Again, the LR p-value is closer to the nominal p-value and more consistent with the evidence from the data.

The conservatism in the SW p-value arises because it essentially imposes a "failure to stop" penalty. Note that in equation (10.14), the p-value is bounded below by the first term, $\sum_{j=1}^{k-1} \alpha_j = p_k^{min}$, which is determined simply by the fact that the boundary was not crossed at any of the first $k - 1$ analysis times. Therefore, no matter how strong the evidence at analysis k, the p-value cannot be smaller than p_k^{min}. Hence, the p-value cannot accommodate a large overshoot, $S_k - c_k$. In the MERIT-HF and COPERNICUS examples, the overshoot is quite large and the "failure to stop" penalty is quite large. The dependence of the p_{LR} on the timing of future analyses is relatively minor and can be easily overcome by maximizing the p-value over a range of possible future analysis times. The conservatism induced in the SW ordering by disallowing dependence on future analysis times is a disadvantage that may not be commensurate with resulting benefit. Based on an informal survey of studies reporting adjusted inference, the SW ordering is currently the most widely used.

10.7.2 Confidence Interval Estimation

In the same way that repeated significance testing increases the overall type I error, confidence intervals derived without accounting for the sequential procedure will not have the correct coverage probability. Confidence intervals with the correct coverage probability can be derived using the orderings considered in the previous section.

In the fixed sample case, confidence intervals can be constructed by inverting hypothesis tests. For example, suppose that $X_1, X_2, \ldots, X_n \sim N(\mu, \sigma^2)$. We reject the null hypothesis $H_0 \colon \mu = \mu_0$ if and only if

$$\frac{|\bar{X} - \mu_0|}{\sqrt{\hat{\sigma}^2/n}} \geq t_{1-\alpha/2, n-1}$$

where $t_{1-\alpha/2, n-1}$ is the $100 \times (1 - \alpha/2)$ percentage point of the t-distribution with $n - 1$ degrees of freedom. A $100 \times (1 - \alpha)\%$ confidence interval can be constructed by including all μ_0 for which we do not reject H_0 at level α. That is, the $100 \times (1 - \alpha)\%$ confidence interval for μ is the set

$$
\begin{aligned}
R &= \left\{ \mu_0 \colon \bar{X} - t_{1-\alpha/2, n-1}\sqrt{\hat{\sigma}^2/n} < \mu_0 < \bar{X} + t_{1-\alpha/2, n-1}\sqrt{\hat{\sigma}^2/n} \right\} \\
&= \left\{ \mu_0 \colon \frac{|\bar{X} - \mu_0|}{\sqrt{\hat{\sigma}^2/n}} < t_{1-\alpha/2, n-1} \right\} \\
&= \left\{ \mu_0 \colon p(\mu_0) > \alpha \right\}
\end{aligned}
$$

where $p(\mu_0)$ is the (two-sided) p-value function for $\bar{X}$ under $H_0 \colon \mu = \mu_0$.

Combining the last equality above with the p-values defined in the previous section provides a procedure for finding valid confidence intervals. For a given ordering, O, and observation, (k^*, S^*), define the (upper) one-sided p-value $p_O(\mu_0) = \Pr\{(k, S) \succ (k^*, S^*)|\mu = \mu_0\}$. The $100 \times (1-\alpha)\%$ confidence region, R, is the set of values of μ_0 satisfying

$$\alpha/2 < p_O(\mu_0) < 1 - \alpha/2.$$

Confidence intervals based on the SW ordering were proposed by Tsiatis et al. (1984). Rosner and Tsiatis (1988) and Emerson and Fleming (1990) investigated the MLE ordering. Chang and O'Brien (1986) consider the LR ordering for the case of binary observations in phase II trials. Rosner and Tsiatis (1988) compared properties of all four orderings. Kim and DeMets (1987a) consider confidence intervals based on the SW ordering for a variety of error spending functions.

For the SW and MLE orderings, the p-value function is a monotone function of μ_0 so R is guaranteed to be an interval. For the LR ordering, monotonicity may not strictly hold and it is possible, although unlikely, for R to not be an interval. For the score ordering, R is frequently not an interval.

Similar to the p-values in the previous section, for the SW ordering, R does not depend on the future interim analyses. It is typically shifted towards zero, relative to the fixed sample interval, but in some instances, it can fail to contain the sample mean. Furthermore, if $k^* = 1$, R coincides with the fixed sample confidence interval.

A desirable property of a method for generating a confidence interval is that it should minimize the probability that the interval covers the wrong values of μ; i.e., $\Pr(\mu' \in I(S_T, T))$ should be as small as possible when $\mu' \neq \mu$. Also a confidence interval should be as short as possible. When μ is near zero, both the LR and SW orderings above give similar results. Neither method dominates uniformly over the parameter space. In general, however, the LR does better than the MLE ordering. Emerson and Fleming (1990) suggest that the MLE ordering is competitive when looking at the average length of the confidence intervals.

10.7.3 Point Estimation

When sequential procedures are used, the naive point estimate of treatment differences, $\hat{\mu} = S^*/I_{k^*}$, is biased. This bias is introduced because sample paths of S fluctuate randomly about their mean, μt, and a path for which S is larger than its expectation is more likely to cross the upper boundary sooner when $\hat{\mu}$ is large and with large variance. Conversely, paths for which S is smaller than expected tend to cross later, if at all, when the variance of $\hat{\mu}$ is smaller, and hence values are less extreme.

Figure 10.11 shows the bias in the maximum likelihood estimate of the treatment difference using the one-sided O'Brien-Fleming boundary with $\alpha =$

0.025, given by (10.7). Note that the bias increases with increasing μ until μ is about 1.7, after which the bias decreases. If μ is sufficiently large, a large proportion of realizations will cross the boundary at the first look, and the procedure begins to approximate a fixed sample test in which $\hat{\mu}$ is unbiased.

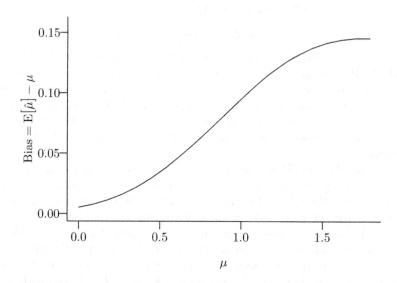

Figure 10.11 *Bias in maximum likelihood estimate of the standardized treatment difference following sequential testing using the one-sided O'Brien-Fleming boundary with 5 looks and $\alpha = 0.025$ (equation (10.7)).*

A number of estimators that reduce or eliminate bias have been proposed and investigated. The case in which $X_1, X_2, \ldots$ are iid $N(\mu, 1)$ and $S_k = X_1 + \cdots + X_k$ was studied by Siegmund (1978). For the repeated significance test of $H_0 \colon \mu = 0$ defined by the continuation region

$$|S_k| > c\sqrt{k},$$

Siegmund proposed the modification $\hat{\mu}_m$ of the maximum likelihood estimator

$$\hat{\mu}_m = \begin{cases} (S^*/k^*)/(1 + 2/c^2), & \text{if } |S^*| > c\sqrt{k^*} \\ S_K/K, & \text{otherwise} \end{cases}$$

where K is the maximum sample size. Siegmund shows that $\hat{\mu}_m$ is unbiased as $c \to \infty$, which is the case for (nearly) continuous monitoring. For group sequential designs with less frequent monitoring, $\hat{\mu}_m$ does not perform well.

Alternatively, letting $b(\mu) = E[\hat{\mu}] - \mu$, if $b(\mu)$ were known, $\hat{\mu} - b(\mu)$ would be unbiased. As $b(\mu)$ is unknown, Whitehead (1986) proposed a bias adjusted estimate, $\tilde{\mu}_W$, defined as the solution to

$$\tilde{\mu}_W = \hat{\mu} - b(\tilde{\mu}_W)$$

which can be solved iteratively for $\tilde{\mu}_W$. Whitehead shows that the bias in $\tilde{\mu}_W$ is quite small and that its standard error is smaller than that of $\hat{\mu}$.

Other bias corrected estimators have been proposed. For S_k above, S_1 is an unbiased estimate of μ, but has large variance. Applying the Rao-Blackwell theorem, Emerson and Fleming (1990) and Liu and Hall (1999) show that among estimators not depending on the stopping boundaries after the terminal analysis, there exists a uniformly minimum variance unbiased estimator of the sample mean defined by

$$\breve{\mu} = E\{S_1|(S^*, k^*)\}.$$

Given an ordering, O, of the sample space, the *median unbiased estimator*, $\tilde{\mu}_0$, (Kim 1989) is defined as the solution to

$$p_O(\mu_0) = \Pr((S_k, k) \succ (S^*, k^*)|\mu = \mu_0) = 0.5. \tag{10.15}$$

All point estimates except for $\breve{\mu}$ and the median unbiased estimate based on the SW ordering require prespecification of the times and frequency of interim analyses. There remains, however, disagreement on the appropriate ordering of the sample space, and no consensus has emerged regarding which point estimator is preferable. The problem has also been studied by other authors (Pinheiro and DeMets 1997; Qu and DeMets 1999; Li and DeMets 1999). The median unbiased estimator based on the SW ordering appears to have been adopted by many investigators and is incorporated into commercial products such as EaSt (Cytel Software Corporation 2000) and PEST (MPS Research Unit 2000).

10.7.4 Inference in MADIT

MADIT was terminated when upper boundary of the triangular test was crossed. The results reported (Moss et al. 1996) were adjusted for the sequential procedure used. The reported p-value, obtained based on the SW ordering, was 0.009. The nominal p-value (estimated from the figure in the primary article) was 0.003. Because the interim analyses are closely spaced, the overshoot is not likely to be large; under each of the SW, LR, and MLE orderings the more extreme values will likely occur at earlier analyses times, and so these orderings will provide similar results. The median unbiased estimate of the hazard ratio using (10.15) was reported to be 0.46, with an adjusted 95% confidence interval based on

$$P_{SW}(\mu_L) = 0.025 \text{ and } P_{SW}(\mu_U) = 0.975$$

of (0.26, 0.82). Other secondary analyses were performed using the Cox proportional hazards regression model.

10.8 Discussion

Data monitoring is a difficult undertaking and not without controversy. We close this chapter with a discussion of issues surrounding interim monitoring.

In this chapter we have focused primarily on efficacy monitoring. Because it is difficult, if not impossible, to prespecify all possible safety issues that might arise, safety monitoring is less amenable to a rigorous statistical approach. A few authors have proposed formal monitoring plans explicitly accommodating safety monitoring (Jennison and Turnbull 1993; Bolland and Whitehead 2000).

10.8.1 Comparison of boundaries

Figure 10.12 shows one-sided O'Brien-Fleming and Pocock boundaries superimposed on the Emerson-Fleming boundary from Figure 10.2 and the MADIT boundary from Figure 10.8, transformed so that $V = 37$ corresponds to full information, and shown on the Z scale. The boundary for the triangular test assuming continuous monitoring is shown without correction to prevent the figure from being too busy. The boundary using the "christmas tree" correction would be pulled into the middle in a fashion similar to that of Figure 10.7. When shown on a common scale, the distinguishing features of the four boundaries are evident. The O'Brien-Fleming boundary is slightly more conservative than the Emerson-Fleming boundary due to the fact that the Emerson-Fleming boundary allows early stopping for lack of benefit, allowing the efficacy boundary to be lowered while preserving the overall type I error rate. The upper triangular boundary appears to be strictly above the Pocock boundary, but this is due to the assumption of continuous monitoring for the triangular test. If the correction for discreteness were shown, the triangular boundary would be slightly below the Pocock boundary after the second analysis. Nonetheless, after the first two interim analyses, the upper triangular boundary has similar behavior to the Pocock boundary in that it is relatively constant, with a relatively large final critical value. It is important to note that for the triangular and Emerson-Fleming boundaries, preservation of the overall type I error requires that the trial be stopped whenever the lower boundary is crossed.

10.8.2 Perspectives Regarding Interim Monitoring

There are (at least) two perspectives regarding interim efficacy monitoring resulting in different approaches. The first view holds that a trial is designed primarily to demonstrate the efficacy of new treatment with the goal that the trial do so as efficiently as possible. From this point of view there is no practical distinction between the interim analyses and the final analysis, hence the phrase "early termination" has no meaning. Once the objective of rejecting H_0 (or rejecting H_1) has been met there is no reason to continue the trial.

The second viewpoint holds that a trial is designed to accrue a predetermined amount of information and early stopping is driven solely by ethical considerations; i.e., the result is so compelling that continuation is unethical. From this viewpoint, if an interim analysis provides convincing evidence of treatment benefit with respect to all-cause mortality or serious, irreversible

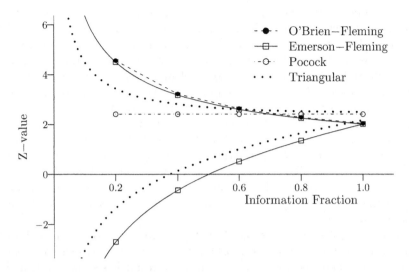

Figure 10.12 *Comparison of (one-sided) monitoring boundaries. The O'Brien-Fleming and Pocock boundaries are one-sided $\alpha = 0.025$ boundaries, the Emerson-Fleming boundary is from Figure 10.2, and the boundary for the triangular test is transformed from the MADIT boundary from Figure 10.8.*

morbidity such as heart attack or stroke, the trial should be stopped to allow both control subjects and future patients access to the more effective treatment as soon as possible. Conversely, if benefit is demonstrated with respect to a nonfatal, non-serious outcome such as quality of life or exercise tolerance (even though these outcomes may be invaluable to the individual subject), then one might argue that there is no ethical imperative to stop, and that the trial should continue to its planned conclusion in order to both strengthen the efficacy result and maximize the amount of other information, especially regarding safety, that is collected.

The former viewpoint suggests that boundaries that satisfy an optimality criterion such as average sample number (ASN) should be preferred because they allow stopping as soon as the result is clear, with the minimum exposure of trial subjects to inferior treatments. Conversely, the latter viewpoint suggests that boundaries should be as conservative as possible while allowing study termination in cases where the evidence is sufficiently compelling. For example, Pocock (2005) commends the Haybittle-Peto boundary which requires a nominal p-value less than 0.001 before termination, and also suggests that interim monitoring not begin too soon when little information regarding both safety and efficacy is available.

For example, the primary outcome in the WIZARD trial (O'Connor et al. 2003; Cook et al. 2006) was a composite of all-cause mortality, recurrent myocardial infarction (MI), revascularization procedure, or hospitalization for angina. This outcome was chosen, in part, to increase study power while maintaining an affordable sample size. Because benefit with respect to revascularization procedures or hospitalizations for angina may not be sufficient to compel study termination on ethical grounds, interim monitoring was conducted using the composite of all-cause mortality and recurrent MI. (Chen, DeMets, and Lan (2003) discuss the problem of monitoring using mortality for interim analyses while using a composite outcome for the final analysis.) Furthermore, even though the overall type I error rate of $\alpha = 0.05$ was used, the monitoring boundary used an O'Brien-Fleming type alpha spending function based on an overall type I error rate of $\alpha = 0.01$. The resulting critical values at the planned information fractions of 1/3 and 2/3 were more conservative than those for the Haybittle-Peto boundary (± 4.46 and ± 3.15 respectively, (Cook et al. 2006)). The effect of interim monitoring on the final critical value using the primary composite outcome was virtually unaffected by the interim monitoring plan.

The ideal probably lies somewhere between these two extremes. For trials involving mortality or serious morbidity, one should be less willing to allow a trial to continue past the point at which the result has shown clear and convincing evidence of benefit sufficient to change clinical practice. For diseases with less serious outcomes, one may be more willing to impose more stringent stopping criteria in order to gain a fuller understanding of the full effect of the treatment. Regardless, early stopping is a complex decision requiring careful consideration of many factors, some of which are outlined in the next section.

10.8.3 Discretion in Data Monitoring

It is important to keep in mind that data monitoring committees must be afforded discretion regarding the recommendation to terminate a trial. For example, although a test statistic may have exceeded a stopping boundary, for a variety of reasons, a DMC may elect not to recommend termination and this decision may affect the statistical properties of the monitoring procedure. Before describing the statistical implications, we present a series of questions, proposed by the Coronary Drug Project Research Group (1981), that should be taken into consideration before making a recommendation to terminate a trial.

1. How has the treatment performed with respect to a host of endpoints and potential side effects? Stated in a different way, what does the totality of the findings indicate about the overall benefit-risk ratio?

2. Can the observed "treatment effects" be explained by differences in the baseline distributions of risk factors or comorbid conditions between the treatment and control groups?

3. Is there a possibility of bias in the recognition or diagnosis of the endpoint(s) of interest (a) due to the study not be double-blind, (b) due to breakdown of the double-blind because of specific side effects, or (c) due to side effects of one or more treatment groups leading to enhanced detailed workup of

some patients and coincidentally leading to enhanced ascertainment of the endpoint? If there is no possibility of biased diagnosis (as, for example, in the case of total mortality), is there a possibility that patients in one group may have received different medical management from those in the other groups(s) as a result of drug side effects or of unblinding?

4. What is the likelihood of a reversal of early adverse or beneficial trends if the study were to be continued to its scheduled conclusion?

5. Are the findings concordant for all identifiable subgroups of the study population or is early termination warranted only in one or more subgroups?

6. If there is more than one active treatment under study, is there a suggestion that the placebo group may be abnormally high or low in incidence of the primary endpoint in comparison to every one of the other treatment groups?

7. If a decision for early stopping were to be made, what would be the anticipated impact of this decision and the ensuing recommendations on the medical community (i.e., physicians) as a whole? For example, if there was an existing strong conviction in favor of a certain treatment in the medical community, would an early decision to stop because of an adverse effect of the treatment provide strong enough data to counteract such physician opinion?

While the answers to these questions require a combination of statistical and medical judgment, the implication is that the decision of a DMC cannot be dictated strictly by formal statistical procedures. Monitoring procedures are not "stopping rules" in the sense that they must be strictly adhered to under all circumstances. On the other hand, statistical procedures are more than "guidelines" in the sense that they form the basis for valid statistical inference and failure to heed them can result in a loss of credibility in the trial results. The latter is more likely in the case where a trial is stopped before a formal monitoring boundary had been crossed.

For example, the U.S. carvedilol program (Fisher and Moyé 1999) comprised four trials undertaken to assess the effect of a beta-blocker, carvedilol, on subjects with heart failure. In three of the trials the primary endpoint was change in exercise tolerance and in the remaining trial the primary outcome was quality of life. A single committee was responsible for simultaneous monitoring of all trials in the program. The program was terminated when it was observed that when the four studies were combined, 31 of 398 (7.8%) subjects in the placebo groups died, compared to 22 of 696 (3.2%) subjects in the carvedilol groups ($p < 0.001$); the hazard ratio was 0.35 (Packer et al. 1996). Because there was no monitoring plan in place for overall mortality, there was no formal statistical basis for the decision to terminate the program. The decision of the DMC was based on the finding that the mortality difference "exceeded all conventional boundaries used to stop clinical trials" (Packer et al. 1996). A controversy arose regarding whether carvedilol should be approved by the FDA on this basis (Fisher 1999; Moyé 1999). The decision ultimately made by the FDA to approve carvedilol was corroborated by subsequent trials that conclusively demonstrated the benefit of beta-blockers for the treatment of heart failure (Packer et al. 2001; MERIT-HF Study Group 1999). Nonetheless, the difficulties could have been avoided had a formal monitoring plan been in place and adhered to by the DMC.

Finally, we note that while most studies are designed and powered for an overall type I error rate of $\alpha = 0.05$, a (two-sided) p-value for benefit of, say, 0.03 or 0.04 may not be sufficient, without supplementary evidence of benefit, either for regulatory approval or to change clinical practice. Thus, another consideration is whether the result, combined with evidence from previous studies or other sources, provides sufficient evidence for benefit. If a trial is terminated early for efficacy, it is unlikely that a second confirmatory trial will be undertaken—the current trial may represent the only opportunity to collect further information. Since it is generally known when the trial is initiated the degree of evidence that is likely to be required, the formal monitoring boundaries should be formulated with this in mind.

10.8.4 Symmetry

As suggested in Section 10.4.2, the stopping problem is not symmetric—the basis for stopping for benefit is different than that of stopping for harm or futility (DeMets, Pocock, and Julian 1999). Our recommendation is that upper and lower boundaries be constructed separately keeping the distinct objectives for each in mind. Furthermore, one must be aware of how the issues discussion in Section 10.8.3 affect the operating characteristics of the monitoring procedures.

We first note that there are two kinds of lower boundaries, boundaries for harm and boundaries for futility. By harm we mean that we reject $H_0: \mu = 0$ in favor of the control arm. By futility we mean either that the probability of rejecting H_0 is low (see Section 10.6), or we can formally reject a particular alternative hypothesis of interest, H_1 (see Section 10.4.2), in favor of the null hypothesis. In the case of boundaries for harm, as indicated in Section 10.4.4, the probability of a sample path crossing both upper and lower boundaries is negligible so the upper and lower boundaries can be independently constructed.

In the case of futility, the boundaries have form similar to those of Figures 10.2 and 10.10. In this setting, the probability of a sample path crossing both boundaries may not be negligible and if the lower futility boundary is used to "buy back" type I error probability, allowing one to lower the upper boundary, then it is possible for the final critical value to be smaller than that for the fixed size test (e.g., nominal p-value > 0.05, even though the overall $\alpha = 0.05$). Additionally, if a DMC chooses to continue after the futility boundary is crossed, then the type I error will be inflated. Therefore, in order to ensure that the error rates are properly controlled, we recommend that the upper and lower boundaries be created independently.

10.8.5 Additional Comments

We close this chapter with two additional comments beginning with a comment regarding p-values. Historically, p-values have served two purposes: first as summary statistics upon which hypothesis tests are based—H_0 is rejected if p is smaller than a prespecified value—and second, as measures of strength of evidence. The latter use is primarily a result of historical practice rather than being based on foundational principles. In the fixed sample setting where there is a monotone relationship between p-values and other measures of evidence such as likelihood ratios, it is somewhat natural for p-values to play both roles. In the sequential setting, however, the p-value, either nominal (unadjusted) or adjusted, is affected by the monitoring procedure, i.e., the sampling distribution of the nominal p-value is no longer uniform under H_0, and consequently, the necessary correction, and therefore, the adjusted p-value, depends on the monitoring procedure. Since there is no theoretical justification for linking measures of evidence to the monitoring plan, the utility of the p-value as a measure of strength of evidence is diminished. Therefore, it may be desirable for an alternative summary of the strength of evidence to be introduced to serve as a measure of strength of evidence. It may be that the likelihood ratio (or equivalently the standardized Z-score) is the best choice, although it should be clear that it does not necessarily have its usual probabilistic interpretation.

Second, we emphasize once again that traditional interim monitoring is based on tests of hypotheses and monitoring procedures are constructed to ensure the validity of these tests. Thus, rejection of H_0 in favor of the experimental treatment implies that either the treatment is beneficial, or a type I error has been made, albeit with a low, controlled, probability. On the other hand, because, as noted previously, the monitoring procedure affects the sampling distributions of the observed summary statistics, formal inference beyond the hypothesis test—construction of p-values, point estimates, and confidence intervals—is difficult. Given that the monitoring procedure provides a valid test of the hypothesis, and in light of the first comment in the previous paragraph, in trials employing such procedures, p-values may be entirely unnecessary, and perhaps undesirable, in sequential trials. Furthermore, as noted in Chapter 2, direct interpretation of an estimate of treatment effect is problematic because it is not clear that the "true" value of the associated parameter has meaning beyond an individual trial. This estimate is based on a sample population that is not a random sample or a representative population. It is based on volunteers who met entry criteria and are treated under more rigorously controlled conditions than is likely in common practice. Thus, the estimate obtained, corrected or not, may not really reflect the population or circumstances in which the intervention may be used. From this point of view, one can argue that bias adjustment serves little purpose, especially since, as shown by Figure 10.11, the bias introduced by sequential monitoring is not likely to be large compared to the variability. This argument may apply equally to the construction of confidence intervals. While the coverage probability of the nominal confidence interval is not quite correct for the "true" parameter, it is not likely to be misleading. Thus, our position is that there is probably little to be gained from formal adjustments to point estimates and confidence intervals and that the unadjusted quantities are generally adequate. This recommendation may be controversial among those who insist on mathematical rigor; however, in light of the complexities of clinical trials, with the opportunity for bias to be introduced at multiple points throughout, it is not clear that such mathematical refinements serve a real purpose.

10.9 Problems

10.1 For each method of analysis, create an example for which deterministic curtailment could be used (if such an example exists). If deterministic curtailment is not possible for the given method, explain.

(a) Single-sample binomial test of $\pi = .5$.

(b) Two-sample binomial test of $\pi_1 = \pi_2$.

(c) Paired t-test of $\mu_1 = \mu_2$ on normal data.

(d) Two-sample t-test of $\mu_1 = \mu_2$ on normal data.

(e) Log-rank test on two groups of possibly censored survival times (no ties).

10.2 Suppose you are testing

$$H_0 \quad : \quad \mu_1 - \mu_2 = 0 \ \text{vs.}$$
$$H_1 \quad : \quad \mu_1 - \mu_2 \neq 0,$$

using two independent groups with normal outcomes and $\sigma = 1$. At the end of the study, which will have 500 patients in each group, you intend to use a standard two-sample, two-tailed test at level $\alpha = .05$. An interim analysis, at which you have only 200 patients in each group, shows a z-value (standardized test statistic) of 2.6 under H_0.

(a) Given the interim information, what is the probability of rejecting H_0 at the end of the trial, given H_0 is true?

(b) Given the interim information, what is the probability of rejecting H_0 at the end of the trial, given H_1 is true ($\mu_1 - \mu_2 = 2$)?

10.3 Take the group sequential boundary implemented by using the usual critical value (e.g., 1.96 for a two-sided test at $\alpha = 0.05$) at the trial's conclusion and a single conservative value (e.g., 3.00) for interim analyses. Suppose we use this method (with the boundary values given above in parentheses) for a trial comparing two proportions (i.e., a two-sample binomial test). There are to be a total of 100 subjects in each arm if the trial does not stop early.

(a) Suppose, at an interim analysis, 90 subjects have been observed in each group. In the experimental treatment group we have observed 25 failures, while in the control group we have observed 44. Calculate the z-statistic. Does its value indicate that the trial should be stopped?

(b) At the end of the trial 30 failures have been observed in the treatment group and 44 failures have been observed in the control group. What is the conclusion of the final test?

(c) What is interesting about this example?

(d) What are the advantages and disadvantages of this sequential method? Would you recommend its use?

CHAPTER 11

Selected Issues in the Analysis

The previous chapters discussed methods in the design and conduct of clinical trials that minimize bias in the comparison of the experimental and control treatments. It is also possible, however, to introduce bias into both hypothesis tests and estimates of treatment effects by flawed analysis of the data. This chapter addresses issues regarding the choice of analysis population, missing data, subgroup and interaction analyses, and approaches to the analysis of multiple outcomes. Methods specific to interim analyses or intended for use after early termination are discussed in Chapter 10 and will not be covered here. Since the underlying goal in most of this material is the minimization of bias in the analysis, we begin with a brief discussion of bias.

11.1 Bias in the Analysis of Clinical Trial Data

We begin by noting that there are two types of bias that are of interest—bias in hypothesis testing, and bias in estimation. A *hypothesis test* is considered to be *unbiased* if the type I error rate is controlled at (no greater than) level α under the null hypothesis and the probability of rejection is greater than α for all alternatives hypotheses. If a hypothesis test is unbiased and we reject H_0 we can be confident that the observed difference is due to either chance (with a low, controlled probability) or an actual treatment effect either across the entire population, or within a subpopulation. Additional analyses may sometimes be used to refine our understanding of the consistency of the treatment effect, although trials are rarely powered to be able to make definitive statements beyond the primary hypothesis. If a test is biased, rejection of H_0 may be due to systematic errors that may be unrelated to a direct effect of treatment on the outcome of interest.

An *estimator* of treatment effect or other parameter is unbiased if its expected value under its sampling distribution is equal to the true value of parameter. Bias in estimation is more difficult to assess or even define. First, the "true effect of treatment" may not itself be well defined because the population in a study may differ from the population in whom the treatment will be used and conditions in the trial may not be representative of conditions under which the treatment may be used. Second, the definition of the outcome of interest in a particular trial may not correspond precisely to definitions used in other settings. Third, the response by a particular subject to a particular treatment may depend on unobservable subject characteristics. Thus it is not clear that the population average effect represents the effect in any particular subject. Finally, there may be subjects who are unable to tolerate or otherwise undergo their assigned treatment, and therefore for these subjects the effect of treatment cannot be defined.

If we can assume that the "true effect of treatment" is well defined, there are still multiple potential sources of bias in its estimation. One source of bias discussed in this chapter is the non-adherence[1] of subjects to their assigned treatment. If the response to a drug is dose dependent and some proportion of subjects in a trial fail to receive the entire dose of the treatment to which they have been assigned, we might expect that the observed benefit will be less than what would be observed had all subjects taken the full dose. In any case, subjects who fail to receive *any* of their assigned treatment cannot receive the benefit of the treatment and this will certainly attenuate the observed treatment difference. Another source of bias, discussed in Chapter 10, is a sequential monitoring procedure that allows a trial to be terminated prior to its planned conclusion because of compelling evidence of benefit. These two sources of bias tend to operate in opposing directions and it may not be possible to know the true extent or even the direction of the overall bias.

11.2 Choice of Analysis Population

If all randomized subjects in a clinical trial meet all of the inclusion criteria and none of the exclusion criteria, remain on their assigned treatment, and are otherwise fully compliant with all study procedures for the duration of the study with no missing data, then the choice of the analysis population at the conclusion of the study as well as their duration of follow-up is obvious. This is rarely, if ever, the case.

The collection of subjects included in a specified analysis, as well as the period of time during which subjects are observed, is referred to as an *analysis set*. Different analysis sets may be defined for different purposes. There is wide agreement that the the most appropriate analysis set for the primary efficacy analyses of any confirmatory (phase III) clinical trial is the *intent-to-treat* population.[2] A commonly used alternative is referred to as the "per protocol" or "evaluable" population, defined as the subset of the subjects who comply sufficiently with the protocol. Outcomes observed after treatment discontinuation may also be excluded from the analysis of this population. As we will see, use of the "per protocol" population can introduce bias of unknown magnitude and direction and is strongly discouraged.

---

[1] As we note in Section 4.3, we use the term *non-adherence* to refer to the degree to which the assigned treatment regimen is followed, rather than *non-compliance* which can refer, more generally, to any deviation from the study protocol.

[2] http://www.fda.gov/cber/gdlns/ichclinical.txt

11.2.1 The Intent-To-Treat Principle

The *Intent-to-Treat* (ITT) principle may be the most fundamental principle underlying the analysis of data from randomized controlled trials. The ITT principle has two elements: all randomized subjects must be included in the analysis according to their assigned treatment groups regardless of their adherence to their assigned treatment, and all outcomes must be ascertained and included regardless of their purported relationship to treatment. The latter element requires that follow-up continue for subjects even if they have discontinued their assigned treatment.

ITT is foundational to the experimental nature of randomized controlled trials. The distinction between RCTs and observational studies is that the randomization ensures that there are no factors other than chance confounding the relationship between treatment and outcome—any differences in outcomes between treatment groups after randomization must be due to either chance or the effect of treatment. Therefore, properly applied, the ITT principle provides unbiased hypothesis tests (see Lachin (2000) for examples). This is in marked contrast to observational studies which are subject to confounding by factors related to the exposure of interest and the outcome (examples of which were provided in Chapter 1).

Confounding similar to that found in observational studies may be introduced in common alternatives to an ITT analysis, for example when subjects or outcomes are excluded from the analysis because of nonadherence to the assigned treatment (discussed in Section 11.2.2) or because of ineligibility (discussed in Section 11.2.3). When adherence is related to both the exposure of interest (assigned treatment) and the outcome, the exclusion of subjects or outcomes from the analysis based on nonadherence will result in confounding and a biased test of the effect of treatment on outcome. This can easily occur, for example, when subjects are more likely to discontinue from one treatment arm because of progression of their disease, which also puts them at higher risk for the outcome of interest. In general, any comparison of treatment groups within a subgroup defined according to observations made after randomization violates the ITT principle and is potentially biased (see also Section 11.4.2). There are circumstances under which such analyses may be useful, for example to help answer questions related to the mechansim of action of the treatment, but the primary assessment of treatment effect should be the ITT analysis.

Objections to ITT

The primary objection to the use of ITT is that subjects who discontinue their study treatment can no longer receive the benefit from the treatment, or that adverse experiences occurring after treatment discontinuation cannot be attributed to the treatment, and, therefore, including these subjects or events inappropriately biases the analysis against the treatment. There is merit to this objection to the extent that the effect of treatment discontinuation is to attenuate the mean difference between treatment groups. In the presence of non-adherence, the ITT estimate of the treatment difference is likely to be smaller than if full adherence were strictly enforced (assuming that full adherence is possible).

We provide three rebuttals to this objection. First, the goal of ITT is to produce unbiased hypothesis tests, and not necessarily unbiased estimates of the treatment effect. Common alternatives to ITT are subject to confounding and result in biased hypothesis tests. Therefore, the overall conclusion regarding whether the treatment is effective can be incorrect.

Second, one can argue that an ITT analysis assesses the overall clinical effectiveness most relevant to the real life use of the therapy. Once a treatment is approved and in general use, it is likely that adherence to the treatment will be no better, and is probably worse, than that in an RCT. Thus, the treatment difference estimated using ITT better reflects the effect that would be expected in actual use than the effect estimated under full adherence. The former has been referred, most commonly in the contraceptive literature, to as *use effectiveness* and the latter *method effectiveness* (Meier 1991). For example, oral contraceptives have been shown to have extremely high method effectiveness, i.e., when used strictly as prescribed. Their use effectiveness is often much lower in certain populations because of poor adherence. Alternative methods with lower method effectiveness may actually more reliably prevent pregnancy if there is greater use effectiveness. Other authors (Schwartz and Lellouch 1967) distinguish between *pragmatic* and *explanatory* trials. Explanatory trials are intended to assess the underlying effect of a therapy, carried out under "optimal" conditions, whereas pragmatic trials are intended to assess the effectiveness to be expected in normal medical practice. Application of ITT corresponds to the pragmatic approach.

Third, just as naive analyses that exclude subjects or events as a function of subject adherence to assigned treatment produce biased hypothesis tests, they also produce biased estimates of treatment benefit. Therefore, such analyses cannot overcome this fundamental objection to the ITT analysis but can only introduce a different kind of bias.

A second objection to ITT, raised by Rubin (1998), is that when there is significant nonadherence, the ITT analysis can lack power and that power can be increased by making use of information regarding adherence. This argument also has merit, although it is not clear that the potential meaningful increases in power can be achieved except in extreme cases or without strong, untestable assumptions. It is likely that cases with sufficiently extreme nonadherence would lack credibility in the scientific community, regardless of the analysis approach.

A third objection to ITT is often raised in the setting of non-inferiority or equivalence trials (see Section 3.3). Because the effect of nonadherence is often to dilute the observed (ITT) treatment difference and thus make treatments look more similar, when the goal is to establish that the experimental treatment is similar to the control, nonadherence may work to the advantage of the experimental treatment. In the extreme case, if no subjects in either group comply with their assigned treatment, there will be no difference between groups and non-inferiority will be established. This leads to the notion that "sloppy" trial conduct, in which little attempt is made to ensure adherence, especially to the control therapy, may be beneficial to the sponsor by making it easier to establish non-inferiority. Again, there is merit to the argument that in this setting the ITT analysis is deficient. The primary difficulty, however, lies less with the analysis than with the design and conduct of the trial. As noted, naive analyses based on, for example, the "per protocol" population do not correctly address the confounding introduced by non-adherence, and simply introduce additional biases of unknown magnitude and direction. There is currently no practical alternative to ITT so it is imperative that all efforts be made to ensure that the protocol is followed as closely as possible.

Additionally, the notion that in non-inferiority/equivalence trials the effect of nonadherence is to attenuate differences between treatment groups is incorrect. A key difference between placebo-controlled trials and non-inferiority trials (and active-controlled trial generally) is that the active control is presumed to be effective and this fact alters the impact of non-adherence. We illustrate with a simplified example. Suppose that treatment A is the experimental treatment and treatment B is the active control. Assume that if untreated, all subjects have (mean) response $y = 0$ and that if given treatment A, the mean response is $y = \mu$ and if given treatment B, the mean response is $y = \mu + \Delta$. Suppose further that nonadherence to assigned treatment is independent of response,[3] and that in group A, a fraction, q_A, of subjects adhere to treatment A, and in group B, a fraction, q_B, adhere to treatment B. Nonadherers receive no treatment. The treatment difference (B-A) from the ITT analysis shows the mean difference to be $q_B(\mu + \Delta) - q_A\mu = q_B\Delta + (q_B - q_A)\mu$. If A is ineffective, $\mu = 0$ and dilution of the true difference Δ does in fact occur. On the other hand, if, for example, A and B are equally effective ($\Delta = 0$) then the ITT difference will depend on the relative adherence between the two groups, and could be either positive or negative. In practice, the situation is likely to be far more complex, making an analytic approach extremely difficult if not impossible.

Implementation of ITT

Strict adherence to the ITT principle has been formally espoused by regulatory authorities at the Food and Drug Administration (FDA), yet remains incompletely applied in practice. On the one hand, the concept remains difficult for many clinicians to understand and accept. It is also possible that an inferior therapy could appear effective if it leads to rapid withdrawal and subsequent treatment with a better therapy. Supplemental analyses of adher-

---

[3] This assumption is almost certainly false. In trials where it can be assessed, poor adherers typically also have poorer outcomes. See, for example, the CDP example on page 344.

ence to treatment and use of concomitant therapies are necessary to ensure the validity and acceptance of the conclusions.

Of course, every subject is free to withdraw their consent to participate in a clinical trial at any time, making subsequent follow-up difficult or even impossible. Consideration should be given to including in the consent form a provision allowing subjects who withdraw consent for study procedures to nevertheless agree to having limited outcome information collected about them.

In double-blind studies, a variation of ITT, sometimes referred to as *modified ITT*, is commonly used. *Modified ITT* excludes subjects who are randomized but fail to receive study drug. The rationale for modified ITT is that, in a double-blind trial, neither the subject nor the investigator know the treatment assignment, and since no drug is taken, there is no opportunity for the subject to experience side-effects of the treatment. Therefore, exclusion of the subject cannot be related to treatment assignment so no confounding is possible. If in fact the blind is secure, then modified ITT should be considered a valid alternative to strict ITT. If modified ITT is used, some rudimentary examination of the data is recommended, for example, ensuring that the number of exclusions is comparable across treatments. An imbalance is evidence that the blind may not be secure.

11.2.2 Nonadherence to Assigned Treatment

Probably the most common reason given for eliminating randomized subjects or their events from the analysis is that the subject did not fully adhere to the study treatment or permanently discontinued the treatment prior to the onset of the event. Indeed, as noted by Meier (1991), the failure of many subjects to take medication in the quantities or on the schedule recommended is one of the most intractable problems in the conduct and interpretation of clinical trials. There are many reasons for nonadherence, including forgetful behavior or other subject characteristics, an adverse experience, a treatment that is unpleasant, or progression of the disease. Few, if any of these, can be assumed to be independent of the treatment or outcome of interest. When nonadherent subjects or events are excluded from the analysis, hypothesis tests are susceptible to bias, even when the number of excluded individuals is comparable between treatment groups.

We begin with some examples.

Examples

The Coronary Drug Project (CDP) (The Coronary Drug Project Research Group 1980) was a randomized placebo-controlled trial conducted to evaluate several cholesterol lowering drugs, including a drug called *clofibrate*, in the long-term treatment of coronary heart disease. Overall, the five-year mortality in 1103 men treated with clofibrate was 20.0% and nearly identical to that of 2789 men given placebo (20.9%), p=0.55 (Table 11.1). Among subjects randomized to clofibrate, the better adherers, defined as those who took

Table 11.1 *5-year mortality in the Coronary Drug Project according to adherence.*

	Clofibrate		Placebo	
	N	% Mortality	N	% Mortality
All Randomized	1103	20.0	2789	20.9
< 80% Adherent	357	24.6	882	28.2
≥ 80% Adherent	708	15.0	1813	15.1

80% or more of the protocol prescription during the five-year period, had a substantially lower five-year mortality than did poor adherers (15.0 vs. 24.6%, $p=0.0001$). One might be tempted to take this as evidence that clofibrate is effective. On the other hand, the mortality difference between adherers and non-adherers is even greater among those subjects assigned to placebo, 15.1% and 28.2%, respectively. Because this latter difference cannot be due to the pharmacologic effect of the placebo, it is most likely due to differences in subject characteristics, such as disease severity, between good and poor adherers.

A second example is from the VA Cooperative Study of Coronary Artery Bypass Surgery.[4] Conducted between 1972 and 1990, this randomized clinical trial was designed to compare the survival time of subjects assigned optimal medical therapy to those assigned coronary artery bypass surgery. A total of 686 subjects were enrolled between 1972 and 1974—354 were assigned to medical therapy and 332 were assigned to surgical therapy. The Kaplan-Meier plots of survival by assigned treatment (ITT analysis), shown in Figure 11.1 (from Peduzzi et al. (1991)), suggest that there is no difference by assigned treatment ($p=$ 0.99). Of those assigned medical therapy, however, 147 eventually received coronary artery bypass surgery during the 14 year follow-up period (after a mean waiting time of 4.8 years), while of those assigned surgery, only 20 refused surgery. Given the high crossover rate from the medical group to the surgical group, there was concern that the ITT analysis did not reflect the true benefit of coronary artery bypass surgery and alternative analyses were sought.

Peduzzi et al. (1991, 1993) considered several alternatives to ITT and we comment on two of them here. The first alternative is a "Treatment Received" analysis. In this analysis subjects are reassigned to treatment groups according to the treatment eventually received—subjects who underwent bypass surgery anytime prior to the end of the study are considered in the surgery group and subjects who never underwent bypass surgery during the study are considered medical subjects—regardless of their assigned treatment groups. The second alternative is an "Adherers Only" analysis. This analysis considers subjects according to their assigned treatment group, but excludes any subjects who

---

[4] The Veterans Administration Coronary Artery Bypass Surgery Cooperative Study Group (1984)

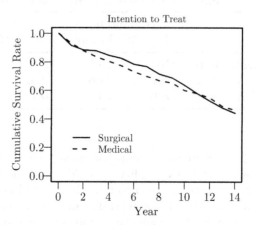

Figure 11.1 *Cumulative survival rates for intention to treat analysis in the VA Cooperative Study of Coronary Artery Bypass Surgery. (Adapted from (Peduzzi et al. 1991)).*

crossed over. The results of these alternative analyses are qualitatively quite similar (Figure 11.2), and both differ substantially from the ITT analysis. These results seem to suggest that, in contrast to the ITT analysis, there is a substantial survival benefit among surgery subjects relative to medical subjects.

Given the apparent contradiction between these two analyses, which should we believe? The first consideration is that the effect of nonadherence is to dilute the effect of treatment so that the observed treatment difference is smaller on average than the true difference. Unless nonadherence is extremely large, however, a proportion of the true treatment effect should remain. In this example, were the "Treatment Received" apparent treatment effect real, we would expect that the residual effect in the ITT analysis would be much larger than what we have seen. Second, subjects crossing over to surgery do not do so immediately. In fact, only about 10% of medical subjects have crossed over by two years. This would suggest that for the ITT analysis, the early portion of the Kaplan-Meier curves, before a meaningful number of medical subjects have crossed over, would be largely free of the influence of crossovers. During this period, however, the Kaplan-Meier curves by assigned treatment are virtually indistinguishable. Conversely, the corresponding curves for the "Treatment Received" analysis diverge immediately. Peduzzi et al. (1993) also conduct an analysis (not shown here) in which subjects begin in their assigned groups, but medical subjects are switched into the surgery group at the time

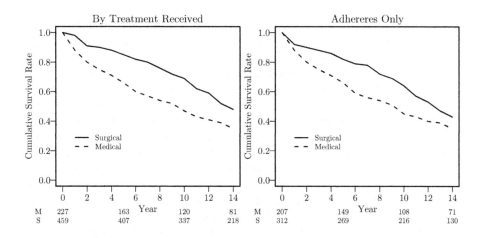

Figure 11.2 *Cumulative survival rates for "Treatment Received" and "Adherers Only" analyses in the VA Cooperative Study of Coronary Artery Bypass Surgery. (Adapted from (Peduzzi et al. 1991)).*

of surgery. This analysis yields results virtually identical to the ITT analysis in Figure 11.1.

Finally, there is a simple model that easily explains most of what we have observed in the VA study. The underlying idea is simple—in order for a medical subject to receive surgery, they must survive long enough to become a candidate for the procedure. Specifically, the crossover time must be before both the death time and the end of follow-up. The model we construct is similar to one constructed in Peduzzi et al. (1993). Under the null hypothesis and using the ITT analysis, the combined 14 year cumulative survival is approximately 45%, so the hazard rate is approximately $\lambda_M = -\log(.45)/14 = 0.057$. Similarly, the cumulative 14 year rate of crossover for medical subjects is approximately 55% ("censoring" subjects at death, assuming independence between death and crossover), so the hazard function for crossover is also approximately $\lambda_C = -\log(1-.55)/14 = .057$. We simulate death times with the common hazard rate of λ_M, and independent crossover times for the medical group with hazard rate λ_C. A medical subject is considered a crossover if the crossover time precedes the death time and is before 14 years. For this simulated data, the Kaplan-Meier curves for the ITT analysis correctly show no difference between groups. The "Treatment Received" and "Adherers Only" analyses for the simulated data, in which the null hypothesis is true, yield Kaplan-Meier curves similar to those shown in Figure 11.2. Thus, the naive alternatives to ITT presented in this example almost certainly yield biased and misleading results. The ITT analysis is the only credible analysis among those considered.

11.2.3 Ineligibility

Another reason given for eliminating randomized subjects from the analysis
is that they are found to be ineligible after randomization (Gent and Sackett
1979; Fisher et al. 1990). In most cases, eligibility criteria can be verified
before the subject is randomized. In other cases, the validation of entry criteria
may take a few hours or days to verify. Consider, for example, a study of
a treatment for subjects experiencing an acute myocardial infarction (heart
attack or MI). The definition of an MI usually involves the assessment of
chest pain, levels of specific enzymes in the blood, and EKG measurements.
An accurate diagnosis may require several hours of observation and repeated
measurements. On the other hand, to be effective, it may be necessary to
start treatment as soon as possible following the MI. In other cases, errors in
judgment or in the recording of measurements may lead to the subject being
erroneously enrolled and treated. Thus, there may be some subjects who are
enrolled and treated, but later found not to have met the specific criteria for
inclusion. One possible effect of having technically ineligible subjects in the
trial, subjects for whom the treatment is not expected to be beneficial, is to
dilute the observed treatment effect and thereby reduce the power of the trial.
The temptation is to remove such subjects from the analysis.

Examples

A well known example involving subject eligibility is the Anturane Reinfarction Trial (ART).[5] This trial was a well-conducted, multi-center randomized
double-blind placebo controlled trial of a drug, *anturane*, whose effect is to
inhibit clotting of blood. The hypothesis was that this drug would reduce the
incidence of all-cause death, sudden death, and cardiovascular death in subjects with a recent myocardial infarction. The trial randomized and followed
1629 subjects but a re-evaluation of eligibility identified 71 subjects who did
not meet the entry criteria. The ineligible subjects were divided almost equally,
38 vs. 33, between the two treatment groups. The primary reasons for being
ineligible were that the heart attack did not occur within the window of time
specified in inclusion/exclusion criteria, that the blood enzymes levels specific
to heart muscle damage were not sufficiently elevated suggesting a very mild
heart attack, and that there were other competing medical conditions.

   The authors of the initial ART publication presented mortality data for only
the eligible subjects. The justification for excluding the ineligible subjects was
that the eligibility criteria were prespecified in the protocol and based on
data measured prior to randomization. Further review of the results by the
FDA revealed that the mortality results differed substantially depending on
whether the analysis included all randomized subjects or only those declared
to be eligible (Temple and Pledger 1980). Final data for the ART study are
shown in Table 11.2. The analysis of all randomized subjects with 74 deaths

---

[5] The Anturane Reinfarction Trial Research Group (1978, 1980)

Table 11.2 *Mortality in the Anturane Reinfarction Trial according to eligibility.*

	Anturane		Placebo		p-value
All Randomized	74/813	(9.1%)	89/816	(10.9%)	0.20
Eligible	64/775	(8.3%)	85/783	(10.9%)	0.07
Ineligible	10/38	(26.3%)	4/33	(12.1%)	0.12
Eligible vs. Ineligible	p=0.0001		p=0.98		

on anturane and 89 on placebo yielded a log-rank p-value of 0.20 which is far short of statistical significance. If only the "eligible" subjects are analyzed, however, a p-value of 0.07 is obtained. In the initial analysis of the ART data[6] that was based on a shorter follow-up period and fewer deaths, the analysis of "eligible" subjects was actually nominally significant at the 0.05 level. While the direction of the treatment difference did not change, the degree of certainty was substantially weakened when all randomized subjects were included.

Of special interest is the comparison of mortality between those eligible and those ineligible within each treatment arm. In the placebo arm, the difference in mortality is minimal. For the anturane arm, however, subjects deemed ineligible had substantially greater mortality (p=0.0001) than those who were eligible. One can only speculate that bias was introduced into the re-evaluation of eligibility of the 1629 randomized subjects. The difference in the two analyses generated considerable discussion and controversy (Kolata 1980) and provided a great deal of motivation to the FDA and the cardiovascular research community to endorse the ITT principle.

Inclusion of ineligible subjects in the analysis does not necessarily reduce study power. An illustration of this is provided by the Beta-blocker Heart Attack Trial (BHAT) whose results are shown in Table 11.3 (Beta-Blocker Heart Attack Trial Research Group 1982). BHAT, like ART, was a randomized

Table 11.3 *Mortality in the Beta-blocker Heart Attack Trial according to eligibility.*

	N	Mortality Propranolol	Placebo
All Randomized	3837	7.2%	9.8%
Eligible	3496	7.3%	9.6%
Ineligible	341	6.7%	11.3%

double-blind multicenter placebo-controlled trial in subjects who had experienced a recent myocardial infarction with mortality as the primary outcome.

[6] The Anturane Reinfarction Trial Research Group (1978)

The treatment being studied was the beta-blocker, propanolol. Examination of eligibility based on the EKG criteria was conducted to evaluate how well the local physicians diagnosed myocardial infarction compared to a centralized evaluation. Those subjects not meeting the centralized criteria were labeled for this exercise as being technically ineligible. As shown in Table 11.3, there was a mortality benefit in both ineligible and eligible subjects, but those considered ineligible had the largest observed benefit of treatment.

While the idea of eliminating from the analysis subjects not meeting the entry criteria has appeal superficially, the process can introduce bias and should be avoided. In a double-blind trial, if one is confident that the blind is secure, then elimination of ineligible subjects prior to the initiation of treatment may be justified on the basis that the assessment of ineligiblity cannot be related to treatment and therefore will not lead to bias. If this is to be done, however, it must be done before the unblinding of the trial results; otherwise, investigators may be able to select and report the more favorable of the results. To ensure the credibility of the result, the best analysis is always the one based on all randomized subjects. Furthermore, the best treatment strategy is to delay the randomization of subjects until immediately before the initiation of treatment whenever possible.

11.2.4 Model-based Alternatives to ITT

Several model-based alternatives to the strict ITT analysis have been proposed. One class of alternatives is part of a broader statistical approach known as *causal inference* and discussed in Chapter 2. Causal inference methods attempt to decompose observed differences into components that are due to the effect of treatment and other confounding factors. The general principle involves estimating the difference between the *potential outcomes* that a subject would experience if they could be given each treatment in turn. Specifically, in a trial with treatments A and B, there are two potential outcomes of interest, Y_A and Y_B. We are interested in the mean difference $\delta = E[Y_A - Y_B]$. If we could observe each subject on each treatment (as we might be able to do in crossover studies), this difference would be directly estimable. Unfortunately, we are in general able only to observe each subject on at most one of A or B. If we have full adherence with assigned treatment in a randomized trial, this difference is also directly estimable as the ITT difference between treatment groups. Unfortunately, when we do not have full adherence, the ITT difference may not represent the causal effect, δ, since adherence may be a confounding factor. While there are many proposed approaches to causal inference, we will briefly discuss two here.

Rubin (1998) promotes an estimand, known as the *Complier average causal effect* (CACE), that can be estimated using a technique known as *principal stratification* (Frangakis and Rubin 2002). The subject population is decomposed into strata defined by treatment adherence, and the treatment effect is estimated within those strata for which such estimates are sensible. Alternatively, Efron and Feldman (1991) attempt to identify subjects in the placebo group whose placebo response would be similar to particular subjects in the active group as a function of relative adherence with assigned treatment. The method of Efron and Feldman relies on a number of untestable assumptions and so may lack credibility. The principal stratification approach requires fewer assumptions and therefore is more likely to find acceptance. We take each of these approaches in turn.

Complier Average Causal Effect

While Rubin's principal stratification approach can be applied to more general situations, we illustrate it using the simple case of *all-or-nothing* adherence with only two available treatments—active and placebo. That is, subjects either receive complete treatment A or complete treatment B—partial adherence is not allowed. Rubin also makes the *exclusion assumption* that simply states that the subject response depends only on the treatment received and not the treatment assigned (the exclusion assumption implies that the placebo response is the same as the no-treatment response, precluding the possibility of a placebo effect).

Under these conditions Rubin defines four strata of subjects: *compliers*,[7] *never-takers*, *always-takers*, and *defiers*. *Compliers* are those subjects who always comply with their assigned treatment. *Never-takers* are subjects who will always receive placebo (or equivalently, no treatment) regardless of treatment assignment. *Always-takers* will always receive active treatment regardless of treatment assignment, and *defiers* will never receive the treatment that they are assigned. Note that for *never-takers* and *always-takers*, the causal effect of treatment, D, is not defined since it is not possible for these subjects to receive both treatments. Rubin makes the additional assumption that there are no *defiers*. Note that in many situations this is an unverifiable assumption and is based on expectations regarding human nature. For simplicity, we will also assume that there are no *always-takers*. When active treatments are unavailable except to subjects explicitly assigned them in the trial, both of these conditions are automatic.

Under these assumptions, among subjects assigned active treatment, we can identify the *compliers* (those who received active treatment) and *never-takers* (those who did not receive active treatment). Among those assigned placebo, we cannot distinguish *compliers* from *never-takers* since this distinction can only be determined by observing adherence to active treatment. (Failure to comply with assigned placebo does not imply failure to comply with active treatment and vice versa.) We can, however, rely on the exclusion assumption to infer that the mean observed response in the placebo group is an unbiased estimate of $E[Y_B]$. By contrast, the mean observed response in the active group is a linear combination of placebo responses and active treatment responses.

---

[7] For consistency with Rubin's terminology, here we will use the term *complier* to refer to subjects who adhere to assigned treatment.

We let μ_{CT} and μ_{NT} denote the mean responses for *compliers* and *never-takers* respectively after receiving treatment T, noting that μ_{NA} is not defined. Then, if the observed proportion of subjects who are *compliers* is q, we have

$$
\begin{aligned}
E[\bar{Y}_B] &= q\mu_{CB} + (1-q)\mu_{NB} \\
E[\bar{Y}_A] &= q\mu_{CA} + (1-q)\mu_{NB}
\end{aligned}
$$

where $\bar{Y}_A$ and $\bar{Y}_B$ are the observed means among subjects assigned A and B respectively. By replacing $E[\bar{Y}_T]$ with the observed $\bar{Y}_T$, an unbiased estimate of $D_C = \mu_{CA} - \mu_{CB}$ is

$$
D_C = \frac{Y_A - Y_B}{q}. \tag{11.1}
$$

The quantity D_C is known as the *complier average causal effect* (CACE). The estimate of the CACE in equation (11.1) is a simple moment estimator. Other more sophisticated estimators are available if one makes distributional assumptions regarding the three unknown distributions (Heitjan 1999; Rubin 1998).

It is important to note that the CACE estimate in (11.1) cannot "rescue" a negative result. That is, since the estimate of the CACE is simply a rescaling of the ITT treatment difference, a test of $H_0 : D_C = 0$ using the estimate in (11.1) is nearly equivalent to the ITT test of $H_0 : D = 0$. Since q in equation (11.1) is estimated from the data, the test of $H_0 : D_C = 0$ would be slightly *less* powerful when the variability in this estimate is accounted for. Heitjan (1999) and Rubin (1998) illustrate how more powerful tests can be constructed, although either extreme non-adherence or strong distributional assumptions are required in order to achieve meaningful improvement.

Efron and Feldman Causal Model

The approach of Efron and Feldman (1991) is similar to the Rubin approach in that it views adherence, z, as a subject characteristic independent of assigned treatment. There are a number of subtleties in their approach that are beyond the scope of this book so we will limit our discussion to a few key issues. The model proposed by Efron and Feldman is intended for situations in which a continuous response is a function of the total dose received and adherence is measured by the proportion of the assigned dose actually received. The goal of the analysis is to estimate the dose response, $\delta(x) = E[Y(x) - Y(0)]$ where x is a hypothetical dose given to a subject and $Y(x)$ is the *potential outcome* for a subject given dose x. For simplicity, we consider x to be the fraction of the maximum possible dose and thus $x \in [0, 1]$. $Y(0)$ is the *placebo response* under the exclusion assumption given previously ($x = 0$ and placebo are assumed to produce identical responses). The available data for each subject are the assigned treatment group, τ, the dose (either active drug or placebo) actually received, z_τ, and the outcome of interest, Y. Since we are considering adherence, z, to be a subject characteristic independent of assigned treatment, we let $z = z_T$, the level of adherence were the subject to be assigned active treatment. For subjects in the experimental arm we observe z directly as z_T. For subjects assigned placebo, we observe z_C, the level of adherence to placebo.

The first key assumption made by Efron and Feldman is that for a given subject, z_T and z_C are related by a monotone increasing function, $z_T = m(z_C)$. The randomization then implies that $F_C(z_C) = F_T(z_T)$ where $F_C(\cdot)$ and $F_T(\cdot)$ are the CDFs for z_C and z_T, and therefore $m(z_C) = F_T^{-1}F_C(z_C)$. The transformation $m(\cdot)$ allows us to impute z for placebo subjects. This assumption may be reasonable if the side-effects of treatment are uniform over subjects and adherence within each treatment group is a function of subject baseline risk only. On the other hand, if side-effects vary widely across subjects, then tolerability of active treatment, and hence adherence, to active treatment may be quite unrelated to adherence to placebo. This assumption must be viewed cautiously in the light of known reasons for non-adherence.

The second key assumption is that the level of adherence is solely a function of the placebo response. If there is evidence (from the placebo group) that there is also association between adherence and baseline covariates, it is possible to incorporate this information into the model, but for simplicity we will not consider this possibility. Together these assumptions allow us to infer the placebo response for subjects in the active treatment arm as a function of their level of adherence, and therefore estimate the treatment difference as a function of adherence z.

Specifically, suppose we model the response as a function of adherence separately for each treatment group: $T(z) = E[Y(z)|z]$, and $C(z) = E[Y(0)|z]$. $T(\cdot)$ and $C(\cdot)$ can be directly estimated using standard regression methods, and can have any functional form. The quantity $D(z) = T(z) - C(z)$ is referred to by Efron and Feldman as the *observed difference* and is the mean treatment difference among subjects with adherence level z who receive dose z. Note that in the setting of Section 11.2.4, $z \in \{0, 1\}$ so $D(1)$ coincides precisely with CACE—the treatment difference among adherers. Interestingly, under the assumptions of Section 11.2.4, the Efron and Feldman estimand, $\delta(x)$, is *not* defined since $Y(1)$ is undefined for *never-takers*. On the other hand, under these assumptions $D(1)$ is directly estimable using equation (11.1), so the two key assumptions of Efron and Feldman are not required.

Note further that because the adherence level z is not randomly assigned, $D(x)$ is *not* the mean response were an arbitrary subject to receive dose x unless the dose response is independent of the placebo response. Hence, Efron and Feldman introduce a correction term, parameterized as $H(z)[Y(0) - EY(0)] = D(z) - \delta(z)$ where $H(z)$ is a function with $H(0) = 0$. The two key assumptions above do not provide a basis for estimating $H(\cdot)$ and Efron and Feldman resort to providing bounds for $H(\cdot)$ that are based on additional assumptions and the degree of variance inflation induced by non-adherence. (See Efron and Feldman (1991) for details of the procedure.)

The most serious difficulty with the EF approach is that it requires that one infer a mean response, $EY(x)$, for subjects whose observed dose, z, is different from x and, hence, has never been observed. To make this precise, suppose we let $\delta_z(x) = E[Y(x) - Y(0)|z]$. $\delta_z(x)$ is the mean response to exposure to dose x in subjects whose adherence level is z. The population average dose response is the average of these over the population, $\delta(x) = E\delta_z(x)$ (the expectation is taken with respect to the distribution of z). Note that the $D(z) = \delta_z(z)$ so that using the two key assumptions we can estimate $\delta_z(z)$. On the other hand, there is an infinite family of $\delta_z(x)$, all of which yield the identical values of $\delta_z(z)$. For example, suppose that $D(z) = az$ for some constant a and that $\delta_z(x) = az^{1-\rho}x^\rho$ for some $\rho > 0$. For each member of this family we have $\delta_z(z) = az$. Nevertheless, $\delta(x) = aE[z^{1-\rho}]x^\rho$, so the shape of the underlying population average dose response varies dramatically as a function of ρ. If we assume further that the distribution of the errors, $Y(x) - \delta(x)$, does not depend on ρ, then it is not possible to estimate ρ from the observed data, and hence, the dose response $\delta(x)$ is not estimable without strong additional, and untestable, assumptions. Specifically, this implies that $H(z)$ is not estimable. Thus, regardless of the estimation procedure, the estimated dose response, $\hat{\delta}(x)$, from this model must be interpreted carefully.

To further assess the robustness of the model to deviations from model assumptions, Albert and DeMets (1994) conducted a study in which they fit the Efron and Feldman model to simulated data in which the key assumptions are violated to varying degrees. They find that the estimation bias can be substantial as the violations become more extreme. Since the underlying structure is unidentifiable, it is impossible to assess the validity of the assumptions in practice.

We have seen that in general, unless one is extremely careful, analyses that deviate from the intent-to-treat principle are fraught with potential biases. Given that most alternatives rely on untestable assumptions or have difficulties in interpretation, the ITT analysis is the cleanest, most acceptable analysis in most situations, especially as the primary analysis and is consistent with the principle of randomization. Alternative analysis may be performed, but their role should be limited to supplementary analysis that support or provide additional insight into the primary results. Since the effect of non-adherence is primarily to dilute the observed treatment difference, thereby reducing study power and undermining the credibility of the results, all attempts must be made during the conduct of the trial to maximize subject adherence.

11.3 Missing Data

Despite our best efforts, data are often missing for one or more of the outcome variables. This may be because a subject did not return for a scheduled follow-up visit, or that the subject was unable or unwilling to complete the outcome assessment. Data may also be missing because a clinical site simply failed to perform the required test or that the equipment necessary to make the measurement was not available or not functioning properly. Whatever the reason, missing data are problematic because of the potential for bias to be introduced either by the exclusion of subjects with missing data, or by incorrect assumptions required for application of statistical methods that account for missing data. For our purposes, we consider data to be *missing* if the value that the observation takes is well defined, but is not observable for reasons such as those suggested above. If an observation is missing because the subject has died, or is otherwise nonsensical, such as the six minute walk distance for a subject who is either a paraplegic or an amputee, we do not consider this to be missing for the purpose of the discussion that follows. This kind of "missingness" is more appropriately viewed in the setting of *competing risks* and will be discussed in Section 11.3.5.

11.3.1 Terminology

Little and Rubin (2002) proposed terminology that is now commonly used for classification of missing data according to the missingness mechanism. Missing data are classified as:

1. *Missing Completely at Random* (MCAR) if the probability that an observation, Y, is missing does not depend on values of the missing or non-missing observations,

2. *Missing at Random* (MAR) if the probability that Y is missing depends on non-missing observations but *not* on the values of the missing observations,

3. *Missing Not at Random* (MNAR) if the probability that Y is missing depends on the value of Y.

For data that are MCAR or MAR, unbiased analyses can be performed—the effect of missing data will be solely to decrease power. For data that are MNAR, unless the missing data mechanism is correctly modeled, unbiased analyses cannot, in general, be performed. When the missing data are MCAR or MAR, we also say that the missing-data mechanism is *ignorable*.

Unfortunately, as with nonadherence, the missing data mechanism is not identifiable from observed data—that is, there are many potential missing data models that produce observed data with a given distribution, so there is no information in the data from which the missing data mechanism can be ascertained ("you don't know what you don't know"). At best, one or more analysis can be performed using different assumptions regarding the missingness mechanism. Regrettably, often the only analysis performed is one that assumes that the missingness is ignorable and without assessment of the sensitivity of the conclusion to deviations from this assumption. By considering a range of potential associations between missingness and response, one can assess the degree to which the conclusion can be influenced by the missingness mechanism. This approach is generally referred to as *sensitivity analysis*. If the conclusion is largely unchanged for plausible alternatives to MAR, the result may be considered robust. Otherwise, the conclusion should be interpreted cautiously and may be misleading. In the following section, we illustrate the use of sensitivity analyses with a simple example.

11.3.2 Sensitivity Analysis

Suppose that we have randomized N subjects to two treatment groups, a control group ($j = 1$) and an experimental group ($j = 2$), with n_j subjects in group j. Let p_j be the true probability of failure, say death, in group j, and y_j be the observed number of deaths in group j. We wish to compare the incidence of failure between the two groups. Suppose that we have vital status for m_j subjects in each group, so that we are missing vital status for $n_j - m_j$ from each group.

A simple, hypothetical example is provided in Table 11.4. In this case, the trial has 170 events observed in the treatment arm and 220 events in the control arm, a trend that favors treatment. There are also 30 subjects with missing data on the treatment arm and 10 on the control arm.

Table 11.4 *Hypothetical trial with missing outcomes.*

Treatment	Dead	Alive	Missing	Total
Control	220	270	10	500
Experimental	170	300	30	500

The naive analysis, assuming that missing vital status is ignorable, might use the Pearson chi-square test for the 2×2 table and only consider the subjects with non-missing outcomes. Two additional naive analyses are *best-case* and *worst-case* analyses. For the best-case analysis we perform a Pearson chi-square test for the 2×2 table obtained by assuming that all missing subjects in the control group are dead, and that all the missing subjects in the experimental group are alive. The worst-case analysis is performed by making the opposite assumption. If the results are consistent for the three analyses, the result is clear. Unless the extent of the missing data is small or the observed difference is extremely large, it is unlikely that the results will be consistent.

If we consider only the observed cases, we have that $Z = -2.75$ ($p=0.0059$). The "best-case" is the one in which none of the 30 missing subjects on treatment died whereas all of the 10 control subjects died, so $Z = -3.87$. In the "worst-case" all of the 30 missing treatment arm subjects died and none of the 10 controls died and $Z = -1.28$. In the "worst-case", the result would no longer reach statistical significance. On the other hand, the "worst-case" is probably not plausible, if only because it is unlikely that the missing data mechanism could differ so dramatically between the two treatment groups.

A more useful assessment examines robustness for a set of plausible deviations from ignorability. To do this, we first propose a model for missingness as a function of the unobserved outcome (vital status). In this simple example, let π_{jy} be the probability that a subject in group j and outcome $y = 0, 1$ is missing. Given the simplicity of the data, this is the most general missingness model that we can propose. The observed data will depend on three probabilities for each treatment group:

$$
\begin{aligned}
\Pr\{\text{Observed to die}|\text{group} = j\} &= p_j(1 - \pi_{j1}) \\
\Pr\{\text{Observed to survive}|\text{group} = j\} &= (1 - p_j)(1 - \pi_{j0}) \\
\Pr\{\text{missing}|\text{group} = j\} &= p_j\pi_{j1} + (1 - p_j)\pi_{j0}
\end{aligned}
$$

Now, we re-parameterize the model as a logistic model, so let

$$
\log \frac{p_j}{1 - p_j} = \alpha + \beta z_j
$$

where $z_1 = 0$ and $z_2 = 1$. Similarly, let $\pi_{j1} = e^{\gamma_j}\pi_{j0}$. The likelihood for the observed data becomes

$$
\begin{aligned}
L(\alpha, \beta) &= \prod_{j=1}^{2} \left(\frac{\exp(\alpha + \beta z_j)}{1 + \exp(\alpha + \beta z_j)}(1 - e^{\gamma_j}\pi_{j0}) \right)^{y_j} \times \\
&\quad \left(\frac{1}{1 + \exp(\alpha + \beta z_j)}(1 - \pi_{j0}) \right)^{m_j - y_j} \times \\
&\quad \left(\frac{\exp(\alpha + \beta z_j)}{1 + \exp(\alpha + \beta z_j)}e^{\gamma_j}\pi_{j0} + \frac{1}{1 + \exp(\alpha + \beta z_j)}\pi_{j0} \right)^{n_j - m_j} \\
&= \prod_{j=1}^{2} e^{(\alpha + \beta z_j)y_j} \left(1 + e^{\alpha + \beta z_j}\right)^{n_j} \left(1 + e^{\alpha + \beta z_j + \gamma_j}\right)^{n_j - m_j} H(\gamma_j, \pi_{j0})
\end{aligned}
$$

where $H(\cdot, \cdot)$ is a function of the (assumed) known parameters γ_j and π_{j0}.

The log-likelihood is

$$
\begin{aligned}
\log L(\alpha, \beta) &= \sum_{j=1}^{2} (\alpha + \beta z_j)y_j - n_j \log\left(1 + e^{\alpha + \beta z_j}\right) + \\
&\quad (n_j - m_j) \log\left(1 + e^{\alpha + \beta z_j + \gamma_j}\right) + \log H(\gamma_j, \pi_{j0}).
\end{aligned}
$$

The components of the vector-valued score function are

$$
\begin{aligned}
U_\alpha(\alpha, \beta) &= \frac{\partial \log L(\alpha, \beta)}{\partial \alpha} \\
&= \sum_{j=1}^{2} y_j - n_j \frac{e^{\alpha + \beta z_j}}{1 + e^{\alpha + \beta z_j}} + (n_j - m_j)\frac{e^{\alpha + \beta z_j + \gamma_j}}{1 + e^{\alpha + \beta z_j + \gamma_j}} \quad (11.2)
\end{aligned}
$$

and

$$
\begin{aligned}
U_\beta(\alpha, \beta) &= \frac{\partial \log L(\alpha, \beta)}{\partial \beta} \\
&= y_2 - n_2 \frac{e^{\alpha + \beta}}{1 + e^{\alpha + \beta}} + (n_2 - m_2)\frac{e^{\alpha + \beta + \gamma_2}}{1 + e^{\alpha + \beta + \gamma_2}}. \quad (11.3)
\end{aligned}
$$

We note several things.

- The score function, and hence inference regarding α and β, depends on the missingness mechanism only through γ_1 and γ_2.

- The first two terms of each of these equations represent the observed minus expected number of deaths if we had complete ascertainment of vital status. The third term adjusts this difference for the number of unobserved deaths that are expected given the proposed missingness model and the parameters α and β.

- If $\gamma_1 = \gamma_2 = 0$, the score function reduces to the score function for just the nonmissing data, and, hence, the missingness is ignorable. In the case $\gamma_j \to +\infty$, all missing subjects for treatment j are dead, effectively adding these $n_j - m_j$ deaths to y_j. Similarly, in the case $\gamma_j \to -\infty$, all missing subjects for treatment j are alive, so there is no contribution from the third term of equations (11.2) and (11.3). Hence $\gamma_1 \to +\infty, \gamma_2 \to -\infty$ coincides with the "best-case" as described above, and $\gamma_1 \to -\infty, \gamma_2 \to +\infty$ coincides with the "worst-case."

The score test for $H_0 : \beta = 0$ is obtained by first finding the solution, $\hat{\alpha}_0$, to $U_\alpha(\alpha, 0) = 0$. Then, under H_0, $U_\beta(\hat{\alpha}, 0)$ has mean zero and variance $V(\hat{\alpha}, 0) = U_{\beta,\beta}(\hat{\alpha}, 0) - U_{\alpha,\beta}(\hat{\alpha}, 0)^2 / U_{\alpha,\alpha}(\hat{\alpha}, 0)$, where $U_{st} = \partial^2 \log L(\alpha, \beta) / \partial s \partial t$ (see Appendix A.2).

The test statistic for H_0 is $Z = U_\beta(\hat{\alpha}, 0) / V(\hat{\alpha}, 0)^{1/2}$. The sensitivity of this test to the missingness mechanism can be ascertained by considering the values of Z for a range of values of γ_1 and γ_2. In the case $\gamma_1 = \gamma_2 = 0$, Z^2 is the usual Pearson chi-square statistic for the no-missing data. In the cases $\gamma_1 \to +\infty, \gamma_2 \to -\infty$ and $\gamma_1 \to -\infty, \gamma_2 \to +\infty$, Z^2 is the usual Pearson chi-square statistic for the best-case and worst-case scenarios.

In Figure 11.3, the value of Z is plotted against $e^{\gamma_2} = \pi_{20}/\pi_{21}$ for several values of $e^{\gamma_1} = \pi_{10}/\pi_{11}$. We see, for example, that if $e^{\gamma_1} = 1/8$, so that in group 1 subjects who survive are eight times more likely to be missing than those who die, in order for Z to be less than 1.96, we would need for $e^{\gamma_2} > 3.2$, so that in group 2, subjects who die are more than 3 times as likely to be missing than those who survive. This requires that in both treatment groups there is a significant deviation from ignorable ($\gamma_j = 0$) and that it is in the opposite direction. The assessment of whether these deviations are plausible involves clinical judgment and additional knowledge regarding the known reasons that subjects' data are missing. It may be that, ultimately, there is disagreement regarding whether or not this result is compelling. See Kenward (1998), Scharfstein et al. (1999), and Verbeke et al. (2001) for applications to more complex models.

11.3.3 Imputation

The "best-case" and "worst-case" scenarios posited in the previous example illustrate a type of *imputation*. That is, we *impute* values for the missing data, and behave as if they were the observed values. For these simple techniques, the imputed values do not depend on the model parameters of interest, and therefore, inference regarding the model parameters can proceed as if the missing responses were known. This result follows directly from the score

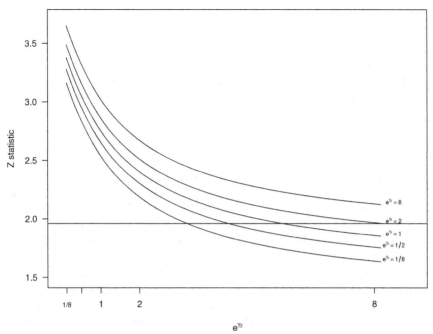

Figure 11.3 *Sensitivity analysis for hypothetical result from Table 11.4.*

function (equations (11.2) and (11.3)) since, in the cases $\gamma_j \to \pm\infty$, α and β drop out of the third term in each equation. If other imputation techniques are used in which the imputed values depend on either the responses or the non-missing data, correct inference can be performed only if the imputation method is taken into account.

Note that the likelihood inference performed in the previous example can be viewed as a kind of imputation. Since inference is based on the likelihood for the observed data under an assumed model for missingness, inference for the treatment effect of interest will be correct if the missingness model is correct. To see how the method used in this example uses a kind of imputation, we can apply Bayes theorem to compute the probability that a missing observation is a death. Letting y_{ij} be the outcome for subject i in group j,

$$
\begin{aligned}
\Pr\{y_{ij} = 1 | y_{ij} \text{ missing}\} &= \frac{\Pr\{y_{ij} \text{ missing}|y_{ij} = 1\}\Pr\{y_{ij} = 1\}}{\Pr\{y_{ij} \text{ missing}\}} \\
&= \frac{\pi_{1j}p_j}{\pi_{1j}p_j + \pi_{0j}(1 - p_j)} \\
&= \frac{e^{\alpha+\beta z_j+\gamma_j}}{1 + e^{\alpha+\beta z_j+\gamma_j}}.
\end{aligned}
\tag{11.4}
$$

Therefore, the third term in each of equations (11.2) and (11.3) is the expected number of deaths in the corresponding treatment group among the subjects with missing responses. Viewing these terms as representing the imputed number of deaths also provides a simple iterative procedure for estimation of α and β. Starting with preliminary estimates of α and β (from the non-missing data, for example), we compute the expected number of deaths among the missing observations using (11.4), impute these values for the missing outcomes, and re-estimate α and β. The process is repeated until sufficient accuracy is achieved. This is a simple application of the *EM algorithm* (Dempster et al. 1977). The EM algorithm is a procedure that alternates between the *E-step* (estimation) and the *M-step* (maximization). Given estimates of the model parameters, the *E-step* fills in the missing observations with their expectations under the estimated model. Given the imputations, for the *M-step* we recompute the maximum likelihood estimates of the model parameters based on complete data. When the observed data likelihood is complex, the EM algorithm is generally a computationally simpler procedure than direct maximization of the likelihood, although the convergence rate for the EM algorithm can be slow, depending on the amount of missing data. In the previous example, only two or three iterations provide adequate accuracy.

It is also clear from this example, that for finite γ_j, the imputed observations depend on the observed data via the parameter estimates. If we impute values based on the fitted model and then assume that they are known, we are likely to underestimate the variance in the test statistic and overstate the statistical significance of the result. By using the variance derived from the observed data likelihood as we did for the score test in the example, this dependence is correctly accounted for.

In more complex situations, the likelihood for the observed data, accounting for the missing data mechanism, can quickly become analytically intractable. While in some cases it may be relatively straightforward to perform the imputation, obtaining correct variances is usually more difficult. Correct inference may require a technique such as *multiple imputation* (see, for example, Rubin (1987), Rubin (1996), Liu and Gould (2002), or Little and Rubin (2002)). Using multiple imputation, imputed values are randomly generated for each subject using the posterior distribution derived using Bayes theorem in a manner similar to what was done in the simple example above. The desired test statistic can be computed from the augmented dataset, and the process repeated many times. The variability among the multiple values of test statistic can be used to adjust the full-data variance (conditional on the imputed values) to account for the method of imputation that was used. This differs from the technique we have used in that we have imputed the expected value for each observation, whereas in multiple imputation one generates imputed values as random samples from the entire posterior distribution. Sensitivity analysis can be conducted in the same way as in the previous example to assess robustness of the result to the potential association between missingness and response.

The critical feature in multiple imputation is that the analysis and the imputation are decoupled so that the same analysis can be applied to datasets

generated by a variety of imputation schemes that are derived from a variety
of missingness models. Liu and Gould (2002) state

> Imputation and statistical inference are carried out separately with the MI ap-
> proach. The MAR assumption needs to apply only for the imputation step; the
> statistical inference will be valid if the imputed values are drawn from a proper
> distribution. Since the model used to impute missing values can differ from the
> model used for inference, the imputation model can include considerably more
> potentially predictive information. ...

> The MI method is generally robust against misspecification of the imputation
> model. The imputation method incorporates the variability that arises because of
> the uncertainty about the missing values. The analysis results from each imputed
> data set also provide a way to assess the influence of the missing observations.
> When the estimates vary within a small range, the missing data are unlikely to
> influence the conclusions dramatically. Otherwise, if the results from the imputed
> data sets differ considerably, the impact of missing data or the imputation model
> may be substantial.

Last Observation Carried Forward

A commonly used method for imputation of missing values when data are collected at prespecified follow-up times is referred to as "last observation carried
forward" or LOCF. Using LOCF, the value of the last non-missing observation
is imputed for future missing observations with the analysis at one or more
prespecified follow-up times proceeding as if the data were complete. The advantages of this approach are that it is simple and allows one to conduct an
analysis at a particular follow-up time that includes data from all randomized
subjects (or at least those with at least one non-missing value). The disadvantages are that there is no theoretical basis for the analysis and the resulting
comparison is largely uninterpretable. In fact, for subjects who have died prior
to the specified time, LOCF is clearly not meaningful. An observed case (OC)
analysis, using only subjects with observations at the specified time, is, in
general, subject to unknown biases resulting from unknown associations between data availability and the treatments and outcome in question. LOCF
does nothing to address this difficulty and simply compounds the problem by
carrying forward trends that may appear in the data collected at earlier times
into later times, and it is likely to do this differentially by treatment. Thus
it is unclear how much of any observed difference (or lack thereof) is due to
either early trends or missingness, both of which may be treatment dependent,
and the actual effect of treatment. Molenberghs et al. (2004) argue that even
strong MCAR conditions cannot guarantee the validity of LOCF (Verbeke
and Molenberghs 2000; Mallinckrodt et al. 2003; Carroll 2004).

LOCF is frequently used in combination with an observed case analysis—
one analysis may be the prespecified primary analysis and the other a "confirmatory" analysis. Again, it is doubtful that this is a meaningful approach.
Whether the LOCF analysis agrees or disagrees with the OC analysis, the fact
that the former is fundamentally flawed sheds no light on the reliability of the

OC analysis. The best solution is, again, to ensure that all efforts are made to maximize completeness of the data.

11.3.4 Censoring in Survival Analyses

The importance of choosing outcome variables that can be ascertained in all subjects was noted in Chapter 2. In this context, outcomes that consist of the occurrence of an event, or the time to the occurrence of an event, generally have an advantage over outcomes that require a specific assessment to be performed on a subject at a specified time during the study. This is because the occurrence and date of an event can often be established without the physical presence of the subject being required (e.g., upon review of medical records), thereby reducing the frequency of missing outcomes.

When survival analysis methods are used, loss to follow-up can be technically handled by censoring the subject follow-up at the time of the loss to follow-up using methods such as the Kaplan-Meier estimate of the survival probabilities or the log-rank test for comparing two survival curves. Under the assumption of ignorable missingness, such estimates and hypothesis tests will be unbiased. In clinical trials, the ignorability assumption is likely to fail except for administrative censoring (i.e, when subjects reach a prespecified follow-up time). It is particularly important, as has been previously noted, that subject follow-up for study outcome events continues after discontinuation of study treatment. If there is a small rate of non-administrative loss to follow-up, the analysis may not be affected to a great extent but interpretation of the results should not ignore the fact that some data are missing.

Within the FDA, the randomized clinical trial has historically played a much larger role in the approval of new drugs—regulated by the Center for Drug Evaluation and Research (CDER)—than it has in the approval of medical devices, the responsibility of the Center for Devices and Radiological Health. The COMPANION study (Bristow et al. 2004) was initiated in 1999 and designed to compare both a pacemaker and a pacemaker-defibrillator combination with phamacologic therapy in subjects with advanced heart failure. COMPANION was one of the first large randomized trials performed for this device class. The primary outcome was a composite of death from any cause or hospitalization for any cause. Because of the nature of the therapy, subjects and their physicians were unblinded to their treatment. During the course of the study pacemakers were approved by the FDA based on shorter term outcome data, resulting in a substantial and unanticipated number of subjects withdrawing from the pharmacologic-therapy group in order to receive commercially available pacemakers. The original protocol and consent process did not specify any follow-up procedures for subjects who discontinued from their assigned treatment. Given the extent of withdrawal and its imbalance between treatment groups, no analysis would be satisfactory. Even though the available data suggested a statistically significant mortality benefit of the devices relative to best drug treatment, it was perceived that results would not be accepted. Thus, the sponsor of the trial implemented a policy, at considerable effort and time, of recontacting subjects who had withdrawn in order to obtain their consent for collection of data on vital status and hospitalizations for the duration of the study. The amount of censored data was dramatically reduced in the control arm. The final results continued to show significant benefit of the device. Much effort would have been saved, however, by anticipating and providing for the continued follow-up of subjects withdrawn from randomized therapy in the original study design.

Even when loss to follow-up is ignorable in theory, it is often not clear exactly when a subject is lost to follow-up. The technically correct censoring date is the latest date such that any event occurring before this date would be reported and any event occurring later than this date would not be reported. Unfortunately, this date is generally not known. For example, if subjects are expected to make regular clinic visits, say every six months, and the subject is lost to follow-up after a particular visit (their *last visit*), then all that is known is that the subject was lost to follow-up sometime *between* their last visit and the scheduled time of the next visit. Unless the subject formally withdraws consent for follow-up at their last visit, if the subject were to fail (e.g., die) the day after the last visit, this event would likely be reported. The further beyond the last visit the event occurs, the greater the likelihood that the event would not be reported. If an analysis includes events after the last visit for subjects known to have these events, but censors remaining subjects lost to follow-up on the date of the last visit, the choice of censoring date has induced a dependence between the censoring and outcome and event rates will be overestimated. This bias may be quite small and have little effect on the test of treatment difference, but to our knowledge, the optimal choice of censoring time in the case of this uncertainty has never been studied.

11.3.5 Competing Risks

As indicated previously, if observations are missing because the subject has died, or if the desired quantity is not well defined because of the state of the subject, we view this as a problem of *competing risks*. For example, a major event (such as death) may preclude the subsequent occurrence of a lesser event (such as hospitalization) or measurement of outcome (such as exercise tolerance) in the same pathologic sequence. In such cases, the later outcome cannot be considered in isolation without potential bias. Otherwise, for example, the therapy that causes a subject's death before they have a chance to be hospitalized would appear to offer benefit in the prevention of hospitalization. Even when the number of preceding events is similar for the treatment groups being compared, a comparison that excludes subjects who experience the event (for example, an analysis of survivors) or censors observations at the time of the preceding event is no longer a randomized comparison. The reasons for experiencing the event might differ for different treatment groups. For example, subjects on active treatment might die because of toxicity, whereas subjects on placebo might die because of worsening disease.

There is a considerable body of research that has been dedicated to developing practical methods for competing risks data, particularly in the setting of failure time models, although very little is directly applicable to assessing the effect of treatment in randomized studies. When the competing risk is mortality, an incontrovertible adverse outcome, and a new therapy is being considered for regulatory approval, avoidance of potential bias is especially important and several relatively simple approaches can be successfully used. As discussed extensively in Section 2.5, for failure time data one can define the outcome to be a composite event that includes death, and analyze the time to failure as the time to the first event within the composite. For continuous or ordered categorical responses, subjects who die prior to assessment can be assigned some 'worst' value of the response. Like nonadherence, some loss of power would be expected if there is no actual effect of treatment on mortality and this should be anticipated in the design.

An alternative analysis for continuous or ordered categorical responses, measured at a specified follow-up time, is again based on the idea of principal stratification (Frangakis and Rubin 2002). The central, conceptually simple, idea is that the only subjects for whom a comparison of, say, respiratory function at one year makes sense are those who would be alive regardless of treatment assignment. This excludes subjects observed to die before one year and also subjects who are alive at one year but who would have died had they been in the other treatment group. Of course, we can't observe these later subjects, so additional modeling and imputation are required. The reader is referred to Frangakis and Rubin (2002) for further discussion of these techniques.

11.4 Subgroup Analyses

Subgroup analyses are common in randomized clinical trials. It is natural to be interested in knowing whether the treatment effect is consistent across various groups of subjects. For example, do subjects who are less ill appear to benefit from the treatment to the same degree as those who are more ill? Do females have the same benefit as males? Such information can provide insight into how the treatment works and can influence the way that the treatment is implemented. Alternatively, when the overall benefit of the treatment appears to be small, it is often of interest to examine whether a particular type of subject might benefit more than others. Interest in subgroup analyses may also be motivated by a desire to maximize the information obtained from a given clinical trial, given the tremendous time and resources expended in conducting a trial.

The primary statistical difficulty is that subgroup results are often unreliable even in large trials. Smaller sample sizes within subgroups lead to greater variances and reduced power relative to the overall clinical trial resulting in an increased risk of a false-negative result, whereas the multiplicity of hypotheses tests that results from examining multiple subgroups will lead to an increased risk of a false-positive result (inflation of type I error).

This does not mean that subgroups should not be examined, but that results within subgroups need to be interpreted with caution. The multiplicity problem can be managed by specifying *a priori* the subgroups that will be examined and a multiple testing procedure (discussed in more detail in Section 11.5) in advance. Often, however, there will be additional subgroup analyses performed. Such analyses are useful for generating hypotheses, but the results will generally require replication. In particular, looking for effects in subgroups is never a good way to rescue a study in which the primary ITT analysis fails to show an overall effect.

Results in subgroups may also be biased when the subgroup is defined by a post-randomization event, for example change in blood pressure with treatment. Another example, the analysis of subgroups defined by adherence, was discussed extensively in Section 11.2.2. Such analyses are in violation of the intent-to-treat principle and subject to confounding by the effect of treatment on the outcome used to define the subgroup.

In the following sections we discuss some examples and analysis considerations with regard to subgroups, distinguishing between subgroups defined by prerandomization characteristics and those that are not.

11.4.1 Baseline Subgroups

Analyses of the estimated treatment effect within subgroups defined by subject characteristics ascertained prior to treatment are consistent with the intent-to-treat principle and are therefore unbiased, although of potentially low power. It is therefore important to examine the consistency of the size of the estimated treatment effect across subgroups rather than to rely on significance testing within subgroups. For example, the COPERNICUS study (Packer et al. 2001) evaluated the effects of carvedilol, a beta-blocker, compared to placebo in 2289 subjects with severe chronic heart failure. The primary outcome was all-cause mortality. All-cause mortality or hospitalization for heart failure (HF), and all-cause mortality or any hospitalization were secondary outcomes. The study was terminated early, based on a highly significant reduction in mortality in the carvedilol group. A previous trial of a different beta-blocker, bucindolol, in patients with severe heart failure (The Beta-Blocker Evaluation of Survival Trial Investigators 2001) resulted in no significant overall survival benefit. The results, however, suggested that bucindolol may be beneficial in non-black but not black patients. The COPERNICUS investigators were therefore interested in the results by racial subgroup. Hazard ratios and 95% confidence intervals by subgroup for each outcome are shown in Table 11.5. Carvedilol reduced the risk of each outcome similarly in black and in non-black patients. Because only a small number of black patients were included in the study, however, the test of significance for all-cause mortality within the black subgroup was not significant ($p=0.41$). It would clearly be inappropriate to conclude, based on this non-significant p-value, that there is no effect of carvedilol in black patients.

Table 11.5 *Effect of treatment in COPERNICUS by race.*

Outcome	Hazard Ratio (95% CI)	
	Black Patients (N=121)	Non-Black Patients (N=2168)
All-cause mortality	0.60 (0.18-2.05)	0.65 (0.52-0.81)
All-cause mortality or HF hospitalization	0.46 (0.25-0.86)	0.71 (0.60-0.84)
All-cause mortality or any hospitalization	0.56 (0.33-0.95)	0.78 (0.68-0.89)

A better approach to formally assess whether there is a difference in treatment effects between subgroups is to perform an interaction test. This considers both the magnitude of the difference between groups and the standard error of the difference.

Two trials, also in congestive heart failure, illustrate the potential to be misled by results within subgroups. The Prospective Randomized Amlodipine Survival Evaluation (PRAISE-I) trial evaluated the effects of amlodipine, a calcium-channel blocker, compared to placebo in subjects with severe heart failure (Packer et al. 1996). The primary outcome was the time to all-cause mortality or cardiovascular hospitalization and a secondary outcome was all-cause mortality. Because it was suspected before the start of the study that amlodipine might have different effects on subjects with different etiologies of heart failure, the randomization was stratified by whether the cause of heart failure was coronary artery disease (ischemic) or nonischemic dilated cardiomyopathy. A total of 1153 subjects were enrolled, 732 subjects with ischemic heart disease and 421 subjects with nonischemic disease. Amlodipine therapy was associated with a non-significant 9 percent overall reduction in the risk of a primary event ($p=0.31$), and a non-significant 16 percent overall reduction in the risk of death ($p=0.07$). There was, however, a statistically significant ($p < 0.05$) interaction between the effect of treatment and the etiology of heart failure, both for the primary outcome ($p=0.04$) and for mortality ($p=0.004$). As a result, the effects of amlodipine were evaluated separately in the two strata (Table 11.6).

Among subjects with ischemic heart disease, there was very little difference between the amlodipine and placebo groups. The hazard ratio for the primary outcome comparison of amlodipine to placebo was 1.04 (95 percent confidence interval, 0.83 to 1.29) and was 1.02 for mortality (95 percent confidence interval, 0.81 to 1.29). In contrast, among subjects with non-ischemic heart disease the hazard ratios for the primary outcome and mortality analyses were 0.69

(95 percent confidence interval, 0.49 to 0.98, $p=0.04$) and 0.54 (95 percent confidence interval, 0.37 to 0.79, $p <0.001$), respectively. The greater beneficial effect of amlodipine in subjects with non-ischemic heart disease was in contrast to the original expectation that subjects with ischemic heart disease would benefit most from amlodipine.

Given the significance of the results for the non-ischemic subgroup, the investigators may have been tempted to conclude that amlodipine was beneficial in subjects with non-ischemic heart disease. Nonetheless, because of the unexpected inconsistency of the subgroup results, the PRAISE-I investigators and sponsor chose a more cautious interpretation. A second trial, using a similar protocol, in non-ischemic heart disease subjects was undertaken in order to confirm the subgroup result. This trial (PRAISE-II) resulted in very nearly identical event rates for the amlodipine and placebo groups, and cast doubt on the results observed for the non-ischemic subgroup in PRAISE-I (Thackray et al. 2000).

In multinational clinical trials the interpretation of differential country- or region-specific treatment differences can also be problematic. Usually there are a large number of countries participating. Comparison of results country by country, or region by region, may be proposed. This can present a multiple testing problem that is difficult to account for, especially if precise subgroups are not predefined. Small numbers of subjects in some countries can lead to arbitrary, or worse, groupings of countries based on observed results. Given that there are often real differences between countries that may affect responses to treatment (e.g., in population ethnicity, socioeconomic status, medical practice patterns, use of concomitant medications) it is also particularly easy to rationalize any differences, real or unreal, that are observed.

The challenges of interpreting subgroup analyses within the multinational Metoprolol Controlled-Release Randomised Intervention Trial in Heart Failure (MERIT-HF) was discussed by Wedel et al. (2001). MERIT-HF was conducted at 313 clinical sites across 14 countries, with a total of 3991 subjects (MERIT-HF Study Group 1999). There were two primary outcomes, time to all-cause mortality and time to all-cause mortality or all-cause hospitalization. Regulatory authorities were concerned that the result for mortality in

Table 11.6 *Effect of treatment in PRAISE-I by etiology of heart failure. P-values correspond to subgroup-by-treatment interactions.*

Outcome	Hazard Ratio (95% CI)		Ischemic vs. Non-ischemic p-value
	Ischemic (N=732)	Non-ischemic (N=421)	
Primary	1.04 (0.83-1.29)	0.69 (0.49-0.98)	0.04
Mortality	1.02 (0.81-1.29)	0.54 (0.37-0.79)	0.004

the United States subjects (hazard ratio=1.05, 95%CI 0.71–1.56, versus 0.55, 95% CI 0.43-0.70, in all other countries combined, interaction p=0.003) indicated that the mortality benefit of treatment was not present in this subgroup. Wedel et al. (2001) discuss the interpretation of this subgroup finding using the causality criteria formulated by Sir Bradford Hill discussed in Chapter 2 (Hill 1965).

1. *The rule of chance/the strength of association.* For the MERIT-HF data, the p-value for the mortality treatment by country interaction test was 0.22 and for mortality plus all-cause hospitalization was 0.70. This suggests that the observed variation among countries is consistent with chance. The interaction test performed by the FDA that compared the United States with all other countries combined was performed after examination of the *observed* treatment differences and does not appropriately adjust for the multiplicity inherent in focusing on this particular comparison.

2. *The biologic gradient.* Wedel et al. (2001) argue that the mortality hazard ratio for U.S. subjects in New York Heart Association class III/IV of 0.80 and one of 2.24 for subjects in NYHA class II is not consistent with causality by biologic gradient (e.g., disease severity).

3. *Consistency (internal/external).* The hazard ratios for the effect of metoprolol on the second primary outcome (death or all-cause hospitalization) and the secondary outcome (death or heart failure hospitalization) in U.S. subjects were both less than 1.0, indicating a positive effect similar to the overall study results. Several other trials of beta-blockers in heart failure have been conducted, all with a remarkably consistent positive effect of beta-blockade on mortality including the U.S. Carvedilol Program.

4. *Confounding.* No differences in baseline characteristics or treatment characteristics could be identified to explain a differential effect on mortality in U.S. subjects.

5. *Coherence/plausibility.* The overwhelmingly significant positive effect and remarkable consistency of results across studies, known predefined risk groups, and multiple outcomes provides a great deal of assurance that beta-blockers are generally effective in heart failure.

Based on these considerations, Wedel et al. conclude that the most likely explanation for the mortality result in the MERIT-HF U.S. subgroup is chance. They recommend that, in general, the best estimate of treatment effect for any given subgroup is the overall estimate of treatment effect, consistent with the advice of Peto et al. (1976).

The examination of observed treatment effect in subgroups should be for the purpose of qualitatively assessing consistency, rather than to obtain quantitative estimates within subgroups. Subgroups are almost always too small to provide definitive and reliable estimates and are subject to chance results. Once an unexpected result has been noticed, retrospective explanations for it may almost always be found. However such results should be viewed skeptically, and require independent verification.

11.4.2 Subgroups Defined by a Post-Randomization Outcome

Results in subgroups may also be biased when the subgroup is defined using characteristics or outcomes observed after randomization. The properties of randomization do not apply for such subgroups, for the same reason they do not apply in the *Treatment Received* and *Adherers Only* analyses discussed in Section 11.2.2. The fact that such subgroup analyses may be specified in advance within the study protocol or in a detailed analysis plan, or that there are no significant baseline imbalances by treatment group within the subgroups, does not mitigate the potential for bias.

One of the early examples of the problem of interpreting results for subgroups defined by a post-randomization event was again demonstrated by the CDP (The Coronary Drug Project Research Group 1980) and the clofibrate arm compared to the placebo arm. Recall that, overall, there was no difference between the clofibrate arm and the placebo arm in the 5-year mortality (20.0% vs. 20.9%). Nonetheless, there was lower mortality in the clofibrate arm among subjects with a baseline cholesterol greater than 250 mg/dl (17.5% vs. 20.6%) and among subjects with a fall in cholesterol from baseline to the last follow-up visit (17.2% vs. 20.7%) but not a rise in cholesterol (22.2% vs. 19.7%). These results are consistent with the assumed mechanism of action of clofibrate—reduce mortality by lowering cholesterol. Table 11.7 shows the 5-year mortality results according to both baseline cholesterol level and change in cholesterol. As shown, there was only modest variation in the placebo arm mortality results according to baseline cholesterol or change in cholesterol. There were notable differences in the clofibrate arm, however. A favorable difference between clofibrate and placebo is observed among subjects with a low baseline cholesterol level and a subsequent reduction in cholesterol. The greatest observed effect of clofibrate, however, is among subjects with a high baseline cholesterol level and a subsequent increase in cholesterol level (21.3% vs. 15.5% in favor of clofibrate). These results are not consistent with scientific expectations and are not sensible. Furthermore, those comparisons that consider subgroups based on post-treatment changes are inconsistent with ITT and should be avoided.

Table 11.7 *5-Year mortality in the CDP by baseline cholesterol and change.*

Baseline Cholesterol	Cholesterol Change	Clofibrate		Placebo	
		N	% Mortality	N	% Mortality
< 250 mg/dl	Fall	295	16.0	614	21.2
< 250 mg/dl	Rise	212	25.5	705	18.7
≥ 250 mg/dl	Fall	385	18.1	762	20.2
≥ 250 mg/dl	Rise	105	15.5	454	21.3

11.5 Multiple Testing Procedures

In its simplest form, a clinical trial is designed to answer a single well-defined question. For example, the primary goal of the COPERNICUS study (Packer et al. 2001) was to determine whether the beta-blocker carvedilol reduced all-cause mortality relative to placebo in subjects with severe heart failure. There was a single treatment (25 mg carvedilol twice a day), a single comparator (placebo), and a single outcome (all-cause mortality). In practice, clinical trials tend to be more complex. There may be multiple doses of the study drug, multiple comparators (active and placebo), or multiple outcomes. In Chapter 2, we discussed primary and secondary questions, noting that the type I error for the primary question should be strictly controlled. This forces us to compromise between the number of primary hypothesis tests and the ability to find differences that exist (i.e., power). Thus, the primary analysis should be confined to the fewest and most clinically relevant questions.

In some settings, it may also be desirable to control the type I error for secondary questions. For example, the FDA may request that a testing procedure be prespecified for secondary outcomes to aid with labeling decisions that need to be made for any approved drug.

In the previous section we discussed the examinination of treatment effect in subgroups and touched on the multiplicity concerns this raises. The fundamental problem is that multiple tests lead to multiple opportunities for rejecting hypotheses as a result of chance alone. For example, if one uses the usual 0.05 criterion for statistical significance and performs five tests each at the 0.05 level, if all the null hypotheses are true, the probability may be as high as 0.25, depending on the extent of correlation among the tests, that at least one test reaches statistical significance by chance alone. In this section we discuss multiple testing procedures for the control of type I error in clinical trials. The repeated testing of an outcome during interim monitoring of a clinical trial was discussed in Chapter 10 and is not considered further here.

Example

Throughout this section we will refer to the following example. Suppose that we have three treatment groups, high dose, low dose, and placebo, and two outcomes, all-cause mortality and subject-assessed global status. If we are interested in comparing both doses of experimental drug to placebo for each of the two outcomes, we have a total of four elementary hypotheses that are enumerated in Table 11.8. Table 11.8 also provides hypothetical observed p-values from the individual hypothesis tests, since the procedures that we will be discussing are based on these p-values.

Additional Notation

In addition to the four hypotheses in Table 11.8, there are others that are potentially of interest. For example, we might want to test the hypothesis that neither dose of drug has an effect on mortality. This hypothesis claims

Table 11.8 *Hypothetical hypotheses used to illustrate multiple testing procedures.*

H_1: no difference in mortality between high dose and placebo.
        $p_1 = .024$
H_2: no difference in mortality between low dose and placebo.
        $p_2 = .23$
H_3: no difference in global status between high dose and
        placebo. $p_3 = .009$
H_4: no difference in global status between low dose and
        placebo. $p_4 = .02$

that both H_1 and H_2 are true, and would be represented by the intersection $H_1 \cap H_2$. Alternatively, the hypothesis that the low dose had no effect on either outcome would be written as $H_2 \cap H_4$. For this example, there are eleven intersection hypotheses in addition to the elementary hypotheses $H_1, \ldots, H_4$, although it is not likely that all of these would be of interest. In general, if we have m elementary hypotheses, and I is a subset of $\{1, 2, \ldots, m\}$, we will let H_I indicate the intersection hypothesis $\cap_{i \in I} H_i$. The goal of the analysis is to test all hypotheses of interest while ensuring that the probability of a type I error is controlled at a prespecified level, α. We will return to this example after providing some background for multiple testing procedures.

One difficulty that arises is that some of the null hypotheses may be true and some may be false. Ideally, a testing procedure would reject the false hypotheses and not reject the true hypotheses; however, both type I and type II errors are inevitable and at best we can only control the rate at which errors occur. To clarify this, some additional terminology is helpful. The *global* null hypothesis is the hypothesis, $H_1 \cap H_2 \cap \ldots \cap H_m$, that asserts that *all* of $H_1, H_2, \ldots, H_m$ are true. A procedure that rejects the global null hypothesis with probability at most α when it is true is said to provide *weak control of the familywise error rate* (FWER). A procedure that weakly controls the FWER not only for the global null hypothesis, but also for all intersections, $H_I = \cap_{i \in I} H_i, I \subset \{1, 2, \ldots, m\}$, of hypotheses is said to provide *strong control of the FWER*.

11.5.1 Bonferroni Procedure

The most commonly used multiple testing procedure is known as the *Bonferroni* procedure. The procedure is based on the Bonferroni inequality that states that for a set of events $A_1, A_2, \ldots, A_m$, $\Pr\{A_1 \cup A_2 \cup \cdots \cup A_m\} \leq \sum_i \Pr\{A_i\}$ (equality holds if the events are pairwise disjoint). Now suppose that we have m hypotheses, $H_1, H_2, \ldots, H_m$, and let A_i be the event that hypothesis H_i is rejected. The event $A_1 \cup A_2 \cup \cdots \cup A_m$ is the event in which at least one of $H_1, H_2, \ldots, H_m$ is rejected.

Using the Bonferroni procedure, we reject H_i if the p-value for the test of H_i, p_i, is less than α/m, so that $\Pr\{A_i\} \leq \alpha/m$. If the test of H_i is based on a continuous test statistic, it is usually possible to conduct a test for which $\Pr\{A_i\} = \alpha/m$. If the test statistic is discrete, based, for example, on binary responses, we cannot in general achieve equality, but can only guarantee that $\Pr\{A_i\} \leq \alpha/m$, or if an asymptotic approximation is used, that $\Pr\{A_i\} \approx \alpha/m$. If *all* the hypotheses are true, then by Bonferroni's inequality the probability that we reject *at least one* of the hypotheses will be at most $\sum_i \Pr\{A_i\} \leq \alpha$. Note that if the tests of $H_1, H_2, \ldots, H_m$ were independent, we could replace α/m by the slightly larger $1 - (1 - \alpha)^{1/m}$, resulting in Sidak's (1967) procedure. Since we are not likely to have independent hypotheses, and the difference between the critical values from the two procedures is quite small, the Bonferroni procedure is generally preferred.

If we had four independent hypotheses, using the Bonferroni procedure and $\alpha = .05$, we would reject H_i if $p_i < 0.05/4 = .0125$. Using Sidak's procedure, we would require $p_i < 1 - (1 - 0.05)^{1/4} = .0127$. Returning to our example, if we reject H_i when $p_i \leq \alpha/4$, then, when all H_i are true, as above, the probability of rejection of the global null hypothesis is at most α.

Note that if we have only weak control of the FWER, and we reject the global null hypothesis, all we know is that at least one of the hypotheses is false, but we may not be able to make more precise inference without strong control of the FWER. In our example, suppose that both high and low dose improve clinical status, but have no effect on mortality. Then H_1 and H_2 are both true, but H_3 and H_4 are false. If we reject the global null hypothesis, it is important that we still have a low probability of erroneously rejecting H_1 and H_2 and concluding that there is a mortality benefit. Hence, if after rejecting the global null hypothesis we test the hypothesis $H_I = H_1 \cap H_2$, then we will require that the testing procedure control the type I error rate for this hypothesis as well as for the singleton hypotheses H_1 and H_2. This kind of type I error control will be guaranteed if the testing procedure strongly controls FWER. As we noted previously, the Bonferroni procedure guarantees this degree of control. On the other hand, the Bonferroni procedure is conservative in the sense that the FWER can be much less than α, especially when some of the hypotheses are false.

11.5.2 Closed Testing Procedures

One approach to ensuring strong FWER control is to use a *closed testing* procedure (Gabriel 1969; Marcus et al. 1976). A set of null hypotheses, $H = \{H^{(1)}, H^{(2)}, \ldots, H^{(k)}\}$, is said to be closed under intersection if $H^{(i)}, H^{(j)} \in H$ implies $H^{(i)} \cap H^{(j)} \in H$. A *closed testing procedure* is a procedure under which a particular null hypothesis $H^{(i)}$ is rejected if and only if all hypotheses in H that are contained in $H^{(i)}$ have been tested and rejected. In our example, one closed set of hypotheses is $\{H_1 \cap H_2 \cap H_3 \cap H_4, H_1 \cap H_2, H_3 \cap H_4\}$. A closed testing procedure is one in which we test the global null hypothesis at level α and if we reject, we proceed to test each of the other two hypotheses also at level α. Note that the tests used for each of these three hypotheses do not have to be related in any way for the FWER to be strongly controlled, so we may specify them in any way that we like, provided that they are specified in advance. In this example, if we were to reject each of these hypotheses, we could conclude that the experimental drug has an effect on both mortality and clinical status; however, we would not be able to identify which of the two doses were efficacious. If we want to test hypotheses regarding individual doses, we will need to expand our set of hypotheses of interest to include single hypotheses.

If our set of hypotheses is expanded to include the elementary hypotheses H_1 and H_3 both of which relate to the effect of the high dose, we would also be required to add the hypotheses $H_1 \cap H_3$, $H_1 \cap H_2 \cap H_3$, and $H_1 \cap H_3 \cap H_4$ in order to ensure that the set of hypotheses under consideration is closed. We would then be able to test hypotheses H_1 provided that we have rejected the global null hypothesis and all hypotheses containing H_1; $H_1 \cap H_2$, $H_1 \cap H_3$, $H_1 \cap H_2 \cap H_3$, and $H_1 \cap H_3 \cap H_4$. The requirement for H_3 is similar. If, in addition, we want to be able to individually test hypotheses H_2 and H_4, then H would be the collection of all combination of two and three hypotheses.

While there are many ways in which closed testing procedures can be implemented, the procedure in which the family H contains all possible combinations of hypotheses and each subset hypothesis is tested using the Bonferroni procedure is known as *Holm's* procedure (Holm 1979). Holm's procedure can also be implemented as a *sequentially rejective procedure* as follows. Let $p_{(1)}, ..., p_{(m)}$ be the ordered (smallest to largest) p-values and $H_{(1)}, ..., H_{(m)}$ be the corresponding null hypotheses. Holm's procedure rejects $H_{(1)}$ if $p_{(1)} \leq \alpha/m$. If $H_{(1)}$ is rejected, testing continues for $H_{(2)}, H_{(3)}, ...$ with each successive test conducted at progressively higher significance levels, $\alpha/(m-1), \alpha/(m-2), ..., \alpha/1$. Once an hypothesis $H_{(i)}$ fails to be rejected, the procedure stops, and we cannot reject any $H_{(j)}$ for $j \geq i$. In general terms, the procedure rejects $H_{(i)}$ when, for all $j = 1, ..., i, p_{(j)} \leq \alpha/(m - j + 1)$.

In our example, let the p-value for hypothesis H_i be denoted by p_i, $i = 1, 2, 3, 4$, and suppose that we want to control FWER at $\alpha = .05$. Given the p-values from Table 11.8, the smallest p-value is $p_3 = 0.009 < 0.05/4 = 0.0125$. Hence, we can reject H_3. The second smallest p-value is $p_4 = 0.02 > 0.05/3 = 0.0167$, and we cannot reject H_4, nor can we reject H_1 and H_2.

To see how this is a closed testing procedure, in order to reject H_3, we need to also reject all hypotheses contained in H_3: $H_1 \cap H_2 \cap H_3 \cap H_4$, $H_1 \cap H_2 \cap H_3 \cap H_4$, $H_1 \cap H_2 \cap H_3$, $H_1 \cap H_3 \cap H_4$, $H_2 \cap H_3 \cap H_4$, $H_1 \cap H_3$, $H_2 \cap H_3$, $H_3 \cap H_4$, and H_3. Because H_3 is an element of each of these hypotheses, and $\alpha/k \geq 0.0125$ for each set, where k is the number of hypotheses considered in a given set, each will be rejected by the corresponding Bonferroni procedure, and thus we can reject H_3. Next, we note that H_4 contains the hypotheses $H_1 \cap H_2 \cap H_4$. The smallest p-value in this set is $p_4 = .03$, and the corresponding Bonferroni test requires at least one p-value be at most $0.05/3 = 0.0167$ in order to reject; therefore, we cannot reject H_4. We also have that H_1 contains the same hypothesis, $H_1 \cap H_2 \cap H_4$, so it cannot be rejected even though all other hypotheses contained in H_1 are rejected.

The procedures discussed to this point are symmetric in the sense that they treat all hypotheses interchangeably. In practice, outcomes often differ in importance and closed testing procedures can also be applied naturally in this setting. Specifically, suppose that hypotheses are ordered by importance, $H_1, H_2, \ldots, H_m$, and we apply the principle of closed testing procedures to construct a testing procedure as follows. Since H_1 is the most important hypothesis, it is natural to begin by testing H_1 at level α. If we reject H_1, we proceed to test H_2, again at level α. If we reject H_2, we proceed to H_3, and so on. To see why this procedure is a closed testing procedure, let $H^{(i)} = H_i \cap H_{i+1} \cap \ldots \cap H_m$. Then if $i < j$, $H^{(i)} \cap H^{(j)} = H^{(i)}$ and we see that the set $\{H^{(1)}, H^{(2)}, \ldots, H^{(m)}\}$ is closed under intersection, and therefore closed testing procedures can be applied. Since no other hypothesis is contained in $H^{(1)}$, we can begin the procedure by testing $H^{(1)}$ at level α. Since, as we indicated previously, we may use any testing procedure we like for this hypothesis, so we choose the one that rejects $H^{(1)}$ if we reject H_1 at level α. In general we test $H^{(i)}$ only if we have rejected $H^{(j)}$ for $j < i$ and if we reject H_j at level α.

In our example, suppose that we consider mortality differences to be more important than differences in clinical status, and given the outcome, effects of the high dose as more important than the effects of low dose. The order of the hypotheses is that given in Table 11.8: H_1, H_2, H_3, H_4. Using the closed procedure, we reject H_1 and conclude that there is a mortality benefit of the high dose, but because we cannot reject H_2, we cannot conclude benefit for any of the remaining hypotheses.

Alternatively, if we consider all high dose comparisons more important than low dose comparisons, we might order the hypotheses H_1, H_3, H_2, H_4. In this case, we would reject both H_1 and H_3 and fail to reject H_2 and H_4.

Another alternative approach is to combine the closed testing procedure based on the importance ordering with Holm's procedure. For example, we may group the hypotheses into mutually exclusive and exhaustive groups, impose an ordering among the groups, and apply Holm's procedure to each group. In our example, let $H^{(1)} = \{H_1, H_3\}$ represent the high dose hypotheses, and $H^{(2)} = \{H_2, H_4\}$ represent the low dose hypotheses, and order the groups by considering $H^{(1)}$ to be more important than $H^{(2)}$. Applying Holm's procedure to $H^{(1)}$, the smallest p-value in this set is 0.009, so we reject $H^{(1)}$. We are then allowed to both test the individual hypotheses within $H^{(1)}$ and apply Holm's procedure to $H^{(2)}$. Within $H^{(1)}$, Holm's procedure allows us to reject H_1 and H_3. Applying Holm's procedure to $H^{(2)}$, we reject only H_4.

The procedures based on the principle of closed testing procedure that we have described provide a good deal of flexibility while strongly controlling FWER. It is also clear using the example from Table 11.8 that the conclusions that we are allowed to draw depend substantially on the procedure employed. Therefore, it is critical that it be understood that the choice of multiple testing procedure be clearly defined in advance of any analysis, preferably in the study protocol.

11.5.3 Other Multiple Testing Procedures

Other procedures have been proposed, but do not strictly control FWER except in special situations, such as when the test statistics for hypotheses are independent. This will not generally be the case in a controlled clinical trial, except when we are considering hypotheses corresponding to a set of prespecified mutually exclusive subgroups defined by baseline characteristics.

Simes (1986) proposed a test of the global null hypothesis that is more powerful than the Bonferroni procedure and maintains the FWER when the test statistics of the hypotheses are jointly independent. Similar to Holm's procedure, let $p_{(1)} \leq p_{(2)} \leq \ldots \leq p_{(m)}$ be the ordered p-values. Using Simes's procedure, we reject the global null hypothesis if for any j, $1 \leq j \leq m$, we have $p_{(j)} \leq j\alpha/m$. Whereas Holm's procedure will not reject the global null hypothesis, and hence will not reject any hypotheses, unless $p_{(1)} \leq \alpha/m$, Simes's procedure only requires that $p_{(j)} \leq j\alpha/m$ holds for some j. On the other hand, Simes's procedure rejects the global null hypothesis whenever Holm's does, and, therefore, when it can be applied, it is strictly more powerful. Besides requiring independence, Simes's procedure does not allow the testing of individual hypotheses, or other intersections of individual hypotheses.

Hochberg (1988) showed, by applying the principle of closed testing procedures, how Simes's procedure can be extended to tests of individual hypotheses. Similar to Holm, the Hochberg procedure rejects an individual hypothesis H_i if all intersection hypotheses contained in H_i can be rejected using Simes's procedure. Hochberg showed that this procedure can be implemented as a sequentially rejective procedure as follows. If $p_{(m)} \leq \alpha$ then reject all H_i. Otherwise, if $p_{(m-1)} \leq \alpha/(m-1)$ reject $H_{(i)}$ for $i \leq m-1$. In general, if j is the largest integer such that $p_{(j)} \leq \alpha/j$, then we reject all $H_{(i)}$ with $i \leq j$. The resulting procedure is similar to Holm's procedure except it begins with the largest p-value instead of the smallest, and proceeds only when we fail to reject.

If the test statistics of the H_i are jointly independent, then Hochberg's procedure does strictly control the FWER and is strictly more powerful than Holm's procedure. In general, however, the Hochberg procedure does not strictly control the FWER, and conclusions based on it may not be readily accepted. Furthermore, in most cases the gains in power are quite small.

Returning to our example, applying the Hochberg procedure, we reject H_1, H_3, and H_4 unlike Holm that rejects only H_3.

11.6 Summary

Clinical trials are inherently complex enterprises, and the results can be difficult to interpret. In this chapter we have tried to point out some of the issues that frequently arise, some of which have clear defined statistical solutions, while others can be ambiguous and subjective. Because "we don't know what we don't know," the effects of non-compliance and missing data are not readily ascertained or accounted for using purely statistical methods. Subjective assessments regarding the degree to which the results are affected may be central to the ultimate interpretation of the result. That is, if we believe it is plausible that the result that we observe could be an artifact of non-compliance or missing data, the credibility of the result is in question and no amount of speculative exploratory analyses can definitively answer the question.

Treatment comparisons adjusted for post-randomization attributes such as adherence to assigned treatment or the presence or absence of adverse responses are inherently problematic and should be avoided. Fundamentally flawed analyses are subject to bias of unknown magnitude and direction and cannot provide a meaningful assessment of the robustness of the overall result. "Per-protocol" or "evaluable" analyses do not answer the questions that one's instinct might suggest. Unless we are extremely careful, once we leave ITT behind, we have left the world of experimentation and reentered the world of observational studies in which confounding is a serious issue. Just as we have been misled by epidemiological studies, we can be easily misled by non-ITT analyses.

11.7 Problems

11.1 If the power of a single two-sided test with $\alpha = 0.05$ is 80%, what is the power of the same test carried out with a Bonferroni correction for 2 outcomes? For 6 outcomes? (Assume normality.)

11.2 Simulate a set of data as described at the end of section 11.2.2. Use the hazard rate given, 0.057, for both death and crossover, starting with the original allocation of subjects: 354 to medical therapy and 332 to surgical therapy. Plot and compare the two Kaplan-Meier curves for each type of analysis: ITT, "Treatment Received", and "Adherers Only."

11.3 In each of the following cases, use the EM algorithm described in section 11.3.3 to impute the missing values in Table 11.4, then perform a Pearson chi-square test and compare the result to the test based on the score equations, (11.2) and (11.3).

   (a) $\gamma_1 = \gamma_2 = 0.9$

   (b) $\gamma_1 = -\gamma_2 = 1.5$

   (c) $\gamma_1 = -\gamma_2 = -1.5$

CHAPTER 12

Closeout and Reporting

We have seen that before enrollment in a trial begins, the protocol, which establishes all trial procedures, outcome measures, and analyses, must be in place. A similar set of procedures must be established to bring the trial project to a close once subject follow-up is complete. There are multiple tasks to be completed at the clinics, by the sponsor and study leadership, and by the statistical or data coordinating center. The literature on these topics is extensive and we will consider only some of the major issues that have important statistical implications. First, we will discuss important issues in the closeout of a clinical trial. We will emphasize those challenges commonly encountered by the statistical center. We will then focus on reporting issues. There are at least three types of reporting activities: presentation of results at professional meetings, publication of results in scholarly journals, and regulatory reporting for product approval. Of these, we will focus on the publication and presentation aspects. Regulatory aspects were briefly discussed in Chapter 1.

12.1 Closing Out a Trial

Each clinical center typically must have a final exit visit for their participants. At the final visit, data will be collected and sent to the data center. Publication of trial results cannot begin until the database is complete and finalized or "locked." In addition, once the final data have been collected, the physician and clinical team must have a plan for sharing the results of the trial with their subjects. This plan may be formulated by the Steering Committee and the Sponsor. It is important that subjects be properly informed. Coordinating the publication, the scientific and public presentations, and the informing of the subject is challenging; the length of time over which each of these constituencies is informed must be minimized. The order in which they are informed must also be considered.

The statistical center also must have a closeout plan that typically will be implemented several months after closure of the trial. There may be several publications that result from the trial and there is generally a period of months, or even years, over which manuscripts are written and accepted for publication. Once the planned publications are complete, the statistical center must archive the trial data so that it can be easily retrieved at a later date if necessary. The data may be required some time later to answer a new question not anticipated in the first group of publications. In some cases, an analysis or hypothesis contained in a previous publication may need to be reexamined.

In other cases, new information or concern about a safety issue may emerge from other studies and further analysis or additional subject follow-up may be required for the trial.

While archiving a trial is not a task that researchers take on eagerly, it will not be achieved if left to normal routine activity. In a few months after the data collection has been completed, memories of key details about the trial and the database fade and the task of retrieving a data set for further analysis can be daunting unless proper documentation has been developed. Thus, a plan for database archiving must be developed well before the end of the trial and worked towards during the course of the trial.

The protocol, an annotated copy of the case report form, the documentation of the database, and the analysis programs should be carefully archived. The database documentation may be the most challenging, as databases usually have several components that have to be linked together.

Statistical programs used for the analysis may be written using a statistical computing language. Software packages change over time, however, and there is no guarantee that previous programs will run exactly as before and may need to be updated. Thus, it is important to document these programs sufficiently, so that a future statistician or programmer could make the appropriate changes and reproduce the original analyses if necessary.

The medium of storage may also change in our rapidly changing technology environment. Thus, the statistical center closeout plans should address long term archiving. Paper will deteriorate over time. Forms, either paper or electronic, are now routinely stored on digital medium as well as the database and programs. However, the ability to read the digital medium may also change. Thus, if a trial is of sufficient importance, the trial archive may require periodic updates.

12.2 Reporting Trial Results

Once the trial is closed and the database finalized, the next task is to present the results of the trial as quickly as possible while being thorough and accurate. Typically, results are presented in two forums, an oral presentation at a professional meeting and a scholarly publication in a relevant medical journal. Sometimes the oral presentation takes place before the scientific publication and, for other trials, the oral presentation does not occur until shortly after a paper is published. These decisions are often made by the sponsor of the trial, the steering committee, the publication committee, or some combination. The oral presentation must be much shorter and cannot cover as much detail as the publication. In either case, the amount of statistical analyses that can be presented will likely be much less than what was conducted. Choices have to be made regarding which results are most important. This can be a challenge because all important information that might affect the interpretation of the trial results must be included. It is important for the statistician to be involved actively in these decisions so that the results presented accurately reflect the overall sense of the analyses.

12.2.1 Oral Presentation

The oral presentation is usually the first opportunity that the investigators have to share the results with a large body of scientific and clinical colleagues who are interested in the results. Given the short period of time allowed at scientific meetings for these presentations, however, only the important highlights can be shared. The selection of material to be presented must give the audience a clear sense of the purpose of the trial, key design assumptions including sample size and power, characteristics of the subjects studied, the treatment administered, and the primary outcome(s), along with any important toxicity or serious adverse events. Interpretation of the results and the relevance to other existing treatments are also presented. Because available time is limited, it is important that the tables and graphs used to present the results are clear and neither confusing nor misleading. The statistical issues in the oral presentation are similar to those in the scientific publication and we will cover those in the next sections.

12.2.2 Scientific Publication

The scientific publication is the most important vehicle for dissemination of clinical trial results because it is the most complete report available to the general medical community. In addition, manuscripts receive peer review prior to publication which adds to the quality and credibility of the report. The total length of such papers is usually 20–25 double spaced typed pages plus figures and tables, so careful selection of results and concise writing is required. In some cases, a separate trial design paper may be published that contains greater detail about the trial protocol and procedures. In the 1990s, an international group of scientists working in clinical trials created a publication called the CONSORT statement (Moher et al. 2001). The purpose of the CONSORT statement is to improve the quality of the reporting of clinical trial results. The CONSORT statement describes each of the components that should be included in a paper. In this section, we give the outline of a study report and discuss the essential elements. The typical scientific results paper has four sections: *Introduction*, *Methods*, *Results*, and *Discussion*. We will examine each of these sections briefly.

Introduction

In the "Introduction", the authors should give the scientific background and describe the rationale for the trial. This should include a very brief review of recent relevant publications or trials that have addressed the same or similar questions. The current trial is likely designed to answer some of the questions left open by previous trials or is testing a new approach to a similar question. The introduction should make it clear why the current trial has been conducted and that it was in fact ethical to do so. For example, the COPER-NICUS (Packer et al. 2001) trial tested the effect of a beta-blocker drug in a population with more severe heart failure (New York Heart Class IV) than the two previous beta-blocker trials, MERIT-HF (MERIT-HF Study Group 1999) and CIBIS-II (CIBIS-II Investigators 1999). Those two trials tested a beta-blocker in a Class II–III heart failure population and demonstrated a 35% reduction in mortality and heart failure hospitalization. Prior to these trials, use of beta-blockers in this type of heart failure population was believed to be harmful. Thus, the potential benefit of a beta-blocker in a more severe, higher risk heart failure population remained an open question and the COPERNICUS trial was designed to answer that very specific question. A brief review of this history was included in the COPERNICUS article and provided the necessary background information to the readers. This review also signals to the readers that the authors are aware of the previous relevant trials.

The "Introduction" should also state clearly the specific hypothesis that is being tested and the outcome measures that will be used to address the hypothesis. In the COPERNICUS trial, the hypothesis stated was that total mortality and mortality plus hospitalization for heart failure would be reduced with the beta-blocker. The trial was designed to compare the best standard of care with the best standard of care plus a beta-blocker (carvedilol).

This section may also refer to the organizational structure, number of clinical centers, and sponsor of the trial.

Methods Section

The "Methods" section is a synopsis of the trial protocol. The methods section briefly conveys the essence of the design. Some trials may have a separate published design paper that can be cited, but otherwise the protocol must be cited for further details.

In this section, the eligibility criteria for the trial should be concisely described. This is often done by listing the main inclusion and exclusion criteria, following a similar list to that provided in the protocol as a guide. This is important because a physician reading the paper must understand how the results pertain to his/her practice. Other researchers may find the results useful when planning further trials. Similarly, the number, type, and location of each clinic at which data were collected should be reported to assist in application of trial results.

In addition, the paper should describe the specific outcome measures that were used to assess the risks and benefits of the intervention and the frequency and timing of those measurements. If cause-specific mortality or morbidity is used as an outcome, then the definition must be included. For example, in COPERNICUS, hospitalization for heart failure was an outcome of interest. To qualify as an event, a hospitalization must have been at least 24 hours long and related to worsening symptoms of heart failure. Treatment in an emergency room for only a few hours would not be considered an outcome event. Trial masking or blinding procedures must also be described, if used, since it is relevant to the interpretation of the results. For example, a trial may have masked tablets to minimize bias in outcome assessment. If the treatment or intervention cannot be masked, then the classification of potential events should be assessed in a masked or double-blind fashion. In some trials, both the treatment and the outcome adjudication are masked. Such details should be clearly described.

The randomization process, or allocation of interventions to participants, must also be described. For example, if the paper states that the intervention was randomly allocated to participants using a permuted block design with varying block sizes (2-6), stratified by clinic or region, then the reader has sufficient information with appropriate references to understand the allocation method. Also the manner in which the allocation was implemented is important. For example, the randomization assignments could be provided in sealed envelopes (which are vulnerable to tampering) or an interactive voice response system (IVRS) could be used. The paper should mention the particular individuals or groups responsible for implementation of randomization. These details can be succinctly described but are important to the interpretation of the results.

The statistician should take responsibility for the sample size summary. Sufficient detail is needed so that the sample size calculation could be replicated by an informed reader. The significance level, whether the test was one sided or two sided, and the power of the design must be specified. In addition, the event rate or the mean level of response, and its variability, and the size of the hypothesized treatment effect must be provided. The latter could be expressed either as a percent change or an absolute change but it is necessary to be clear which metric is presented. For example, in COPERNICUS, the paper states that the trial was designed for a two sided 0.05 significance level with 90% power to detect a 25% change in mortality, assuming an annual mortality of 20% in the control arm. From this information, we can estimate the sample size independently. If adjustments were made for non-compliance, either drop-out or drop-in, these should be stated as well as the effect on the final sample size. References to the statistical methods should be included. Inclusion of the sample size methods is important because it tells the reader the significance level that was used as the criterion for success, whether the trial had adequate power, whether the assumed control group response rate was actually observed, and whether the effect size specified was reasonable.

The methods for analysis must also be presented. Based on the issues described in Chapter 11, the primary outcome measures must be analyzed on an intent to treat basis where all subjects who are randomized and all events occurring during the follow up period are accounted for. Any supplementary analyses that will be presented, such as "per protocol" analyses, must be defined as well. The description of methods also includes the statistical test(s) that were used. This can be done succinctly by naming the statistical tests with appropriate references. For example, for time to event outcome measures such as mortality or death plus hospitalization, the Kaplan-Meier method might be used to estimate the time-to-event curves and the log-rank test used to compare them. A simple sentence with references can convey the necessary information. Generally a summary measure of effect size, accompanied by an assessment of variability, will be included. This might be a mean difference, relative risk, odds ratio, or hazard ratio estimate, along with, for example, a corresponding 95% confidence interval. If missing data are anticipated, then the protocol should address how this was to be handled and this should also be summarized briefly in the methods section. If any covariate adjustment was done, such as adjustment for clinic or baseline risk factors, this should be stated along with the statistical methods with references and the list of covariates utilized. Enough detail about the analysis plan should be given so that another researcher with access to the original data would be able to reproduce the main results. Some trials, especially those used for regulatory purposes, have a separate analysis plan document that can be cited.

Most trials conducted in the United States must now have a monitoring plan, and trials with serious outcomes such as death or irreversible morbidity should have an independent data monitoring committee (DMC), as described in Chapter 10. Membership on the DMC might be reported in an appendix, for example. In order to protect against false positive claims of treatment effect, either for benefit or harm, many DMCs use a statistical procedure to account for interim analyses, and these should be reported with appropriate references. For example, COPERNICUS used an independent DMC with a Lan-DeMets alpha spending function of the O'Brien-Fleming type (Lan and DeMets 1983) with an overall 0.05 significance level. This informs the reader how the trial was monitored, and guides the interpretation of the primary results. This is especially important for trials that terminate early for either benefit or harm. If adjustments to the estimate of the effect size were made to account for interim monitoring, the specific methods should be referenced.

Subgroups that were predefined in the protocol should also be described. If there were numerous subgroups, indications of which were primary are useful. If this was not done in the protocol, adjustments made for multiple testing of many subgroups, as discussed in Chapter 11, must be described. Lack of any such description may leave the reader to assume that the authors do not appreciate the issue and may minimize any subgroup results, potentially leading readers to ignore an important subgroup result.

Results Section

The "Results" section of the scientific paper is typically the primary focus and must be carefully prepared. This section must not include any editorial opinions or comments; those should be included in the "Discussion" section. Here, the results must be presented in a complete, clear, and concise manner. We must report the results as observed in the trial, not as we might have wished them to be or after we have "cleaned them up." We might, within reason, have alternative results to share in the "Discussion" section.

There are typically more analyses conducted than can be summarized in the standard scientific publication. Thus, the results presented must be consistent with the goals stated in the protocol and described in the "Methods" section. Still, difficult choices regarding which analyses to present will have to be made. It may be that not all of the important results can be presented in one manuscript. The MERIT-HF trial, for example, presented the two primary outcome results in two separate papers, published almost a year apart (MERIT-HF Study Group 1999; Hjalmarson et al. 2000). One reason for this was that the mortality paper (MERIT-HF Study Group 1999) could be completed and verified more quickly. The second paper focused on the second primary outcome of death and heart failure hospitalization and came later because it took much longer to collect, validate, and adjudicate the cause-specific hospitalization data (Hjalmarson, Goldstein, Fagerberg, et al. 2000). By separating the results into two papers, the mortality results could be more rapidly disseminated and both papers could include more detailed analyses than if these two outcomes had been combined in one single manuscript.

We will now describe some of the typical, and necessary, results of the trial that are to be presented. Some of these results may best be presented in a graphical display, and others as tables. In some cases, either is acceptable. As we go through the elements, we will comment on those for which we have a recommendation regarding the style of display.

One of the first tables or figures is a summary of the screening process, typically shown in the format of the "CONSORT diagram" (Moher et al. 2001). While the subjects enrolled are rarely a representative sample (nor do they need to be), it is still useful for the reader and practicing physician to see how many subjects were screened but did not qualify or volunteer for the trial. There cannot be great detail in this table but it is useful to know how many subjects were excluded for some of the major entry criteria and the number of subjects who did not consent. This type of information gives physicians a sense of how the results might pertain to their own practice. This table should also clearly present the exact number of subjects randomized. The reader can judge how close the trial came to the recruitment goal and then knows how much data to expect for any given variable, based on the accompanying tables. An example from the MERIT-HF study is shown in Figure 12.1.

The interpretation of trial results may depend heavily on the time frame in which the trial took place. Medical practice, and even population attributes, can change over this period. The "Results" section should report important dates including the dates on which subject accrual began and ended, as well as the ending date of follow-up.

The next standard table (see Table 12.1) describes the major baseline characteristics, as defined in the protocol, by treatment arm with an indication of where, if at all, imbalances occurred. This table is important for two primary reasons. First, it describes in some detail the characteristics of the subjects or

Figure 1. Patient Flow in the Randomized
Controlled Trial

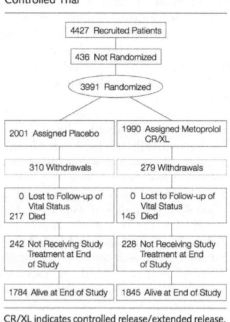

CR/XL indicates controlled release/extended release.

Figure 12.1 *CONSORT diagram (Figure 1) from MERIT-HF study report (Hjal-*
marson et al. 2000). Copyright © 2000 American Medical Association. All rights
reserved.

participants that actually received intervention. This includes demographics,
known risk factors, and, perhaps, risk factors that proved to be important
during the conduct of the trial and can be compared to what the inclusion
and exclusion criteria in the protocol might have predicted. Even among subjects meeting eligibility criteria, the actual participants entered may have been
younger, sicker, or had more prior exposure to other medications than anticipated.

The second use for the baseline table is to establish that the two treatment
groups were comparable with respect to important factors that were measured
at baseline. In addition to descriptive statistics, many readers want to quantify
the observed baseline differences using p-values in order to identify imbalances
that might confound the treatment comparison. We know with certainty that
any differences we see are due to chance and that comparing a greater number of baseline variables means a greater likelihood of imbalance. Thus, the
usual measures of "statistical significance" such as p-values are not meaningful for baseline comparisons in randomized trial. While not recommended,
if p-values are included at the request of journals or other co-authors, they

should be interpreted cautiously. If potential covariate imbalances are noted, covariate adjustment methods for the major outcomes may be appropriate, and presented in either later tables or in the text. As shown in Table 12.1 from MERIT-HF, the baseline covariates are extremely well balanced for both demographics and heart failure risk factors.

Table 12.1 *Baseline table (Table 1) from MERIT-HF study report (Hjalmarson et al. 2000). Copyright © 2000 American Medical Association. All rights reserved.*

Table 1. Baseline Characteristics of the Randomization Groups*		
	Treatment Group	
Characteristics	Metoprolol CR/XL (n = 1990)	Placebo (n = 2001)
Age, mean, y	63.9	63.7
Sex, % female	23	22
White, %	94	94
Ischemic etiology of heart failure, %	65	66
NYHA class, %		
II	41	41
III	56	55
IV	3.4	3.8
Ejection fraction, mean	0.28	0.28
Previous myocardial infarction, %	48	49
Time since last myocardial infarction <1 y, %	8	7
Hypertension, %	44	44
Diabetes mellitus, %	25	24
Medications, %		
Diuretics	91	90
ACE inhibitor	89	90
A-II–blocker	7	6
ACE inhibitor or A-II–blocker	95	96
Digitalis	63	64
Spironolactone	7	8

*CR/XL indicates controlled release/extended release; NYHA, New York Heart Association; ACE, angiotensin-converting enzyme; and A-II, angiotensin II.

Once the balance across treatment arms among baseline covariates has been established, a description of treatment and protocol compliance should be presented. The reader needs to know how much of the treatment that was specified in the protocol was received. If a trial demonstrates a statistically significant positive benefit but the compliance was less than anticipated, the interpretation is still that the treatment is beneficial. On the other hand, if a trial comparing standard care plus an experimental treatment to standard care alone produced a neutral outcome with poor compliance, the result could be due either to an ineffective experimental treatment or to poor adherence to assigned treatment.

The publication should also report the relevant concomitant medication that subjects in each treatment arm received. This can be important if subjects in one of the arms received more of a particular or key concomitant medication or therapy than those in the others. It is ethically mandated that all subjects receive the best available care. This may result in differences in concomitant care between treatment groups and these differences may affect the interpretation of the results. For example, if subjects in the experimental treatment arm received more of a particular concomitant medication, it may be difficult to distinguish the effect of the experimental treatment from that of the concomitant medication. This can be especially problematic in unblinded trials. Because most concomitant medication is reported on a log-form (see Chapter 6), it is often of poorer quality and reliability than other data. Nonetheless, the use of any important concomitant medications should be reported.

Compliance to the protocol beyond concomitant medication and experimental medication should also be reported for each treatment arm. For example, the completeness of subject clinic visits, the percent of subject visits within the prescribed time window, and the completeness of prescribed procedures and measurements are important. The number of participants lost to follow-up should be reported. If protocol compliance is not as expected or not acceptable, then the results may not be easily understood. Because non-compliance with the protocol procedures is likely not to happen at random, it is important that this information be presented.

The primary outcome(s) and major secondary outcomes are the next results to present. If the trial has identified a single primary outcome, then this result should be highlighted. If there is more than one primary outcome, all primary outcomes should be clearly identified as such. Secondary outcomes may be shown in the same table as the primary outcomes as long as they are clearly identified.

If the outcomes are summarized by sample means, the tables should indicate, for each treatment arm, the sample size, the mean value, and the standard deviation or standard error. In addition, the standardized test statistic or the corresponding p-value (or both) should be shown. Also, it is helpful to show the estimated treatment difference and the 95% confidence interval. There has been debate whether p-values or confidence intervals should be presented in published reports. Our recommendation is that both should be presented since they convey different information, but we agree with some authors that the confidence intervals are preferred since they contain more useful information.

A time-to-event outcome should include Kaplan-Meier (Kaplan and Meier 1958) survival or mortality plots that also indicate the number of subjects at risk at selected time points in the follow-up. In addition, a table should also be included summarizing the number of events in each arm and the statistic used

Table 12.2 *Composite outcome table (Table 2) from MERIT-HF study report (Hjal-marson et al. 2000). Copyright © 2000 American Medical Association. All rights reserved.*

Table 2. Effect of Metoprolol CR/XL and Placebo on Combined End Points*

Combined End Points	Metoprolol CR/XL Group, No. of Patients (n = 1990)	Placebo Group, No. of Patients (n = 2001)	Total	Risk Reduction, % (95% Confidence Interval)
Total mortality or all-cause hospitalization	641	767	**1408**	19 (10-27)
Total mortality or hospitalization due to worsening heart failure	311	439	**750**	31 (20-40)
Death or heart transplantation	150	218	**368**	32 (16-45)
Cardiac death or nonfatal acute myocardial infarction	139	225	**364**	39 (25-51)
Total mortality or hospitalization or emergency department visit due to worsening heart failure	318	455	**773**	32 (21-41)

*Only the first end point that occurred in each patient was counted. $P<.001$ for all comparisons. CR/XL indicates controlled release/extended release.

for comparing the survival curves, typically the log-rank test statistic, and its corresponding p-value. The table should also include a summary statistic such as a relative risk, odds ratio, or hazard ratio with a 95% confidence interval. Examples of these presentations from MERIT-HF (MERIT-HF Study Group 1999) are shown in Table 12.2 and Figure 12.2.

After the primary and secondary outcomes have been presented, most trial reports present subgroup analyses to assess the consistency of the results across the range of patients the practicing physician might encounter. The important point is not that each subgroup result be "statistically significant" but that the results are generally consistent. While absolute consistency might seem to be the ideal, it should not be expected. The size of the observed treatment differences can vary considerably because of random variation due to the smaller sample sizes in most baseline subgroups. Real differences in treatment effect might be present, but it is difficult to distinguish real differences from random differences. One convenient way to represent subgroup results is illustrated by Figure 12.3, taken from the MERIT-HF trial (Hjalmarson et al. 2000). In this figure, each hazard ratio is plotted with a 95% confidence interval for several standard subgroups of interest in the treatment of heart failure. The results are remarkably consistent in direction of treatment benefit with relatively small variations in the size of the effect. Tests for treatment-by-subgroup interactions can be provided as part of the figure if desired, or described in the text for subgroups for which a qualitative interaction is of interest.

In order to understand and assess the risk-to-benefit ratio for a new treatment, the publication must present serious adverse events (SAEs) in a table. An example from MERIT-HF is shown in Table 12.3. SAEs are usually defined

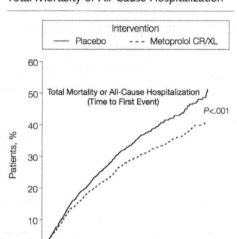

Figure 2. Cumulative Percentages (Time to First Event) for the Combined End Point of Total Mortality or All-Cause Hospitalization

Figure 12.2 *Composite outcome figure (Figure 2) from MERIT-HF study report (Hjalmarson et al. 2000) (modified slightly from the original). Copyright © 2000 American Medical Association. All rights reserved.*

as adverse events that are either life-threatening, result in permanent damage, or require hospitalization. Trials also collect information on less serious adverse events (AEs) and some of these may also be reported. Many of these are often of very low frequency and not of great interest. Some AEs, however, may reflect how well a patient may tolerate the new treatment. The tables of the primary and secondary outcomes combined with SAE results form the basis for assessing the risk-to-benefit ratio and thus the overall interpretation of the results. Thus, it is important that the SAEs and relevant AEs be reported completely and accurately.

There are many other results that trials might report such as the results from sub-studies or ancillary studies. These are often presented in separate publications. Major trials often yield numerous papers subsequent to the main results paper(s). These subsequent publications may expand on particular results appearing in the primary paper, or address new questions not covered in initial publication.

Figure 4. Absolute Numbers and Relative Risks (Time to First Event) for Total Mortality or All-Cause Hospitalization and for Total Mortality or Hospitalization Due to Worsening Heart Failure in Predefined Subgroups According to Baseline Characteristics

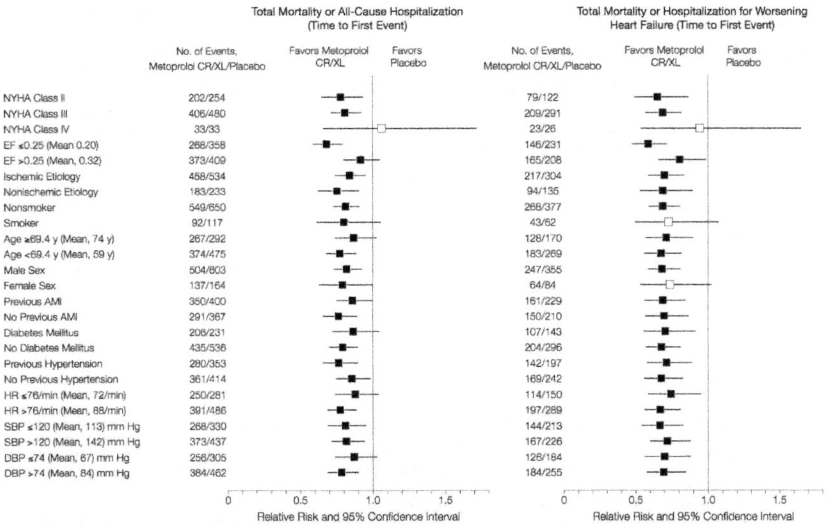

Filled squares indicate subgroups with a total of 180 events or more; open squares, subgroups with a total of less than 180 events (low power); CR/XL, controlled release/extended release; NYHA, New York Heart Association; EF, ejection fraction; AMI, acute myocardial infarction; HR, heart rate; SBP, systolic blood pressure; and DBP, diastolic blood pressure.

Figure 12.3 *Subgroup analyses figure (Figure 4) from MERIT-HF study report (Hjalmarson et al. 2000). Copyright © 2000 American Medical Association. All rights reserved.*

Discussion Section

While the "Methods" section of the paper should present the trial design and the "Results" section should provide the trial results with little or no interpretation or editorial comment, the "Discussion" section offers the authors the opportunity to give their interpretation of the results. The authors may summarize in the opening paragraphs what they believe the results mean. For some trials, this may be obvious, but for others it may take considerable effort and insight. The "Discussion" section should comment on how the actual trial conduct and results were relative to what was expected in the protocol and the planning process. Few trials turn out exactly as expected so authors should not be defensive or apologetic. Mistakes and disappointments should also be discussed.

The "Discussion" section should put the results of the current trial in the context of previous trials. Each trial contributes important information. For example, are the results scientifically consistent with previous knowledge about the treatment and are the results consistent with previous relevant trials? Perhaps the current trial focused on a higher risk group or one of the subgroups identified in a previous trial. For example, the MERIT-HF and

Table 12.3 *Adverse event table (Table 4) from MERIT-HF study report (Hjalmarson et al. 2000). Copyright © 2000 American Medical Association. All rights reserved.*

Table 4. Cause-Specific Adverse Events Leading to Withdrawal of Study Drug According to Absolute Value for Net Difference Between the Randomization Groups*

Adverse Events†	Metoprolol CR/XL, No. (%)	Placebo, No. (%)	Net Difference, % per First Year
Heart failure	78 (3.9)	117 (5.8)	−2.2
Atrial fibrillation	2 (0.1)	17 (0.8)	−0.8
Angina pectoris	9 (0.5)	20 (1.0)	−0.6
Bradycardia‡	16 (0.8)	5 (0.2)	0.6
Hypotension‡	12 (0.6)	5 (0.2)	0.4
Dizziness‡	12 (0.6)	6 (0.3)	0.3
Fatigue	14 (0.7)	9 (0.4)	0.3
Dyspnea	15 (0.8)	12 (0.6)	0.2
Myocardial infarction§	11 (0.6)	15 (0.7)	−0.2
All patients with any adverse event	196 (9.8)	234 (11.7)	−2.2

*CR/XL indicates controlled release/extended release. Adverse events that led to withdrawal of study drug are specified if the frequency of the cause-specific adverse event was greater than 0.5% in either group. The net difference (metoprolol CR/XL – placebo) refers to the percentage of patients treated during the first year of treatment (1836 vs 1819 patient-years of follow-up until withdrawal of study medicine or death in the metoprolol CR/XL group and placebo group, respectively).
†Patients may have had more than 1 reason for withdrawal.
‡The cumulative net difference for bradycardia, dizziness, and hypotension in the metoprolol CR/XL group was 0.9%.
§The total number of patients who had a myocardial infarction during follow-up was 35 vs 41 in the metoprolol CR/XL and placebo groups, respectively.

CIBIS-II (CIBIS-II Investigators 1999) trials demonstrated that two drugs in the beta-blocker class reduced mortality and mortality/heart failure hospitalization in subjects with Class II and III heart failure. While there were Class IV subjects in these two trials, there were not enough to adequately answer whether beta-blocker drugs should be used in this more severe class of patients. The COPERNICUS trial (Packer et al. 2001) was designed and conducted to address this question. The results were consistent with previous, but limited, data and established convincingly that this class of drugs reduced both mortality and mortality/heart failure hospitalization in a wide range of patients.

It is also important to note inconsistencies, either internally or with previous results. A small, early trial of an inotropic drug, vesnarinone, in subjects with heart failure suggested a 50% reduction in mortality in the low dose arm compared to the placebo arm (Feldman, Bristow, Parmley, et al. 1993). A high dose arm, however, had been discontinued earlier because of apparent toxicity. This inconsistency resulted in failure to receive regulatory approval and led investigators to conduct a second, much larger trial (Cohn et al. 1998) called the Vesnarinone Trial (VesT). In VesT, the mortality rates were significantly higher for subjects on vesnarinone than for those on placebo. The inconsistency observed in the earlier trial proved to be an important result prompting further research and discovery.

The authors should also describe how the results of the trial pertain to clinical practice based on their experience in the trial. In particular, they should discuss the generalizability of the current results to the general practice of medicine. The current trial may be a rigorous test of the new experimental treatment in a select group of subjects, but the results may or may not be relevant to all patients with the same diagnosis. For example, some future potential patients may not be eligible because of the need for contraindicated treatments, or because there are not enough subjects of that type in the current trial. Until COPERNICUS was completed, physicians were uncertain about whether Class IV heart failure patients should be treated with beta-blockers or not. Given the limited experience with these patients, MERIT-HF and CIBIS-II investigators[1] could only speculate about the potential benefit of beta-blockers in this population, but such speculation is important as it can motivate future research.

The statistician associated with the trial should play an active role in not only preparing the analysis, tables, and figures, but also in the interpretation. As discussed in Chapter 11, results can easily be interpreted inappropriately. Some analyses are more definitive in answering a question while others are less definitive. The difference between these types of analyses must be made clear.

Authorship/Attribution

A clinical trial obviously requires contributions from many individuals, not all of which can be authors of the primary or later publications. Two practices have emerged over the past decades to address this problem. One practice is to publish manuscripts using a group authorship such as the "Coronary Drug Project Research Group."[2] Many components of the trial research group, including the actual writing team, are then identified in the appendix. This practice has recently met with some resistance from medical journals, preferring to have specific individuals identified and accountable for the contents of the article. In response, more recent trial reports have identified selected individuals to be authors, along with the trial research group name. The entire trial research group is then enumerated as before in the appendix. A principal investigator with perhaps one or two associates may be listed for each of the participating clinical centers. Often the study chair, the steering committee, and other key committees are also identified. The Data Monitoring Committee, if there was one, should be identified, as well as the statistical center or data coordinating center. The study statistician might well be one of the lead authors since that individual has contributed to the trial design and much of the technical analysis and has participated in the drafting of the primary and secondary papers. This does, however, require special effort by the statistician, but this effort is necessary for the publication to be of the highest quality.

It is important that agreement regarding authorship be reached and doc-

---

[1] MERIT-HF Study Group (1999), Hjalmarson, Goldstein, Fagerberg, et al. (2000), CIBIS-II Investigators (1999)

[2] The Coronary Drug Project Research Group (1975, 1980)

umented in the protocol or another planning document before the trial is complete. For those in academia as well as for government and industry, recognition of scholarly achievement, as measured by authorship on publications, is important. Allowance should also be made for those investigators who have either successfully recruited the most subjects or made extraordinary efforts on key committees. Our experience is that these issues can be addressed most satisfactorily if done in advance.

12.3 Problems

12.1 Find an article in a medical journal that reports the results of a randomized clinical trial. Try to identify the components of a good clinical trial publication as discussed in this chapter. Discuss which elements were included by the authors and which are missing or inadequate.

APPENDIX A

Delta Method, Maximum Likelihood Theory, and Information

A.1 Delta Method

One simple technique commonly used for deriving variance estimators for functions of random variables is called the *delta method*. Suppose that a random variable X has mean μ and variance σ^2. Suppose further that we construct a new random variable Y by transforming X, $Y = g(X)$, for a continuously differentiable function $g(\cdot)$. Then, by Taylor's theorem, $g(X) = g(\mu) + g'(\mu)(X - \mu) + O((X - \mu)^2)$. Ignoring the higher order terms, we have that

$$E[Y] = E[g(X)] \approx g(\mu)$$

and

$$\begin{aligned} \mathrm{Var}[Y] &= E[g(X) - g(\mu)]^2 \\ &\approx g'(\mu)^2 E[X - \mu]^2 \\ &= \sigma^2 g'(\mu)^2. \end{aligned}$$

This simple approximation to the variance of Y is often referred to as the *delta method*.

Example A.1. Suppose $Y = \log(X)$, then $g'(x) = 1/x$, so $\mathrm{Var}(Y) \approx \sigma^2/\mu^2$.
□

A.2 Asymptotic Theory for Likelihood Based Inference

Suppose that Y is a random variable with the p.d.f. $f_Y(y; \theta)$ where θ is an unknown parameter of dimension p, and $f_Y(y; \theta)$ is twice differentiable in a neighborhood of the true value of θ. The *likelihood function*, $L_Y(\theta)$, is the density function for the observed values of Y viewed as a function of the parameter θ. If $Y_i, Y_2, \ldots, Y_n$ are an i.i.d. sample, then, letting $\boldsymbol{Y} = (Y_1, Y_2, \ldots, Y_n)$,

$$L_{\boldsymbol{Y}}(\theta) = \prod_{j=1}^{n} f_Y(y_j; \theta). \tag{A.1}$$

The *maximum likelihood estimate* (MLE) of θ is the value of θ, $\hat{\theta}$, that maximizes $L_Y(\theta)$, or equivalently, the value of θ for which

$$U_Y(\theta) = \frac{\partial \log L_Y(\theta)}{\partial \theta} = 0.$$

For the cases we will consider, this equation will have a unique solution. The function $U_Y(\theta)$ is known as the *efficient score* for θ. It can be shown that $E_\theta U_Y(\theta) = 0$ where E_θ denotes expectation when Y has distribution $f_Y(y; \theta)$.

An important special case is the one in which $f_Y(y; \theta)$ is part of an *exponential family*. That is, $f_Y(y; \theta) = \exp(\eta(x, \theta)T(y) - A(\eta(x, \theta)))$ where x is a subject level covariate (possibly vector valued), $\eta(x, \theta)$ is a function of the covariate and the parameter θ, and $A(\eta)$ is a function of η which forces $f_Y(y; \theta)$ to integrate to one. In this case, $A'(\eta) = ET(y)$ and the score function has the form $U_Y(\theta) = \sum_i B(x, \theta)(T(y) - A'(\eta))$, where $B(x, \theta) = \partial \eta(x, \theta)/\partial \theta$. Hence, the score function is a linear combination of the centered, transformed observations $T(y) - ET(x)$ and the solution to the score equations (A.1) satisfies $\sum_i B(x, \theta)T(y) = \sum_i B(x, \theta)ET(y)$.

Example A.2. Suppose we have the Gaussian linear model $y_i = x_i^T \beta + \epsilon_i$ where x_i and β are p-dimensional vectors and the ϵ_i are i.i.d. $N(0, \sigma^2)$. For simplicity we will assume that σ^2 is known. The log-likelihood is

$$\log L_Y(\beta) = -n\log(2\sigma^2)/2 - \sum_i (y_i - x_i^T \beta)^2/2\sigma^2$$

$$= -\frac{1}{2\sigma^2} \sum_i y_i x_i^T \beta - (x_i^T \beta)^2 + y_i^2 - n\log(2\sigma^2)/2. \quad (A.2)$$

The score equations are

$$U_Y(\beta) = -\sum x_i(y_i - x_i^T \beta)/\sigma^2 = 0.$$

Since, in general, x_i is a vector, the score function is vector valued, so the score equations are a linear system of p equations in p unknowns. If the model has an intercept term, β_1, so that $x_i = (1, x_{2i}, x_{3i}, \ldots, x_{pi})^T$, then we have that the sum of all the observations equals the sum of their expected values, $\sum_i y_i = \sum_i x_i^T \beta$. If we have two treatment groups and one of the covariates is the indicator of treatment, letting R_j be the set of indices of subjects in treatment group $j = 1, 2$, we have

$$\sum_{i \in R_j} y_i = \sum_{i \in R_j} x_i^T \beta.$$

In some settings it may be computationally simpler to fit the model by computing the expected values directly by forcing the required marginal totals to equal the expected totals, rather than by direct estimation of model parameters. □

The expected value of the derivative of $-U_Y(\theta)$ with respect to θ is known as the *Fisher information*, $\mathcal{I}(\theta)$. In the one dimensional case it can be shown that

$$
\begin{aligned}
\mathcal{I}(\theta) &= -E_\theta\left[\frac{\partial^2 \log L_{\mathbf{Y}}(\theta)}{\partial \theta^2}\right] \\
&= E_\theta[U_{\mathbf{Y}}(\theta)^2] \\
&= \mathrm{Var}_\theta[U_{\mathbf{Y}}(\theta)].
\end{aligned}
$$

In many situations, we cannot compute $\mathcal{I}(\theta)$ directly, but will need to use an estimate obtained from the data. It can be shown that under modest regularity conditions, $\hat{\theta} \overset{a}{\sim} N(\theta, \mathcal{I}^{-1}(\theta))$ where $\overset{a}{\sim}$ indicates the asymptotic distribution, e.g., asymptotically $\hat{\theta}$ has a normal distribution with mean θ and variance $\mathcal{I}^{-1}(\theta)$. Note that $\mathcal{I}(\theta)$ is of the expected curvature of the log-likelihood function at the true value of θ. Larger values of $\mathcal{I}(\theta)$ indicate that the likelihood function is more sharply peaked, and therefore, estimates of θ are more precise.

These results can be generalized to the case where θ is a p-dimensional vector with no difficulty. In this case the score, $U_{\mathbf{Y}}(\theta)$ is a p-dimensional vector of partial derivatives, and the Fisher information, $\mathcal{I}(\theta)$, is a matrix of partial derivatives. The asymptotic covariance matrix of $\hat{\theta}$ is the matrix inverse $\mathcal{I}^{-1}(\theta)$.

A.3 Hypothesis Testing

Three commonly used approaches for testing $H_0: \theta = \theta_0$ are as the *likelihood ratio test*, the *score test*, and the *Wald test*. Here we assume that θ has dimension p. In general there may be other unknown parameters, known as *nuisance parameters*, that are not of interest but need to be taken into account.

Example A.3. Suppose that we have two binomial samples, $y_i \sim \mathrm{Bin}(n_i, \pi_i)$, $i = 1, 2$, with y_i the number of successes, n_i the number of trials and π_i the success probability in each sample. If the null hypothesis is $H_0: \pi_1 = \pi_2$, we can let $\Delta = \pi_2 - \pi_2$ so that H_0 is equivalent to $H_0: \Delta = 0$. We may write the joint distribution of y_1 and y_2 in terms of Δ and either π_1 or π_2. We may say that Δ is the parameter of interest and π_1 is the nuisance parameter. $\qquad\square$

In general, if we let ν be the (possibly vector valued) nuisance parameter and $L_{\mathbf{Y}}(\theta, \nu)$ be the likelihood function, then the score function has two components, $U_{\mathbf{Y}}(\theta, \nu) = (U_{\theta,\mathbf{Y}}(\theta, \nu), U_{\nu,\mathbf{Y}}(\theta, \nu))$, where $U_{\theta,\mathbf{Y}}(\theta, \nu) = \partial \log L_{\mathbf{Y}}(\theta, \nu)/\partial\theta$ and $U_{\nu,\mathbf{Y}}(\theta, \nu) = \partial \log L_{\mathbf{Y}}(\theta, \nu)/\partial\nu$. Under $H_1: \theta \neq \theta_0$ let $(\hat{\theta}, \hat{\nu})$ be the solution to $U_{\mathbf{Y}}(\theta, \nu) = 0$ while under H_0, let $\tilde{\nu}$ be the solution to $U_{\theta,\mathbf{Y}}(\theta_0, \nu) = 0$.

The Fisher information can be written in partitioned matrix form as

$$
\mathcal{I}(\theta, \nu) = -\begin{bmatrix} U_{\theta,\theta,\mathbf{Y}}(\theta,\nu) & U_{\theta,\nu,\mathbf{Y}}(\theta,\nu) \\ U_{\nu,\theta,\mathbf{Y}}(\theta,\nu) & U_{\nu,\nu,\mathbf{Y}}(\nu,\nu) \end{bmatrix} = \begin{bmatrix} \mathcal{I}_{\theta,\theta} & \mathcal{I}_{\theta,\nu} \\ \mathcal{I}_{\nu,\theta} & \mathcal{I}_{\nu,\nu} \end{bmatrix}
$$

where

$$
U_{s,t,\mathbf{Y}}(\theta, \nu) = \frac{\partial \log L_{\mathbf{Y}}(\theta, \nu)}{\partial s \partial t}.
$$

The covariance matrix of the vector $(\hat{\theta}, \hat{\nu})$ can be written

$$\mathrm{Var}(\hat{\theta}, \hat{\nu}) = \mathcal{I}(\theta, \nu)^{-1}$$
$$= \begin{bmatrix} (\mathcal{I}_{\theta,\theta} - \mathcal{I}_{\theta,\nu}\mathcal{I}_{\nu,\nu}^{-1}\mathcal{I}_{\nu,\theta})^{-1} & -(\mathcal{I}_{\theta,\theta} - \mathcal{I}_{\theta,\nu}\mathcal{I}_{\nu,\nu}^{-1}\mathcal{I}_{\theta,\nu})^{-1}\mathcal{I}_{\theta,\nu}\mathcal{I}_{\nu,\nu}^{-1} \\ \mathcal{I}_{\nu,\nu}^{-1}\mathcal{I}_{\nu,\theta}(\mathcal{I}_{\theta,\theta} - \mathcal{I}_{\theta,\nu}\mathcal{I}_{\nu,\nu}^{-1}\mathcal{I}_{\theta,\nu})^{-1} & (\mathcal{I}_{\nu,\nu} - \mathcal{I}_{\nu,\theta}\mathcal{I}_{\theta,\theta}^{-1}\mathcal{I}_{\nu,\theta}) \end{bmatrix}$$

The three tests can now be described.

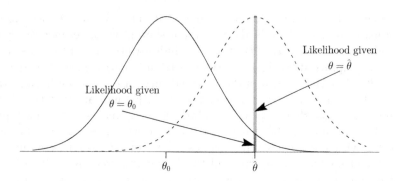

Figure A.1 *Graphical illustration of likelihood ratio test.*

1. Likelihood Ratio Test (LRT). The test statistic is twice the log-likelihood ratio:

$$2\log\frac{L_{\boldsymbol{Y}}(\hat{\theta}, \hat{\nu})}{L_{\boldsymbol{Y}}(\theta_0, \tilde{\nu})} \overset{a}{\sim} \chi_p^2 \text{ under } H_0$$

where χ_p^2 is the χ^2 distribution with p degrees of freedom. Figure A.1 illustrates the principle underlying the LRT when there are no nuisance parameters. Since $(\hat{\theta}, \hat{\nu})$ is the MLE, the likelihood evaluated at $(\hat{\theta}, \hat{\nu})$ is at least as large as the likelihood evaluated at $(\theta_0, \hat{\nu})$. If the likelihood ratio is large enough, there is strong evidence from the data that the observations do not arise from the distribution $f_Y(y; \theta_0)$.

2. Wald test. Since the upper left block of the matrix $\mathcal{I}(\theta)^{-1}$ is the asymptotic covariance matrix of $\hat{\theta}$, we have that

$$(\hat{\theta} - \theta_0)^T(\mathcal{I}_{\theta,\theta} - \mathcal{I}_{\theta,\nu}\mathcal{I}_{\nu,\nu}^{-1}\mathcal{I}_{\nu,\theta})(\hat{\theta} - \theta_0) \overset{a}{\sim} \chi_p^2 \text{ under } H_0,$$

where the $\mathcal{I}_{s,t}$ are evaluated at $(\hat{\theta}, \tilde{\nu})$.

3. Score (Rao) test. We have under H_0, $U_{\boldsymbol{Y}}(\theta_0, \hat{\nu}) \overset{a}{\sim} N(0, \mathcal{I}(\theta_0, \nu))$. Hence the test statistic is

$$U_{\boldsymbol{Y}}(\theta_0, \tilde{\nu})\mathcal{I}(\theta_0, \tilde{\nu})^{-1}U_{\boldsymbol{Y}}(\theta_0, \tilde{\nu}) \overset{a}{\sim} \chi_p^2 \text{ under } H_0.$$

In the exponential family case, the score test assesses the difference between the (possibly transformed) observed data, and its expectation. Since the second component of $U_{\boldsymbol{Y}}(\theta_0, \tilde{\nu})$ is zero, this can also be written

$$U_{\theta,\boldsymbol{Y}}(\theta_0, \nu)^T (\mathcal{I}_{\theta,\theta} - \mathcal{I}_{\theta,\nu}\mathcal{I}_{\nu,\nu}^{-1}\mathcal{I}_{\nu,\theta})^{-1} U_{\theta,\boldsymbol{Y}}(\theta_0, \nu) \overset{a}{\sim} \chi_p^2 \text{ under } H_0,$$

where the $\mathcal{I}_{s,t}$ are evaluated at $(\theta_0, \tilde{\nu})$. Note that unlike the LRT and the Wald test, there is no need to compute the MLE $\hat{\theta}$. The score test is often used to assess the association between the outcome and large numbers of covariates without the need to fit many different models.

Under modest assumptions, these tests are asymptotically equivalent. For ordinary linear regression models with i.i.d. Gaussian errors and known variance, these tests are in fact identical. For other models, the Wald and score tests are quadratic approximations to the likelihood ratio test. The Wald test is based on a quadratic approximation to the LRT at the MLE, while the score test is an approximation at θ_0. These approximations are illustrated by figure A.2.

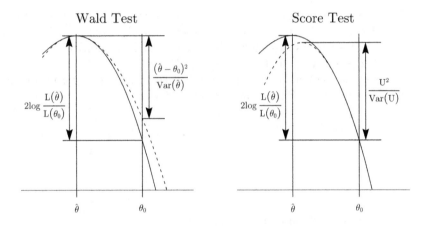

Figure A.2 *Illustrations showing Wald and score tests as quadratic approximations to the likelihood ratio test. The solid line represents the log-likelihood function and the dashed line represents the quadratic approximation.*

Example A.4. Returning to the binomial example, we have

$$L_{\boldsymbol{Y}}(\Delta, \pi_1) = K(y_1, n_1, y_2, n_2)\pi_1^{y_1}(1 - \pi_1)^{n_1 - y_1}(\pi_1 + \Delta)^{y_2}(1 - \pi_1 - \Delta)^{n_2 - y_2}$$

for a function $K(\cdot)$ which does not depend on the unknown parameters. The components of the score function are

$$U_{\Delta,\boldsymbol{Y}}(\Delta, \pi_1) = \frac{y_2}{\pi_1 + \Delta} - \frac{n_2 - y_2}{1 - \pi_1 - \Delta}$$

$$U_{\pi_1,\boldsymbol{Y}}(\Delta, \pi_1) = \frac{y_1}{\pi_1} - \frac{n_1 - y_1}{1 - \pi_1} + \frac{y_2}{\pi_1 + \Delta} - \frac{n_2 - y_2}{1 - \pi_1 - \Delta}.$$

It is easy to show that, under $H_0: \Delta = 0$, the MLE for π_1 is the overall mean $\tilde{\pi}_1 = (y_1 + y_2)/(n_1 + n_2)$, and, under $H_1: \Delta \neq 0$, $\hat{\pi}_1 = y_1/n_1$ and $\widehat{\Delta} = y_2/n_2 - y_1/n_1$.

The log-likelihood ratio is:

$$
\begin{aligned}
\log\left(\frac{L_Y(\widehat{\Delta}, \hat{\pi}_1)}{L_Y(0, \tilde{\pi}_1)}\right) &= y_1 \log \hat{\pi}_1 + (n_1 - y_1)\log(1 - \hat{\pi}_1) \\
&\quad + y_2 \log(\hat{\pi} + \widehat{\Delta}) + (n_2 - y_2)\log(1 - \hat{\pi}_1 - \Delta) \\
&\quad - y_1 \log \tilde{\pi}_1 - (n_1 - y_1)\log(1 - \tilde{\pi}_1) \\
&\quad - y_2 \log \tilde{\pi}_1 - (n_2 - y_2)\log(1 - \tilde{\pi}_1) \\
&= y_1 \log \frac{\hat{\pi}_1}{\tilde{\pi}_1} + (n_1 - y_1)\log(\frac{1 - \hat{\pi}_1}{1 - \tilde{\pi}_1}) \\
&\quad + y_2 \log(\frac{\hat{\pi}_1 + \widehat{\Delta}}{\tilde{\pi}_1}) + (n_2 - y_2)\log(\frac{1 - \hat{\pi}_1 - \Delta}{1 - \tilde{\pi}_1}) \\
&= \sum O \log \frac{O}{E} \quad\quad\quad\quad\quad\quad \text{(A.3)}
\end{aligned}
$$

where the sum in equation (A.3) is over the four cells in the two-by-two table of survival status by treatment, O represents the observed value in a given cell and E represents its expected value under H_0. Asymptotically, the statistic $2 \sum O \log \frac{O}{E}$ has a χ_1^2 distribution under H_0.

To perform the Wald and score tests, we need the Fisher information matrix. The elements of the Fisher information matrix are

$$
\begin{aligned}
\mathcal{I}_{\Delta,\Delta} = \mathcal{I}_{\Delta,\pi_1} = \mathcal{I}_{\pi_1,\Delta} &= E\left[\frac{y_2}{(\pi_1 + \Delta)^2} + \frac{(n_2 - y_2)}{(1 - \pi_1 - \Delta)^2}\right] \\
&= \frac{n_2}{(\pi_1 + \Delta)} + \frac{n_2}{(1 - \pi_1 - \Delta)} \\
&= \frac{n_2}{(\pi_1 + \Delta)(1 - \pi_1 - \Delta)}
\end{aligned}
$$

where the expectation is taken under H_1.

Similarly,

$$
\mathcal{I}_{\pi_1,\pi_1} = \frac{n_1}{(\pi_1)(1 - \pi_1)} + \frac{n_2}{(\pi_1 + \Delta)(1 - \pi_1 - \Delta)}.
$$

The variance of $\widehat{\Delta}$ is, therefore,

$$
\begin{aligned}
\text{Var}\widehat{\Delta} &= (\mathcal{I}_{\Delta,\Delta} - \mathcal{I}_{\Delta,\pi_1}\mathcal{I}_{\pi_1,\pi_1}^{-1}\mathcal{I}_{\pi_1,\Delta})^{-1} \\
&= \frac{\pi_1(1 - \pi_1)}{n_1} + \frac{(\pi_1 + \Delta)(1 - \pi_1 - \Delta)}{n_2}.
\end{aligned}
$$

Note that this is identical to the variance obtained directly using the binomial variance, $\text{Var } y_i/n_i = \pi_i(1 - \pi_i)/n_i$. The variance estimate is obtained by replacing π_1 and Δ by their estimates.

Therefore, the Wald test statistic for H_0 has form

$$
\frac{(y_2/n_2 - y_1/n_1)^2}{\hat{\pi}_1(1 - \hat{\pi}_1)/n_1 + (\hat{\pi}_1 + \widehat{\Delta})(1 - \hat{\pi}_1 - \widehat{\Delta})/n_2}.
$$

The score test is similar. Under H_0, we have

$$U_{\Delta,Y}(0,\tilde{\pi}_1) = \frac{y_2}{\tilde{\pi}_1} - \frac{n_2 - y_2}{1 - \tilde{\pi}_1}$$

$$= \frac{1}{\tilde{\pi}_1(1 - \tilde{\pi}_1)}(y_2 - n_2\tilde{\pi}_1)$$

which is proportional to the observed number of events in group 2 minus the expected number under H_0. Under H_0, the variance of $U_{\Delta,Y}(0,\tilde{\pi}_1)$ is $\mathcal{I}_{\Delta,\Delta} - \mathcal{I}_{\Delta,\pi_1}\mathcal{I}^{-1}_{\pi_1,\pi_1}\mathcal{I}_{\pi_1,\Delta} = (1/n_1 + 1/n_2)^{-1}/\pi_1(1 - \pi_1)$, so the score test statistic is

$$\left(\frac{y_2 - n_2\tilde{\pi}_1}{\tilde{\pi}_1(1 - \tilde{\pi}_1)}\right)^2 \tilde{\pi}_1(1 - \tilde{\pi}_1)(\frac{1}{n_1} + \frac{1}{n_2})$$

$$= \frac{(y_2 - n_2(y_1 + y + 2)/(n_1 + n_2))^2(n_1 + n_2)^3}{n_1 n_2(y_1 + y_2)(n_1 + n_2 - y_1 - y_2)}$$

which is the (uncorrected) Pearson χ^2 test statistic. It can be shown that the score statistic can also be written $\sum(O - E)^2/E$, where O and E are as in equation (A.3).

Note that the Wald test and the score test have similar form; the difference between them is that the Wald test uses the variance computed under H_1, while the score test uses the variance computed under H_0.   □

A.4 Computing the MLE

In most situations there is no closed form solution for the MLE, $\hat{\theta}$, but finding the solution requires an iterative procedure. One commonly used method for finding $\hat{\theta}$ is the *Newton-Raphson* procedure.

We begin with an initial guess $\hat{\theta}_0$, from which we generate a sequence of estimates $\hat{\theta}_1, \hat{\theta}_2, \hat{\theta}_3, \ldots$ until convergence is achieved. For $i = 1, 2, 3, \ldots$, $\hat{\theta}_i$ is derived from $\hat{\theta}_{i-1}$ by first applying Taylor's theorem. We have that

$$U_Y(\theta) = U_Y(\hat{\theta}_{i-1}) + U_{\theta,Y}(\hat{\theta}_{i-1})(\theta - \hat{\theta}_{i-1}) + \text{ higher order terms.}$$

Ignoring the higher order terms, we set the above equal to zero and solve for θ yielding

$$\hat{\theta}_i = \hat{\theta}_{i-1} - U_{\theta,Y}(\hat{\theta}_{i-1})^{-1}U_Y(\hat{\theta}_{i-1}). \tag{A.4}$$

Iteration stops once consecutive values of $\hat{\theta}_i$ differ by a sufficiently small amount.

Note that if θ is a vector of length p, the score function $U_Y(\theta)$ will be a vector of partial derivatives of length p, and $U_{\theta,Y}(\hat{\theta}_{i-1})$ will be the matrix of second order partial derivatives. Equation (A.4) will be an equation involving vectors and matrices.

A.5 Information

There are many different ways of assessing statistical information. Probably the most common information measure, and the one most important for our purposes, is the one we have already seen, *Fisher information*. In this section we discuss the features of Fisher information that play an important role in clinical trial design—specifically, for sample size determination and defining sequential monitoring procedures.

We introduce the concept of information with two simple examples.

Example A.5. Suppose that y_i are independent Gaussian random variables with mean μ and variance σ_i^2, so that they have a common mean but possibly different variances. Such data might arise, for example, if subjects have varying numbers of follow-up observations. For simplicity, we will assume that the σ_i^2 are known. The log-likelihood is $\log L_Y(\mu) = \sum_i -(y_i - \mu)^2/2\sigma_i^2$, the score function is $U_Y(\mu) = \sum_i (y_i - \mu)/\sigma_i^2$, and the Fisher information is $\mathcal{I}(\mu) = \sum_i 1/\sigma_i^2$. Let the null hypothesis be $H_0 : \mu = \mu_0$. The expected value of the score function under an alternative is $E_\mu U_Y(\mu_0) = \sum_i (\mu - \mu_0)/\sigma_i^2 = (\mu - \mu_0)\mathcal{I}(\mu)$, so $E_\mu U_Y(\mu_0)$ factors into a parameter associated with the difference of interest, $\Delta = \mu - \mu_0$, and the Fisher information. Hence, each subject contributes information regarding the true value of μ to the score function in proportion to its contribution to the Fisher information. $\qquad\square$

Example A.6. Second, suppose we have a time-to-failure outcome with constant hazard rate, $\lambda = \exp(\mu)$. Subjects are followed for maximum of C_i years, and let T_i be the minimum of the failure time and C_i. Let y_i be the indicator of failure at time T_i. The log-likelihood for μ_i is $\log L_Y(\mu) = \sum_i \mu y_i - \exp(\mu)T_i$. Hence, $U_Y(\mu) = \sum_i y_i - \exp(\mu)T_i$ and the Fisher information is $\mathcal{I}(\mu) = \exp(\mu)\sum_i ET_i = \sum_i 1 - \exp(-\lambda C_i)$. Under an alternative hypothesis,

$$
\begin{aligned}
E_\mu U_Y(\mu_0) &= \sum_i E_\mu y_i - e^{\mu_0} E_\mu T_i \\
&= \sum_i (1 - e^{-\lambda C_i})(1 - e^{\mu_0 - \mu}) \\
&= \mathcal{I}(\mu)(1 - e^{\mu_0 - \mu}) \\
&= \mathcal{I}(\mu)\Delta,
\end{aligned}
$$

a form similar to the Gaussian example above. Note that if $|\mu_0 - \mu|$ is small, then $\Delta = 1 - e^{\mu_0 - \mu} \approx \mu - \mu_0$, and the forms are identical. We also note that $\mathcal{I}(\mu)$ is the expected number of subjects experiencing events given the censoring times, C_i. In practice, this would be estimated by the total number of subjects observed to experience an event. $\qquad\square$

Another property of the score function, important in sequential monitoring, is the *independent increments* property. Suppose $U_{Y_1}(\mu)$ is the score function given the full data Y_1 at time t_1, and $U_{Y_2}(\mu)$ is the score function at a later time, t_2, given the full data $\boldsymbol{Y}_2$ (including $\boldsymbol{Y}_1$) observed at time t_1. For most test statistics of interest, when μ is the true value of the parameter, $U_{\boldsymbol{Y}_1}(\mu)$ and $U_{\boldsymbol{Y}_2}(\mu) - U_{\boldsymbol{Y}_1}(\mu)$ are independent with variances $\mathcal{I}_1(\mu)$ and $\mathcal{I}_2(\mu) - \mathcal{I}_1(\mu)$ when $\mathcal{I}_j(\mu)$ is the variance of $U_{\boldsymbol{Y}_j}(\mu)$. The independent increments property implies that $\mathrm{Cov}(U_{\boldsymbol{Y}_1}(\mu), U_{\boldsymbol{Y}_2}(\mu)) = \mathrm{Var}(U_{\boldsymbol{Y}_1}(\mu))$ and, hence, that $\mathrm{Cor}(U_{\boldsymbol{Y}_1}(\mu), U_{\boldsymbol{Y}_2}(\mu)) = \sqrt{\mathcal{I}_1(\mu)/\mathcal{I}_2(\mu)}$. Thus the entire asymptotic distribution of a vector of test statistics, $(U_{\boldsymbol{Y}_1}(\mu), U_{\boldsymbol{Y}_2}(\mu), \ldots, U_{\boldsymbol{Y}_K}(\mu))^T$ is characterized by the information, $(\mathcal{I}_1(\mu), \mathcal{I}_2(\mu), \ldots, \mathcal{I}_K(\mu))^T$. Specifically, $(U_{\boldsymbol{Y}_1}(\mu), U_{\boldsymbol{Y}_2}(\mu), \ldots, U_{\boldsymbol{Y}_K}(\mu))^T$ has mean zero and variance-covariance matrix

$$
\begin{bmatrix}
\mathcal{I}_1(\mu) & \mathcal{I}_1(\mu) & \cdots & \mathcal{I}_1(\mu) \\
\mathcal{I}_1(\mu) & \mathcal{I}_2(\mu) & \cdots & \mathcal{I}_2(\mu) \\
\vdots & \vdots & \ddots & \vdots \\
\mathcal{I}_1(\mu) & \mathcal{I}_2(\mu) & \cdots & \mathcal{I}_K(\mu)
\end{bmatrix}.
$$

Note that under alternative hypotheses, the score process no longer strictly satisfies the independent increments property, but for alternatives close to the null hypothesis the independent increments property is approximately satisfied.

Example A.7. Continuing Example A.6 above, suppose that T_{ij} and y_{ij} are observed for subject i at times t_1 and t_2, respectively, $t_1 < t_2$. Note that if $y_{i1} = 1$, then $y_{i2} = 1$ and $T_{i2} = T_{i1}$. Furthermore, if additional subjects are enrolled between times t_1 and t_2, we can consider all subjects to be observed at time t_1 by letting $y_{i1} = 0$ and $T_{i1} = 0$ for these subjects.

Therefore,

$$
\begin{aligned}
U_{\boldsymbol{Y}_2}(\mu) - U_{\boldsymbol{Y}_1}(\mu) &= \sum_i (y_{i2} - \exp(\mu)T_{i2}) - \sum_i (y_{i1} - \exp(\mu)T_{i1}) \\
&= \sum_i y_{i2} - y_{i1} - \exp(\mu)(T_{i2} - T_{i1}).
\end{aligned}
$$

To establish the independent increments property, we need to show that $E_\mu[(y_{i2} - y_{i1} - \exp(\mu)(T_{i2} - T_{i1}))(y_{i1} - \exp(\mu)T_{i1})] = 0$. If $y_{i1} = 1$, then $y_{i2} - y_{i1} - \exp(\mu)(T_{i2} - T_{i1}) = 0$. Therefore, $y_{i1}(y_{i2} - y_{i1} - \exp(\mu)(T_{i2} - T_{i1})) = 0$. Furthermore, we also have that

$$
\begin{aligned}
&E_\mu[e^\mu T_{i1}(y_{i2} - y_{i1} - e^\mu(T_{i2} - T_{i1}))] \\
&= e^\mu C_{i1} E_\mu[(y_{i2} - e^\mu(T_{i2} - C_{i1}))|y_{i1} = 0]\Pr\{y_{i1} = 0\}.
\end{aligned}
$$

Finally, $E_\mu[(y_{i2} - e^\mu(T_{i2} - C_{i1}))|y_{i1} = 0] = 0$ follows because the exponential distribution is "memoryless."[1]

$\square$

---

[1] If X is an exponential random variable with density $f(x) = \lambda e^{-\lambda x}$, the conditional density of the failure time X given that $X \geq x_0$ is $\lambda e^{-\lambda(x - x_0)}$.

The following example illustrates the case in which the parameter of interest is the effect of treatment and we also have a nuisance parameter.

Example A.8. Two sample exponential survival data. Suppose, in the setting of Example A.6, that we have a treatment variable, $z_i = 0, 1$, so that the likelihood is

$$\log L_{\boldsymbol{Y}}(\mu, \beta) = \sum_i (\mu + \beta z_i) y_i - e^{\mu + \beta z_i} T_i.$$

Under $H_0: \beta = 0$, $\hat{\mu} = \log(\sum_i y_i / \sum_i T_i)$, and $U_{\beta, \boldsymbol{Y}}(\hat{\mu}) = \sum_i z_i (y_i - e^{\hat{\mu}} T_i)$ which is the sum of the observed minus expected under H_0 in the group $z_i = 1$. The Fisher information for the parameter β has the form given by the inverse of the upper left entry of the partitioned matrix in equation (A.3). We have $\mathcal{I}_{\beta, \beta} = \mathcal{I}_{\beta, \mu} = \mathcal{I}_{\mu, \beta} = \sum_i z_i \exp(\hat{\mu}) E T_i = \sum_i z_i (1 - e^{-\hat{\lambda} C_i})$ and $\mathcal{I}_{\beta, \mu} = \sum_i 1 - e^{-\hat{\lambda} C_i}$, so

$$
\begin{aligned}
\mathcal{I}(\beta | \hat{\mu}) &= \mathcal{I}_{\beta, \beta} - \mathcal{I}_{\beta, \mu}^2 / \mathcal{I}_{\mu, \mu} \\
&= \frac{\left(\sum_i z_i (1 - e^{-\hat{\lambda} C_i})\right)\left(\sum_i (1 - z_i)(1 - e^{-\hat{\lambda} C_i})\right)}{\sum_i 1 - e^{-\hat{\lambda} C_i}}.
\end{aligned}
$$

In a trial in which a proportion, ξ, of subjects are randomized to $z_i = 1$, under H_0, asymptotically, $\sum_i z_i e^{\hat{\mu}} T_i / \sum_i e^{\hat{\mu}} T_i \approx \xi$ and so $\mathcal{I}(\beta | \hat{\mu}) \approx \xi(1 - \xi) \sum_i 1 - e^{-\hat{\lambda} C_i}$, which is proportional to the total expected number of subjects with an event.   □

Example A.9. Repeated measures data. Suppose that we have repeated measures data with compound symmetry correlation structure (see Chapter 8, page 236) with common mean μ for all observations. We can write the variance-covariance matrix for the vector of m_j observations, y_j, for the jth subject as $\sigma^2 (I_{m_j} + \rho J_{m_j} J_{m_j}^T)$ where I_m is the m-dimensional identity matrix, J_m is a m-dimensional vector of ones, and ρ is the common correlation. We assume that σ^2 and ρ are known. Using the fact that the inverse of the variance-covarance matrix is

$$\left(\sigma^2 (I_{m_j} + \rho J_{m_j} J_{m_j}^T)\right)^{-1} = \frac{1}{\sigma^2}\left(I_{m_j} - \frac{\rho}{1 + m_j \rho} J_{m_j} J_{m_j}^T\right),$$

the log-likelihood is

$$
\begin{aligned}
\log L_{\boldsymbol{Y}}(\mu) = \\
-K(\sigma^2, \rho) - \sum_j \tfrac{1}{2\sigma^2}(y_j - \mu J_{m_j})^T \left(I_{m_j} - \tfrac{\rho}{1 + m_j \rho} J_{m_j} J_{m_j}^T\right)(y_j - \mu J_{m_j}).
\end{aligned}
$$

The score function is

$$
U_Y(\mu) = \sum_j \frac{1}{\sigma^2} J_{m_j}^T \left(I_{m_j} - \frac{\rho}{1 + m_j\rho} J_{m_j} J_{m_j}^T \right) (y_j - \mu J_{m_j})
$$

$$
= \sum_j \frac{1}{\sigma^2(1 + m_j\rho)} J_{m_j}^T (y_j - \mu J_{m_j})
$$

and the Fisher information is

$$
\mathcal{I}(\mu) = \sum_j \frac{m_j}{\sigma^2(1 + m_j\rho)}.
$$

Now, suppose that at time t_1 we have m_j observations, y_j, for subject j and at a future time, t_2, we have m_j' observations, y_j', so that $m_j \le m_j'$, and y_j is a sub-vector of y_j'. Then the score function will satisfy the independent increments property if $\mathrm{Cov}(U_Y(\mu), U_{Y'}(\mu)) = \mathrm{Var}(U_Y(\mu))$, where Y' represents the full data at time t_2. We have

$$
\mathrm{Cov}\left(\frac{J_{m_j}^T y_j}{1 + m_j'\rho}, \frac{J_{m_j'}^T y_j'}{1 + m_j'\rho} \right) = \frac{\sigma^2 m_j m_j' \rho + m_j}{(1 + m_j\rho)(1 + m_j'\rho)}
$$

$$
= \frac{\sigma^2 m_j}{(1 + m_j\rho)}
$$

$$
= \mathrm{Var}\left(\frac{J_{m_j}^T y_j}{1 + m_j'\rho} \right).
$$

By summing over subjects we see that $U_Y(\mu)$ satisfies the independent increments property.   □

A.6 Brownian Motion

One dimensional Brownian motion is a continuous time stochastic process, $W(t)$, defined on $t \ge 0$, with $W(0) = 0$. Increments $W(t_2) - W(t_1)$ and $W(t_3) - W(t_2)$ are independent for $0 \le t_1 < t_2 < t_3$ and $W(t) \sim N(0, t)$. Thus, $\mathrm{Cor}(W(t_2), W(t_1)) = \sqrt{t_1/t_2}$.

We note several properties of Brownian motion processes:

1. $W(t)$ is continuous but nowhere differentiable. (The variance of the first divided difference is $\mathrm{Var}[(W(t + \Delta t) - W(t))/\Delta t] = 1/\Delta t$, so the limit does not exist).

2. It can also be shown (see Billingsley (1995), page 513) that if $M(t) = \sup_{0 \le s \le t} W(s)$, then $\Pr\{M(t) \ge m\} = 2(1 - \Phi(m/\sqrt{t}))$ where $\Phi(\cdot)$ is the CDF of the standard normal distribution.

3. $W(at)/\sqrt{a}$ is a Brownian motion process.

Brownian motion is useful in the clinical trial setting because a score process that satisfies the independent increments property can (asymptotically)

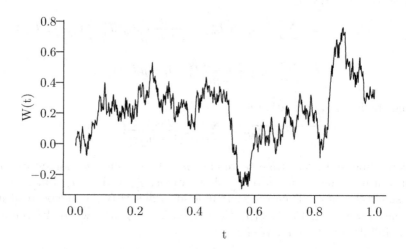

Figure A.3 *A sample Brownian motion path.*

be embedded in a Brownian motion process. Specifically, there is a Brownian motion process, $W(t)$, such that at any time during the trial the observed score function satisfies $U_{\boldsymbol{Y}}(\mu) = W(\mathcal{I}(\mu))$. Thus Fisher information plays a role in a score process equivalent to that of time, t, in a Brownian motion process. In practice, we generally re-scale the information based on the expected information at the end of the trial (see item 3. above). If we observe $U_{\boldsymbol{Y}_k}(\mu)$ at times t_k, $k = 1, 2, \ldots, K$, with information $\mathcal{I}_1, \mathcal{I}_2, \ldots, \mathcal{I}_K$, the *information fraction* (or *information time*) at time t_k is $\mathcal{I}_k/\mathcal{I}_K$. The so-called *B-value* (Lan and Wittes 1988), defined as $B = U_{\boldsymbol{Y}_k}(\mu)/\sqrt{\mathcal{I}_K}$, so that $B(t)$ with $t = \mathcal{I}_k/\mathcal{I}_K$, can be (asymptotically) embedded in a Brownian motion process.

References

Acquadro, C., R. Berzon, D. Dubois, N. Leidy, P. Marquis, D. Revicki, and M. Rothman (2003). Incorporating the patient's perspective into drug development and communication: an ad hoc task force report of the patient-reported outcomes (pro) harmonization group meeting at the food and drug administration. *Value Health 6*(5), 522–531.

Albers, G. W. on behalf of the SPORTIF Investigators (2004). Stroke prevention in atrial fibrillation: pooled analysis of SPORTIF III and V trials. *The American Journal of Managed Care 10*, s462–s473.

Albert, J. M. and D. L. DeMets (1994). On a model-based approach to estimating efficacy in clinical trials. *Statistics in Medicine 13*, 2323–2335.

ALLHAT Collaborative Research Group (2000). Major cardiovascular events in hypertensive patients randomized to doxazosin vs chlorthalidone: the antihypertensive and lipid-lowering treatment to prevent heart attack trial (allhat). *JAMA 283*, 1967–1975.

Alling, D. W. (1963). Early decision in the Wilcoxon two-sample test. *Journal of the American Statistical Association 58*, 713–720.

Altman, D. G., J. J. Deeks, and D. L. Sackett (1998). Odds ratios should be avoided when events are common. [letter]. *BMJ 317*, 1318.

Amberson Jr., J., B. McMahon, and M. Pinner (1931). A clinical trial of sanocrysin in pulmonary tuberculosis. *Am Rev Tuberc 24*, 401–435.

Anderson, T. (1960). A modification of the sequential probability ratio test to reduce the sample size. *Annals of Mathematical Statistics 31*, 165–197.

Angell, M. (1997). The ethics of clinical research in the third world. *N Engl J Med 337*, 847–849.

Anscombe, F. (1954). Fixed sample-size analysis of sequential observations. *Biometrics 10*, 89–100.

Antman, E. (2001). Clinical trials in cardiovascular medicine. *Circulation 103*, e101–e104.

Armitage, P., C. McPherson, and B. Rowe (1969). Repeated significance tests on accumulating data. *Journal of the Royal Statistical Society, Series A 132*, 235–244.

Aspirin Myocardial Infarction Study (AMIS) Research Group (1980). AMIS, a randomized controlled trial of aspirin in persons recovered from myocardial infarction. *JAMA 243*, 661–669.

Babb, J. and A. Rogatko (2004). Bayesian methods for cancer phase I clinical trials. In N. Geller (Ed.), *Advances in Clinical Trial Biostatistics*. Marcel-Dekker, NY.

Babb, J., A. Rogatko, and S. Zacks (1998). Cancer phase I clinical trials: Efficient dose escalation with overdose control. *Statistics in Medicine 17*, 1103–1120.

Barrett-Connor, E. and D. Grady (1998). Hormone replacement therapy, heart disease, and other considerations. *Ann Rev Pub Health 19*, 55–72.

Bartlett, R., D. Roloff, R. Cornell, A. Andrews, P. Dillon, and J. Zwischenberger

(1985). Extracorporeal circulation in neonatal respiratory failure: A prospective randomized study. *Pediatrics 76*, 479–487.

Beresford, S., B. Thompson, Z. Feng, A. Christianson, D. McLerran, and D. Patrick (2001). Seattle 5 a day worksite program to increase fruit and vegetable consumption. *Preventive Medicine 32*, 230–238.

Bergner, M., R. Bobbit, W. Pollard, D. Martin, and B. Gilson (1976). The sickness impact profile: validation of health and status measure. *Med Care 14*, 57–67.

Beta-Blocker Heart Attack Trial Research Group (1982). A randomized trial of propranolol in patients with acute myocardial infarction. *Journal of American Medical Association 247*, 1707.

Billingham, L., K. Abrams, and D. Jones (1999). Methods for the analysis of quality-of-life and survival data in health technology assessment. *Health Technol Assess 3*(10), 1–152.

Billingsley, P. (1995). *Probability and Measure*. John Wiley & Sons.

Blackwell, D. and J. Hodges Jr. (1957). Design for the control of selection bias. *Ann Math Stat 28*, 449–460.

Bolland, K. and J. Whitehead (2000). Formal approaches to safety monitoring of clinical trials in life-threatening conditions. *Statistics in Medicine 19*(21), 2899–2917.

Bollen, K. (1989). *Structural Equations with Latent Variables*. New York: Wiley.

Box, G. E. P. and N. R. Draper (1987). *Empirical Model-building and Response Surfaces*. John Wiley & Sons.

Bracken, M. B. and J. C. Sinclair (1998). When can odds ratios mislead? Avoidable systematic error in estimating treatment effects must not be tolerated. [letter; comment]. *BMJ 317*(7166), 1156–7.

Breslow, N. E. and N. E. E. Day (1980). *Statistical Methods in Cancer Research Volume I: The Analysis of Case-Control Studies*. OxfordUniv:Oxf.

Breslow, N. E. and N. E. E. Day (1988). *Statistical Methods in Cancer Research Volume II: The Design and Analysis of Cohort Studies*. OxfordUniv:Oxf.

Bristow, M., L. Saxon, J. Boehmer, S. Krueger, D. Kass, T. DeMarco, P. Carson, L. CiCarlo, D. DeMets, B. White, D. DeVries, and A. Feldman (2004). Cardiac-resynchronization therapy with or without an implantable defibrillator in advanced chronic heart failure. *New England Journal of Medicine 350*, 2140.

Bristow, M., L. Saxon, et al., and for the COMPANION Investigators (2004). Resynchronization therapy for patients with and without an implantable defibrillator in patients with advanced chronic heart failure. *N Engl J Med 350*, 2140–2150.

Brown, B. (1980). The crossover experiment for clinical trials. *Biometrics 36*, 69.

Bull, J. (1959). The historical development of clinical therapeutic trials. *J Chron Dis 10*, 218–248.

Burzykowski, T., G. Molenberghs, and M. Buyse (Eds.) (2005). *The Evaluation of Surrogate Endpoints*. New York: Springer.

Byar, D. P., A. M. Herzberg, and W.-Y. Tan (1993). Incomplete factorial designs for randomized clinical trials. *Statistics in Medicine 12*, 1629–1641.

Byar, D. P., R. M. Simon, M. D. Friedewald, J. J. Schlesselman, D. L. DeMets, J. H. Ellenberg, M. H. Gail, and J. H. Ware (1976). Randomized clinical trials, perspectives on some recent ideas. *New England Journal of Medicine 295*, 74–80.

Califf, R., S. Karnash, and L. Woodlief (1997). Developing systems for cost-effective auditing of clinical trials. *Controlled Clinical Trials 18*, 651–660.

Cardiac Arrhythmia Suppression Trial II Investigators (1992). Effects of the antiarrhythmic agent moricizine on survival after myocardial infarction. *N Engl J Med* *327*, 227–233.

Carmines, E. and R. Zeller (1979). *Reliability and Validity Assessment Series: Quantitative applications in the social sciences*, Volume 17. Sage University Press.

Carriere, K. (1994). Crossover designs for clinical trials. *Statistics in Medicine 13*, 1063–1069.

Carroll, R. J. (2004). Discussion of two important missing data issues. *Statistica Sinica 14*(3), 627–629.

Carroll, R. J. and D. Ruppert (1988). *Transformation and Weighting in Regression*. Chapman & Hall Ltd.

Carson, P., C. O'Connor, A. Miller, S. Anderson, R. Belkin, G. Neuberg, J. Wertheimer, D. Frid, A. Cropp, and M. Packer (2000). Circadian rhythm and sudden death in heart failure: results from prospective randomized amlodipine survival trial. *J Am Coll Cardiol 36*, 541–546.

Case, L. and T. Morgan (2001). Duration of accrual and follow-up for two-stage clinical trials. *Lifetime Data Analysis 7*, 21–38.

CASS Principal Investigators and their Associates (1983). Coronary artery surgery study (CASS): a randomized trial of coronary artery bypass surgery. *Circulation 68*, 939.

Cella, D., D. Tulsky, G. Gray, B. Sarafin, E. Lin, A. Bonomi, et al. (1993). The functional assessment of cancer therapy scale: development and validation of the general measure. *Journal of Clinical Oncology 11*(3), 570–579.

Chalmers, T., P. Celano, H. Sacks, and H. Smith Jr. (1983). Bias in treatment assignment in controlled clinical trials. *N Engl J Med 309*, 1358–1361.

Chalmers, T., R. Matta, H. Smith, and A. Kunzier (1977). Evidence favoring the use of anticoagulants in the hospital phase of acute myocardial infarction. *N Engl J Med 297*, 1091–1096.

Chang, M. and P. O'Brien (1986). Confidence intervals following group sequential tests. *Controlled Clinical Trials 7*, 18–26.

Chang, M. N., A. L. Gould, and S. M. Snapinn (1995). *P*-values for group sequential testing. *Biometrika 82*, 650–654.

Chassan, J. (1970). A note on relative efficiency in clinical trials. *J Clin Pharmacol 10*, 359–360.

Chen, J., D. DeMets, and K. Lan (2000). Monitoring multiple doses in a combined phase II/III clinical trial: Multivariate test procedures (dropping the loser designs). Technical Report 155, Department of Biostatistics and Medical Informatics, University of Wisconsin, Madison.

Chen, J., D. DeMets, and K. Lan (2003). Monitoring mortality at interim analyses while testing a composite endpoint at the final analysis. *Controlled Clinical Trials 23*, 16–27.

Cheung, K. and R. Chappell (2000). Sequential designs for phase I clinical trials with late-onset toxicities. *Biometrics 56*, 1177–1182.

Chi, Y.-Y. and J. G. Ibrahim (2006). Joint models for multivariate longitudinal and multivariate survival data. *Biometrics 62*(2), 432–445.

Chi, Y.-Y. and J. G. Ibrahim (2007). Bayesian approaches to joint longitudinal and survival models accommodating both zero and nonzero cure fractions. *Statistica Sinica 17*, 445–462.

CIBIS-II Investigators (1999). The Cardiac Insufficiency Bisoprolol Study II (CIBIS-II): a randomised trial. *Lancet 353*, 1–13.

Cochran, W. and G. Cox (1957). *Experimental Designs: 2nd Ed.* New York: John Wiley and Sons.

Cohn, J., S. Goldstein, B. Greenberg, B. Lorell, R. Bourge, B. Jaski, S. Gottlieb, F. McGrew, D. DeMets, and B. White (1998). A dose-dependent increase in mortality with vesnarinone among patients with severe heart failure. *New England Journal of Medicine 339*, 1810–1816.

Cook, T. D. (2000). Adjusting survival analysis for the presence of non-adjudicated study events. *Controlled Clinical Trials 21*(3), 208–222.

Cook, T. D. (2002a). *P*-value adjustment in sequential clinical trials. *Biometrics 58*(4), 1005–1011.

Cook, T. D. (2002b). Up with odds ratios! a case for the use of odds ratios when outcomes are common. *Academic Emergency Medicine 9*, 1430–1434.

Cook, T. D. (2003). Methods for mid-course corrections in clinical trials with survival outcomes. *Statistics in Medicine 22*(22), 3431–3447.

Cook, T. D., R. J. Benner, and M. R. Fisher (2006). The WIZARD trial as a case study of flexible clinical trial design. *Drug Information Journal 40*, 345–353.

Cook, T. D. and M. R. Kosorok (2004). Analysis of time-to-event data with incomplete event adjudication. *JASA 99*(468), 1140–1152.

Coronary Drug Project Research Group (1981). Practical aspects of decision making in clinical trials: the coronary drug project as a case study. *Controlled Clinical Trials 1*, 363–376.

Coumadin Aspirin Reinfarction Study (CARS) Investigators (1997). Randomised double–blind trial of fixed low–dose warfarin with aspirin after myocardial infarction. *Lancet 350*, 389–96.

Cox, D. (1958). *Planning of Experiments.* New York: John Wiley and Sons.

Cox, D. (1972). Regression models and life tables (with discussion). *Journal of the Royal Statistical Society, Series B 34*, 187–220.

Cox, D. R. and D. Oakes (1984). *Analysis of Survival Data.* Chapman & Hall Ltd.

Crosby, R., R. Kolotkin, and G. Williams (2003). Defining clinically meaningful change in health-related quality of life. *Journal of Clinical Epidemiology 56*, 395–407.

Cui, L., H. M. J. Hung, and S.-J. Wang (1999). Modification of sample size in group sequential clinical trials. *Biometrics 55*, 853–857.

Cusick, M., A. Meleth, E. Agron, M. Fisher, G. Reed, F. Ferris III, E. Chew, and the Early Treatment Diabetic Retinopathy Study Research Group (2005). Associations of mortality and diabetes complications in patients with Type 1 and Type 2 Diabetes. Early Treatment Diabetic Retinopathy Study Report No. 27. *Diabetes Care 28*, 617–625.

Cytel Software Corporation (2000). *EaSt-2000: Software for the Design and Interim Monitoring of Group Sequential Clinical Trials.* Cambridge, MA.

D'Agostino, R. B. (1990). Comments on "Yates's correction for continuity and the analysis of 2 × 2 contingency tables". *Statistics in Medicine 9*, 377–378.

Dahlstrom, W., G. Welsh, and L. Dahlstrom (1972). *An MMPI Handbook, Vol I.* University of Minnesota, Minneapolis.

Davies, H. T. O., I. K. Crombie, and M. Tavakoli (1998). When can odds ratios mislead? *BMJ 316*, 989–91.

Dawber, T., G. Meadors, and F. Moore (1951). Epidemiological approaches to heart disease: the Framingham study. *Am J Public Health 41*, 279–286.

Deeks, J. J. (1998). When can odds ratios mislead? Odds ratios should be used only in case-control studies and logistic regression analyses. [letter; comment]. *BMJ 317*(7166), 1156–7.

DeGruttola, V., P. Clax, D. DeMets, G. Downing, S. Ellenberg, L. Friedman, M. Gail, R. Prentice, J. Wittes, and S. Zeger (2001). Considerations in the evaluation of surrogate endpoints in clinical trials: Summary of a National Institutes of Health workshop. *Control Clin Trials 22*, 485–502.

DeMets, D., T. Fleming, R. Whitley, et al. (1995). The Data and Safety Monitoring Board and Acquired Immune Deficiency Syndrome (AIDS) clinical trials. *Controlled Clinical Trials 16*(6), 408–421.

DeMets, D. and M. Halperin (1982). Early stopping in the two-sample problem for bounded random variables. *Controlled Clinical Trials 3*, 1.

DeMets, D., R. Hardy, L. Friedman, and K. Lan. (1984). Statistical aspects of early termination in the beta-blocker heart attack trial. *Control Clin Trials 5*(4), 362–372.

DeMets, D. and J. Ware (1980). Group sequential methods for clinical trials with a one-sided hypothesis. *Biometrika 67*, 651–60.

DeMets, D. and J. Ware (1982). Asymmetric group sequential boundaries for monitoring clinical trials. *Biometrika 69*, 661–663.

DeMets, D. L. and R. M. Califf (2002). Principles from clinical trials relevant to clinical practice: Part I. *Circulation 106*(8), 1115–1121.

DeMets, D. L., S. J. Pocock, and D. G. Julian (1999). The agonizing negative trend in monitoring of clinical trials. *Lancet 354*, 1983–88.

Dempster, A., N. Laird, and D. Rubin (1977). Maximum likelihood from incomplete data via the em algorithm. *Journal of the Royal Statistical Society, Series B 39*, 1–38.

Diabetes Control and Complications Trial Research Group (1993). The effect of intensive treatment of diabetes on the development and progression of long-term complications in insulin-dependent diabetes mellitus. *N Engl J Med 329*, 977–986.

Diabetic Retinopathy Study Research Group (1976). Preliminary report on effects of photocoagulation therapy. *Amer J Ophthal 81*, 383.

Dickstein, K., J. Kjekshus, the OPTIMAAL Steering Committee, et al. (2002). Effects of losartan and captopril on mortality and morbidity in high-risk patients after acute myocardial infarction: the OPTIMAAL randomised trial. *The Lancet 360*(9335), 752–760.

Diggle, P. and M. Kennward (1994). Informative drop-out in longitudinal data analysis. *Applied Statistics 43*, 49–93.

Diggle, P., K. Liang, and S. Zeger (1994). *Analysis of Longitudinal Data.* New York: Oxford Science Publications.

Domanski, M., G. Mitchell, M. Pfeffer, J. Neaton, J. Norman, K. Svendsen, R. Grimm, J. Cohen, J. Stamler, and for the MRFIT Research Group (2002). Pulse pressure and cardiovascular disease-related mortality: Follow-up study of the Multiple Risk Factor Intervention Trial (MRFIT). *JAMA 287*, 2677–2683.

Ederer, F., T. R. Church, and J. S. Mandel (1993). Sample sizes for prevention trials have been too small. *American Journal of Epidemiology 137*(7), 787–796.

Efron, B. (1971). Forcing a sequential experiment to be balanced. *Biometrika 58*, 403–417.

Efron, B. (1982). *The Jackknife, the Bootstrap and Other Resampling Plans.* SIAM [Society for Industrial and Applied Mathematics].

Efron, B. and D. Feldman (1991). Compliance as an explanatory variable in clinical trials (with discussion). *Journal of the American Statistical Association 86*, 9–26.

Eisenstein, E. L., P. W. Lemons II, B. E. Tardiff, K. A. Schulman, M. K. Jolly, and R. M. Califf (2005). Reducing the costs of phase III cardiovascular clinical trials. *American Heart Journal 149*(3), 482–488.

Ellenberg, S., T. Fleming, and D. DeMets (2002). *Data Monitoring Committees in Clinical Trials: A Practical Perspective*. Wiley.

Ellenberg, S. and R. Temple (2000). Placebo-controlled trials and active-control trials in the evaluation of new treatments. Part 2: Practical issues and specific cases. *Ann Int Med 133*, 464–470.

Emerson, S. and T. Fleming (1989). Symmetric group sequential test designs. *Biometrics 45*, 905–923.

Emerson, S. and T. Fleming (1990). Parameter estimation following group sequential hypothesis testing. *Biometrika 77*, 875–892.

Fairbanks, K. and R. Madsen (1982). *P* values for tests using a repeated significance test design. *Biometrika 69*, 69–74.

Fairclough, D. (2002). *Design and Analysis of Quality of Life Studies in Clinical Trials*. Chapman and Hall/CRC.

Fairclough, D., H. Peterson, and V. Chang (1998). Why are missing quality of life data a problem in clinical trials of cancer therapy? *Statistics in Medicine 17*, 667–677.

Fayers, P. and D. Hand (1997). Factor analysis, causal indicator and quality of life. *Quality of Life Research 8*, 130–150.

Fayers, P. and R. Hays (Eds.) (2005). *Assessing Quality of Life in Clinical Trials: Methods and Practice (2nd edition)*. Oxford University Press.

Fayers, P. and D. Machin (2000). *Quality of Life: Assessment, Analysis and Interpretation*. Chichester, England: John Wiley & Sons.

Feldman, A. M., M. R. Bristow, W. W. Parmley, et al. (1993). Effects of vesnarinone on morbidity and mortality in patients with heart failure. *New England Journal of Medicine 329*, 149–155.

Fienberg, S. E. (1980). *The Analysis of Cross-classified Categorical Data*. MIT Press.

Fisher, B., S. Anderson, C. Redmond, N. Wolmark, D. Wickerham, and W. Cronin (1995). Reanalysis and results after 12 years of follow-up in a randomized clinical trial comparing total mastectomy with lumpectomy with or without irradiation in the treatment of breast cancer. *N Engl J Med 333*, 1456–1461.

Fisher, B., J. Constantino, D. Wickerham, C. Redmond, M. Kavanah, W. Cronin, V. Vogel, A. Robidoux, N. Dimitrov, J. Atkins, M. Daly, S. Wieand, E. Tan-Chiu, L. Ford, N. Wolmark, other National Surgical Adjuvant Breast, and B. P. Investigators (1998). Tamoxifen for prevention of breast cancer: Report of the National Surgical Adjuvant Breast and Bowel Project P-1 study. *JNCI 90*, 1371–1388.

Fisher, L. (1999). Carvedilol and the Food and Drug Administration (FDA) approval process: the FDA paradigm and reflections on hypothesis testing. *Control Clin Trials 20*(1), 16–39.

Fisher, L., D. Dixon, J. Herson, R. Frankowski, M. Hearron, and K. Peace (1990). Intention to treat in clinical trials. In K. Peace (Ed.), *Statistical Issues in Drug Research and Development*. Marcel Dekker, Inc., New York.

Fisher, L. and L. Moyé (1999). Carvedilol and the Food and Drug Administration approval process: an introduction. *Control Clin Trials 20*, 1–15.

Fisher, L. D. (1998). Self-designing clinical trials. *Statistics in Medicine 17*, 1551–1562.

Fisher, M. R., E. B. Roecker, and D. L. DeMets (2001). The role of an independent statistical analysis center in the industry-modified National Institutes of Health model. *Drug Information Journal 35*, 115–129.

Fisher, R. (1925). *Statistical Methods for Research Workers*. Edinburgh: Oliver and Boyd.

Fisher, R. (1926). The arrangement of field experiments. *J Min Agric G Br 33*, 503–513.

Fisher, R. (1935). *The Design of Experiments*. Edinburgh: Oliver and Boyd.

Fitzmaurice, G. M., N. M. Laird, and J. H. Ware (2004). *Applied longitudinal analysis*. Wiley-Interscience.

Fleiss, J. L., J. T. Bigger Jr., M. McDermott, J. P. Miller, T. Moon, A. J. Moss, D. Oakes, L. M. Rolnitzky, and T. M. Therneau (1990). Nonfatal myocardial infarction is, by itself, an inappropriate end point in clinical trials in cardiology. *Circulation 81*(2), 684–685.

Fleming, T. (1982). One-sample multiple testing procedures for phase II clinical trials. *Biometrics 38*, 143–151.

Fleming, T. (1990). Evaluation of active control trials in aids. *Journal of Acquired Immune Deficiency Syndromes 3 Suppl*, S82–87.

Fleming, T. (1992). Evaluating therapeutic interventions: some issues and experiences. *Statistical Science 7*, 428–441.

Fleming, T. (1994). Surrogate markers in AIDS and cancer trials. *Statistics in Medicine 13*, 1423–1435.

Fleming, T. (2000). Design and interpretation of equivalence trials. *Amer Heart J 139*, S171–S176.

Fleming, T. (2007). Design and interpretation of equivalence trials. *Statistics in Medicine 26, to Appear*.

Fleming, T. and D. DeMets (1996). Surrogate endpoints in clinical trials: Are we being misled? *Ann Intern Med 125*, 605–613.

Fleming, T. R. and D. P. Harrington (1991). *Counting Process and Survival Analysis*. New York: Wiley.

Fowler, F. (1995). *Improving Survey Questions. Applied Social Research Methods Series*, Volume 38. Sage Publications.

Fowler, F. (2002). *Survey Research Methods. Applied Social Research Methods Series (3rd Edition)*. Sage Publications.

Franciosa, J. A., A. L. Taylor, J. N. Cohn, et al. (2002). African-American Heart Failure Trial (A-HeFT): rationale, design, and methodology. *Journal of Cardiac Failure 8*(3), 128–135.

Frangakis, C. E. and D. B. Rubin (2002). Principal stratification in causal inference. *Biometrics 58*(1), 21–29.

Freedman, L., B. Graubard, and A. Schatzkin (1992). Statistical validation of intermediate endpoints for chronic diseases. *Statistics in Medicine 11*, 167–178.

Freireich, E. J., E. Gehan, E. Frei III, et al. (1963). The effect of 6-mercaptopurine on the duration of steroid-induced remissions in acute leukemia: a model for evaluation of other potentially useful therapy. *Blood 21*, 699–716.

Friedman, L., C. Furberg, and D. DeMets (1985). *Fundamentals of Clinical Trials* (2 ed.). PSG Pub. Co.

Friedman, L. M., C. Furberg, and D. L. DeMets (1998). *Fundamentals of Clinical*

Trials. Springer-Verlag Inc.

Frison, L. and S. J. Pocock (1992). Repeated measures in clinical trials: Analysis using mean summary statistics and its implications for design. *Statistics in Medicine 11*, 1685–1704.

Gabriel, K. R. (1969). Simultaneous test procecdures – some theory of multiple comparisons. *The Annals of Mathematical Statistics 40*, 224–250.

Gallo, P., C. Chuang-Stein, V. Dragalin, B. Gaydos, M. Krams, and J. Pinheiro (2006). Adaptive designs in clinical drug development—an executive summary of the pharma working group. *J Biopharm Stat 16*, 275–283.

Gange, S. J. and D. L. DeMets (1996). Sequential monitoring of clinical trials with correlated responses. *Biometrika 83*, 157–167.

Gao, P. and J. Ware (To appear). Assessing non-inferiority: a combination approach. *Statistics in Medicine*.

Garrett, E.-M. (2006). The continual reassessment method for dose-finding studies: a tutorial. *Clinical Trials 3*, 57–71.

Gart, J., D. Krewski, P. Lee, R. Tarone, and J. Wahrendorf (Eds.) (1986). *Statistical Methods in Cancer Research 3: the Design and Analysis of Long-Term Animal Experiments*. Oxford University Press, Oxford.

Gehan, E. (1961). The determination of the number of patients required in a preliminary and a follow-up trial of a new chemotherapeutic agent. *Journal of Chronic Diseases 13*, 346–353.

Gehan, E. (1984). The evaluation of therapies: historical control studies. *Statistics in Medicine 3*, 315–324.

Gent, M. and D. Sackett (1979). The qualification and disqualification of patients and events in long-term cardiovascular clinical trials. *Thromb Haemost 41*(1), 123–134.

Gillen, D. L. and S. S. Emerson (2005). A note on P-values under group sequential testing and nonproportional hazards. *Biometrics 61*(2), 546–551.

Goldberg, P. (2006). Phase 0 trials signal FDA's new reliance on biomarkers in drug development. *The Cancer Letter 32*, 1–2.

Goldhirsch, A., R. Gelber, R. Simes, P. Gasziou, and A. Coates (1989). Costs and benefits of adjuvant therapy in breast cancer: a quality-adjusted survival analysis. *Journal of Clinical Oncology 7*, 36–44.

Gooley, T., P. Martin, L. Fisher, and M. Pettinger (1994). Simulation as a design tool for phase I/II clinical trials: an example from bone marrow transplantation. *Control Clin Trials 15*, 450–462.

Grady, D., W. Applegate, T. Bush, C. Furberg, B. Riggs, and S. Hulley (1998). Heart and estrogen/progestin replacement study (HERS): Design, methods, and baseline characteristics. *Control Clin Trials 19*, 314–335.

Grambsch, P. M. and T. M. Therneau (1994). Proportional hazards tests and diagnostics based on weighted residuals. *Biometrika 81*, 515–526.

Grambsch, P. M., T. M. Therneau, and T. R. Fleming (1995). Diagnostic plots to reveal functional form for covariates in multiplicative intensity models. *Biometrics 51*, 1469–1482.

Grizzle, J. (1965). The two-period change-over design and its use in clinical trials. *Biometrics 21*, 467.

Grizzle, J. and D. Allen (1969). Analysis of growth and dose response curves. *Biometrics 25*, 357–382.

Gruppo Italiano per lo Studio Della Sopravvivenze Nell'Infarcto Miocardico (GISSI)

(1986). Effectiveness of intravenous thrombolytic treatment in acute myocardial infarction. *Lancet I*, 397–402.

Halperin, J. and Executive Steering Committee, SPORTIF III and V Study Investigators (2003). Ximelagatran compared with warfarin for prevention of thromboembolism in patients with nonvalvular atrial fibrillation: rationale, objectives, and design of a pair of clinical studies and baseline patient characteristics (SPORTIF III and V). *American Heart Journal 146*, 431–438.

Halperin, M., Lan, KKG, N. Johnson, and D. DeMets (1982). An aid to data monitoring in long-term clinical trials. *Controlled Clinical Trials 3*, 311–323.

Halperin, M. and J. Ware (1974). Early decision in a censored Wilcoxon two-sample test for accumulating survival data. *Journal of the American Statistical Association 69*, 414–422.

Hardwick, J., M. Meyer, and Q. Stout (2003). Directed walk designs for dose-response problems with competing failure modes. *Biometrics 59*, 229–236.

Hareyama, M., K. Sakata, A. Oouchi, H. Nagakura, M. Shido, M. Someya, and K. Koito (2002). High-dose-rate versus low-dose-rate intracavitary therapy for carcinoma of the uterine cervix: a randomized trial. *Cancer 94*, 117–124.

Harrington, D. and T. Fleming (1982). A class of rank test procedures for censored survival data. *Biometrika 69*, 553–566.

Haybittle, J. (1971). Repeated assessment of results in clinical trials of cancer treatment. *Brit. J. Radiology 44*, 793–797.

HDFP Cooperative Group (1982). Five-year findings of the hypertension detection and follow-up program. III. Reduction in stroke incidence among persons with high blood pressure. *JAMA 247*, 633–638.

Healy, B., L. Campeau, R. Gray, J. Herd, B. Hoogwerf, D. Hunninghake, G. Knatterud, W. Stewart, and C. White (1989). Conflict-of-interest guidelines for a multicenter clinical trial of treatment after coronary-artery bypass-graft surgery. *N Engl J Med 320*, 949–951.

Heart Special Project Committee (1998). Organization, review, and administration of cooperative studies (Greenberg Report). A report from the Heart Special Project Committee to the National Advisory Heart Council, May 1967. *Control Clin Trials 9*, 137–148.

Heitjan, D. F. (1999). Causal inference in a clinical trial: A comparative example. *Controlled Clinical Trials 20*, 309–318.

Hennekens, C., J. Buring, J. Manson, M. Stampfer, B. Rosner, N. Cook, C. Belanger, F. LaMotte, J. Gaziano, P. Ridker, W. Willett, and R. Peto (1996). Lack of effect of long-term supplementation with beta-carotene on the incidence of malignant neoplasms and cardiovascular disease. *N Engl J Med 334*, 1145–1149.

Hill, A. (1971). *Principles of Medical Statistics* (9 ed.). New York: Oxford University Press.

Hill, S. A. B. (1965). The environment and disease: Association or causation. *Proceedings of the Royal Society of Medicine 58*, 295–300.

Hills, M. and P. Armitage (1979). The two-period cross-over clinical trial. *Br J Clin Pharmacol 8*, 7–20.

Hjalmarson, Å., S. Goldstein, B. Fagerberg, et al. (2000). Effects of controlled-release metoprolol on total mortality, hospitalizations, and well-being in patients with heart failure: The metoprolol CR/XL randomized intervention trial in congestive heart failure (MERIT-HF). *JAMA 283*, 1295–1302.

Hochberg, Y. (1988). A sharper Bonferroni procedure for multiple tests of significance. *Biometrika* 75, 800–802.

Hodges, J. L. and E. L. Lehmann (1963). Estimates of location based on rank tests (Ref: V42 p1450-1451). *The Annals of Mathematical Statistics* 34, 598–611.

Holland, P. W. (1986). Statistics and causal inference. *Journal of the American Statistical Association* 81, 945–960.

Holm, S. (1979). A simple sequentially rejective multiple test procedure. *Scandinavian Journal of Statistics* 6, 65–70.

Hughes, M. (2002). Commentary: Evaluating surrogate endpoints. *Control Clin Trials* 23, 703–707.

Hulley, S., D. Grady, T. Bush, C. Furberg, D. Herrington, B. Riggs, E. Vittinghoff, and for the Heart and Estrogen/progestin Replacement Study (HERS) Research Group (1998). Randomized trial of estrogen plus progestin for secondary prevention of coronary heart disease in postmenopausal women. *JAMA* 280, 605–613.

Hung, H., S. Wang, and R. O'Neil (2005). A regulatory perspective on choice of margin and statistical inference issue in non-inferiority trials. *Journal of AIDS* 3, 82–87.

Hung, H., S. Wang, Y. Tsong, J. Lawrence, and R. O'Neil (2003). Some fundamental issues with non-inferiority testing in active controlled trials. *Stat in Med* 22, 213–225.

Hürny, C., J. Bernhard, R. Joss, Y. Willems, F. Cavalli, J. Kiser, K. Brunner, S. Favre, P. Alberto, A. Glaus, H. Senn, E. Schatzmann, P. Ganz, and U. Metzger (1992). Feasibility of quality of life assessment in a randomized phase III trial of small cell lung cancer. *Ann Oncol* 3, 825–831.

Hypertension Detection and Follow-up Program Cooperative Group (1979). Five-year findings of the hypertension detection and follow-up program. I. Reduction in mortality of persons with high blood pressure, including mild hypertension. *JAMA* 242, 2562–2571.

Jennison, C. and B. W. Turnbull (1993). Group sequential tests for bivariate response: interim analyses of clinical trials with both efficacy and safety endpoints. *Biometrics* 49, 741–752.

Jennison, C. and B. W. Turnbull (2000). *Group Sequential Methods with Applications to Clinical Trials*. CRC Press Inc.

Jennison, C. and B. W. Turnbull (2006). Efficient group sequential designs when there are several effect sizes under consideration. *Statistics in Medicine* 25(6), 917–932.

Jöreskog, K. and D. Sörbom (1996). *LISREL 8: User's Reference Guide*. Chicago: Scientific Software International.

Jung, S., M. Carey, and K. Kim (2001). Graphical search for two-stage designs for phase II clinical trials. *Control Clinical Trials* 22, 367–372.

Kalbfleisch, J. and R. Prentice (1980). *The Statistical Analysis of Failure Time Data*. New York: Wiely.

Kaplan, E. L. and P. Meier (1958). Nonparametric estimation from incomplete observations. *Journal of the American Statistical Association* 53, 457–481.

Kaplan, R., T. Ganiats, W. Sieber, and J. Anderson (1998). The quality of well-being scale: critical similarities and differences with sf-36. *International Journal for Quality in Health Care* 10, 509–520.

Karrison, T., D. Huo, and R. Chappell (2003). A group sequential, response-adaptive design for randomized clinical trials. *Controlled Clin Trials* 24(5), 506–522.

Kempthorne, O. (1977). Why randomize? *Journal of Statistical Planning and In-*

ference 1, 1–25.

Kenward, M. G. (1998). Selection models for repeated measurements with non-random dropout: An illustration of sensitivity. *Statistics in Medicine 17*, 2723–2732.

Kim, K. (1989). Point estimation following group sequential tests. *Biometrics 45*, 613–617.

Kim, K. and D. DeMets (1987a). Confidence intervals following group sequential tests in clinical trials. *Biometrics 43*, 857–864.

Kim, K. and D. DeMets (1987b). Design and analysis of group sequential tests based on the type I error spending rate function. *Biometrika 74*, 149–154.

Klein, R., M. Davis, S. Moss, B. Klein, and D. DeMets (1985). The Wisconsin Epidemiologic Study of Diabetic Retinopathy. A comparison of retinopathy in younger and older onset diabetic persons. *Advances in Experimental Medicine & Biology 189*, 321–335.

Klein, R., B. Klein, K. Linton, and D. DeMets (1991). The Beaver Dam Eye Study: visual acuity. *Opthalmology 98*, 1310–1315.

Klotz, J. (1978). Maximum entropy constrained balanced randomization for clinical trials. *Biometrics 34*, 283.

Koch, G., I. Amara, B. Brown, T. Colton, and D. Gillings (1989). A two-period crossover design for the comparison of two active treatments and placebo. *Statistics in Medicine 8*, 487–504.

Kolata, G. (1980). FDA says no to anturane. *Science 208*, 1130–1132.

Korn, E. (1993). On estimating the distribution function for quality of life in cancer clinical trials. *Biometrika 80*, 535–542.

Koscik, R., J. Douglas, K. Zaremba, M. Rock, M. Spalingard, A. Laxova, and P. Farrell (2005). Quality of life of children with cystic fibrosis. *Journal of Pediatrics 147*(3 Suppl), 64–8.

Krum, H., M. Bailey, W. Meyer, P. Verkenne, H. Dargie, P. Lechat, and S. Anker (2006). Impact of statin therapy on clinical outcomes in chronic heart failure patients according to beta-blocker use: Results of CIBIS-II. *Cardiology 108*, 28–34.

Lachin, J. (1988a). Properties of simple randomization in clinical trials. *Controlled Clinical Trials 9*, 312.

Lachin, J. (1988b). Statistical properties of randomization in clinical trials. *Controlled Clinical Trials 9*, 289.

Lachin, J. (2000). Statistical considerations in the intent-to-treat principle. *Controlled Clin Trials 21*, 167.

Lachin, J. M. (2005). Maximum information designs. *Clinical Trials 2*, 453–464.

Laird, N. and J. Ware (1982). Random effects models for longitudinal data. *Biometrics 38*, 963–974.

Lakatos, E. (1986). Sample size determination in clinical trials with time-dependent rates of losses and noncompliance. *Controlled Clinical Trials 7*, 189.

Lakatos, E. (1988). Sample size based on logrank statistic in complex clinical trials. *Biometrics 44*, 229.

Lakatos, E. (2002). Designing complex group sequential survival trials. *Statistics in Medicine 21*(14), 1969–1989.

Lan, K. and D. DeMets (1983). Discrete sequential boundaries for clinical trials. *Biometrika 70*, 659–663.

Lan, K., R. Simon, and M. Halperin (1982). Stochastically curtailed testing in long-term clinical trials. *Communications in Statistics, Series C 1*, 207–219.

Lan, K. and J. Wittes (1988). The *B*-value: a tool for monitoring data. *Biometrics* *44*, 579–585.

Lan, K. K. G. and D. C. Trost (1997). Estimation of parameters and sample size re-estimation. In *ASA Proceedings of the Biopharmaceutical Section*, pp. 48–51. American Statistical Association (Alexandria, VA).

Lan, K. K. G. and D. M. Zucker (1993). Sequential monitoring of clinical trials: the role of information and Brownian motion. *Statistics in Medicine 12*, 753–765.

Landgraf, J., L. Abetz, and J. Ware (1996). *The CHQ User's Manual 1st ed.* Boston, MA: The Health Institute, New England Medical Center.

LaRosa, J., S. Grundy, D. Waters, C. Shear, P. Barter, J. Fruchart, et al. (2005). Intensive lipid lowering with atorvastatin in patients with stable coronary disease. *N Engl J Med 352*, 1425–1435.

Lawless, J. F. (2003). *Statistical Models and Methods for Lifetime Data.* John Wiley & Sons.

Lee, E. T. (1992). *Statistical Methods for Survival Data Analysis.* John Wiley & Sons.

Lee, J. W. and D. L. DeMets (1991). Sequential comparison of changes with repeated measurements data. *Journal of the American Statistical Association 86*, 757–762.

Lewis, R. J., D. A. Berry, H. Cryer III, N. Fost, R. Krome, G. R. Washington, J. Houghton, J. W. Blue, R. Bechhofer, T. Cook, and M. Fisher (2001). Monitoring a clinical trial conducted under the FDA regulations allowing a waiver of prospective informed consent: The DCLHb traumatic hemorrhagic shock efficacy trial. *Annals of Emergency Medicine 38*(4), 397–404.

Li, Z. and D. L. DeMets (1999). On the bias of estimation of a Brownian motion drift following group sequential tests. *Statistica Sinica 9*, 923–938.

Lin, D., T. Fleming, and V. DeGruttola (1997). Estimating the proportion of treatment effect explained by a surrogate marker. *Statistics in Medicine 16*, 1515–1527.

Lind, J. (1753). *A Treatise of the Scurvy.* Edinburgh: University Press (reprint).

Lipid Research Clinics Program (1984). The Lipid Research Clinics Coronary Primary Prevention Trial results. 1. Reduction in incidence of coronary heart disease. *JAMA 251*, 351–364.

Little, R. and T. Raghunathan (1999). On summary measures analysis of the linear mixed effects model for repeated measures when data are not missing completely at random. *Statistics in Medicine 18*, 2465–2478.

Little, R. J. A. and D. B. Rubin (2002). *Statistical Analysis with Missing Data.* John Wiley & Sons.

Liu, A. and W. J. Hall (1999). Unbiased estimation following a sequential test. *Biometrika 86*, 71–78.

Liu, G. and A. L. Gould (2002). Comparison of alternative strategies for analysis of longitudinal trials with dropouts. *Journal of Biopharmaceutical Statistics 12*(2), 207–226.

Louis, P. (1834). *Essays in clinical instruction.* London, U.K.: P. Martin.

Love, R. and N. Fost (1997). Ethical and regulatory challenges in a randomized control trial of adjuvant treatment for breast cancer in Vietnam. *J Inv Med 45*, 423–431.

Love, R. and N. Fost (2003). A pilot seminar on ethical issues in clinical trials for cancer researchers in Vietnam. *IRB: a Review of Human Subjects Research 25*, 8–10.

Lytle, L., M. Kubik, C. Perry, M. Story, A. Birnbaum, and D. Murray (2006). Influencing healthful food choices in school and home environments: results from the TEENS study. *Preventive Medicine 43*, 8–13.

Machin, D. and S. Weeden (1998). Suggestions for the presentation of quality life data from clinical trials. *Statistics in Medicine 17*, 711–724.

MADIT Executive Committee (1991). Multicenter automatic defibrillator implantation trial (madit): design and clinical protocol. *Pacing Clin Electrophysiol 14* (5 Pt 2), 920–927.

Mallinckrodt, C. H., W. S. Clark, R. J. Carroll, and G. Molenberghs (2003). Assessing response profiles from incomplete longitudinal clinical trial data under regulatory considerations. *Journal of Biopharmaceutical Statistics 13* (2), 179–190.

Mantel, N. (1966). Evaluation of survival data and two new rank order statistics arising in its consideration. *Cancer Chemotherapy Reports 50*, 163–170.

Marcus, R., E. Peritz, and K. R. Gabriel (1976). On closed testing procedures with special reference to ordered analysis of variance. *Biometrika 63*, 655–660.

Mark, E., E. Patalas, H. Chang, R. Evans, and S. Kessler (1997). Fatal pulmonary hypertension associated with short-term use of fenfluramine and phentermine. *N Engl J Med 337*, 602–606.

Matts, J. and J. Lachin (1988). Properties of permuted-block randomization in clinical trials. *Controlled Clinical Trials 9*, 327.

McCulloch, C. and S. Searle (2001). *Generalized, Linear, and Mixed Models*. New York: Wiley.

McGinn, C., M. Zalupski, I. Shureiqi, et al. (2001). Phase I trial of radiation dose escalation with concurrent weekly fulldose gemcitabine in patients with advanced pancreatic cancer. *J Clin Oncol 19*, 4202–4208.

McIntosh, H. (1995). Stat bite: Cancer and heart disease deaths. *J Natl Cancer Inst 87* (16), 1206.

McPherson, C. and P. Armitage (1971). Repeated significance tests on accumulating data when the null hypothesis is not true. *Journal of the Royal Statistical Society, Series A 134*, 15–26.

Medical Research Council (1944). Clinical trial of patulin in the common cold. *Lancet 2*, 373–375.

Medical Research Council (1948). Streptomycin treatment of pulmonary tuberculosis. *BMJ 2*, 769–782.

Meier, P. (1981). Stratification in the design of a clinical trial. *Control Clin Trials 1*, 355–361.

Meier, P. (1991). Comment on "compliance as an explanatory variable in clinical trials". *Journal of the American Statistical Association 86*, 19–22.

Meinert, C. (1996). *Clinical trials dictionary: usage and recommendations*. Harbor Duvall Graphics, Baltimore, MD.

MERIT-HF Study Group (1999). Effect of metoprolol CR/XL in chronic heart failure: Metoprolol CR/XL randomised intervention trial in congestive heart failure (MERIT-HF). *Lancet 353*, 2001.

Mesbah, M., B. Cole, and M. Lee (2002). *Statistical Methods for Quality of Life Studies Design, Measurements, and Analysis*. Springer.

Miller, A., C. Baines, T. To, and C. Wall (1992). Canadian National Breast Cancer Study: breast cancer detection and death rates among women aged 40 to 49 years. *Canadian Medical Association Journal 147*, 1459–1476.

Moertel, C. (1984). Improving the efficiency of clinical trials: a medical perspective. *Statistics in Medicine 3*, 455–465.

Moher, D., K. F. Schulz, D. G. Altman, and the CONSORT Group (2001). The CONSORT statement: revised recommendations for improving the quality of reports of parallel-group randomized trials. *Ann Intern Med 134*, 657–662.

Molenberghs, G., M. Buyse, H. Geys, D. Renard, T. Burzykowski, and A. Alonso (2002). Statistical challenges in the evaluation of surrogate endpoints in randomized trials. *Control Clin Trials 23*, 607–625.

Molenberghs, G., H. Thijs, I. Jansen, C. Beunkens, M. Kenward, C. Mallinkrodt, and R. Carroll (2004). Analyzing incomplete longitudinal clinical trial data. *Biostatistics 5*, 445–464.

Montori, V. M., G. Permanyer-Miralda, I. Ferreira-González, J. W. Busse, V. Pacheco-Huergo, D. Bryant, J. Alonso, E. A. Akl, A. Domingo-Salvany, E. Mills, P. Wu, H. J. Schünemann, R. Jaeschke, and G. H. Guyatt (2005). Validity of composite end points in clinical trials. *BMJ 330*(2), 594–596.

Moss, A., W. Hall, D. Cannom, J. Daubert, S. Higgins, H. Klein, J. Levine, S. Saksena, A. Waldo, D. Wilber, M. Brown, M. Heo, and for the Multicenter Automatic Defibrillator Implantation Trial Investigators (1996). Improved survival with an implanted defibrillator in patients with coronary disease at high risk for ventricular arrhythimia. *N Engl J Med 335*, 1933–1940.

Moss, A., W. Hall, D. Cannom, J. Daubert, S. Higgins, J. Levine, S. Saksena, A. Waldo, D. Wilber, M. Brown, and M. Heo (1996). Improved survival with an implanted defibrillator in patients with coronary disease at high risk for ventricular arrhythmia. *N Engl J Med 335*, 1933–1940.

Moyé, L. (1999). End-point interpretation in clinical trials: the case for discipline. *Control Clin Trials 20*(1), 40–49.

Moyé, L. A. (2003). *Multiple Analyses in Clinical Trials: Fundamentals for Investigators*. New York: Springer-Verlag.

MPS Research Unit (2000). *PEST 4: Operating Manual*. The University of Reading.

Multiple Risk Factor Intervention Trial Research Group (1982). Multiple Risk Factor Interventional Trial: Risk factor changes and mortality results. *JAMA 248*, 1465–1477.

Murray, D., S. Varnell, and J. Blitstein (2004). Design and analysis of group-randomized trials: a review of recent methodological developments. *Am J Public Health 94*, 423–432.

Muthén, B. and L. Muthén (1998). *Mplus User's Guide*. Los Angeles: Muthen & Muthen.

National Commission for the Protection of Human Subjects of Biomedical and Behavioral Research (1979). The Belmont Report: ethical principles and guidelines for the protection of human subjects of research. *Fed Regist 44*, 23192–23197.

Neaton, J. D., G. Gray, B. D. Zuckerman, and M. A. Konstam (2005). Key issues in end point selection for heart failure trials: composite endpoint. *Journal of Cardiac Failure 11*(8), 567–575.

Nocturnal Oxygen Therapy Trial Group (1980). Continuous and nocturnal oxygen therapy in hypoxemic chronic obstructive lungdisease: a clinical trial. *Ann Intern Med 93*, 391–398.

O'Brien, P. C. (1984). Procedures for comparing samples with multiple endpoints. *Biometrics 40*, 1079–1087.

O'Brien, P. C. and T. R. Fleming (1979). A multiple testing procedure for clinical trials. *Biometrics 35*, 549–556.

O'Connor, C. M., M. W. Dunne, M. A. Pfeffer, J. B. Muhlestein, L. Yao, S. Gupta, R. J. Benner, M. R. Fisher, and T. D. Cook (2003). A double-blind, randomized, placebo controlled trial of azithromycin for the secondary prevention of coronary heart disease: the WIZARD trial. *JAMA 290*(11), 1459–1466.

Olschewski, M. and M. Schumacher (1990). Statistical analysis of quality of life data in cancer clinical trials. *Statistics in Medicine 9*, 749.

Omenn, G., G. Goodman, M. Thornquist, J. Balmes, M. Cullen, A. Glass, J. Keogh, F. Meyskens, B. Valanis, J. Williams, S. Barnhart, and S. Hammar (1996). Effects of a combination of beta-carotene and vitamin A on lung cancer and cardiovascular disease. *New Engl J Med 334*, 1150–1155.

Omenn, G., G. Goodman, M. Thornquist, J. Grizzle, L. Rosenstock, S. Barnhart, J. Balmes, M. Cherniack, M. Cullen, A. Glass, and et al. (1994). The beta-carotene and retinol efficacy trial (caret) for chemoprevention of lung cancer in high-risk populations: smokers and asbestos-exposed workers. *Cancer Research 54*, 2038s–2043s.

O'Quigley, J., M. Pepe, and L. Fisher (1990). Continual reassessment method: a practical design for phase I clinical trials in cancer. *Biometrics 46*, 33–48.

Packer, M. (2000). COPERNICUS (Carvedilol Prospective Randomized Cumulative Survival): evaluates the effects of carvedilol top-of-ACE on major cardiac events in patients with heart failure. European Society of Cardiology Annual Congress.

Packer, M., M. R. Bristow, J. N. Cohn, et al. (1996). The effect of carvedilol on morbidity and mortality in patients with chronic heart failure. *The New England Journal of Medicine 334*(21), 1349–1355.

Packer, M., J. Carver, R. Rodeheffer, R. Ivanhoe, R. DiBianco, S. Zeldis, G. Hendrix, W. Bommer, U. Elkayam, M. Kukin, et al. (1991). Effect of oral milrinone on mortality in severe chronic heart failure. *N Engl J Med 325*, 1468–1475.

Packer, M., A. Coats, M. Fowler, H. Katus, H. Krum, P. Mohacsi, J. Rouleau, M. Tendera, A. Castaigne, E. Roecker, M. Schultz, and D. DeMets (2001). Effect of carvedilol on the survival of patients with severe chronic heart failure. *New England Journal of Medicine 344*(22), 1651–1658.

Packer, M., C. O'Connor, J. Ghali, M. Pressler, P. Carson, R. Belkin, A. Miller, G. Neuberg, D. Frid, J. Wertheimer, A. Cropp, and D. DeMets (1996). Effect of amlodipine on morbidity and mortality in severe chronic heart failure. *New England Journal of Medicine 335*, 1107–1114.

Pampallona, S. and A. Tsiatis (1994). Group sequential designs for one-sided and two-sided hypothesis testing with provision for early stopping in favor of the null hypothesis. *Journal of Statistical Planning and Inference 42*, 19–35.

Peduzzi, P., K. Detre, J. Wittes, and T. Holford (1991). Intention-to-treat analysis and the problem of crossovers: an example from the Veterans Affairs randomized trial of coronary artery bypass surgery. *Journal of Thoracic and Cardiovascular Surgery 101*, 481–487.

Peduzzi, P., J. Wittes, K. Detre, and T. Holford (1993). Analysis as-randomized and the problem of non-adherence: an example from the Veterans Affairs randomized trial of coronary artery bypass surgery. *Statistics in Medicine 12*, 1185–1195.

Peto, R., M. Pike, P. Armitage, N. Breslow, D. Cox, S. Howard, N. Mantel, K. McPherson, J. Peto, and P. Smith (1976). Design and analysis of randomised clinical trials requiring prolonged observation on each patient: I. Introduction and design. *British Journal of Cancer 34*, 585–612.

Pinheiro, J. and D. Bates (2000). *Mixed Effects Models in S and S-PLUS*. Springer.

Pinheiro, J. C. and D. L. DeMets (1997). Estimating and reducing bias in group sequential designs with Gaussian independent increment structure. *Biometrika 84*, 831–845.

Pitt, B. (2005). Low-density lipoprotein cholesterol in patients with stable coronary heart disease — is it time to shift our goals? *The New England Journal of Medicine 352*(14), 1483–1484.

Pocock, S. (1977a). Group sequential methods in the design and analysis of clinical trials. *Biometrika 64*, 191–199.

Pocock, S. (1977b). Randomised clinical trials. *Br Med J 1*, 1661.

Pocock, S. and I. White (1999). Trials stopped early: too good to be true? *Lancet 353*, 943–944.

Pocock, S. J. (2005). When (not) to stop a clinical trial for benefit. *JAMA 294*(17), 2228–2230.

Pocock, S. J., N. L. Geller, and A. A. Tsiatis (1987). The analysis of multiple endpoints in clinical trials. *Biometrics 43*, 487–498.

Pocock, S. J. and R. Simon (1975). Sequential treatment assignment with balancing for prognostic factors in the controlled clinical trial (Corr: V32 p954-955). *Biometrics 31*, 103–115.

Prentice, R. (1989). Surrogate endpoints in clinical trials: definition and operation criteria. *Statistics in Medicine 8*, 431.

Prorok, P., G. Andriole, R. Bresalier, S. Buys, D. Chia, E. Crawford, R. Fogel, E. Gelmann, F. Gilbert, et al. (2000). Design of the Prostate, Lung, Colorectal and Ovarian (PLCO) Cancer Screening Trial. *Control Clin Trials 21*, 273–309S.

Proschan, M., K. Lan, and J. Wittes (2006). *Statistical Monitoring of Clinical Trials: A Unified Approach*. Statistics for Biology and Health. USA: Springer USA.

Qu, R. P. and D. L. DeMets (1999). Bias correction in group sequential analysis with correlated data. *Statistica Sinica 9*, 939–952.

Quittner, A. (1998). Measurement of quality of life in cystic fibrosis. *Curr Opin Pulm Med 4*(6), 326–31.

Quittner, A., A. Buu, M. Messer, A. Modi, and M. Watrous (2005). Development and validation of the cystic fibrosis questionnaire in the United States: A health-related quality-of-life measure for cystic fibrosis. *Chest 128*, 2347–2354.

R Development Core Team (2005). *R: A language and environment for statistical computing*. Vienna, Austria: R Foundation for Statistical Computing. ISBN 3-900051-07-0.

Rea, L. and R. Parker (1997). *Designing and Conducting Survey Research: A Comprehensive Guide* (2 ed.). Jossey-Bass.

Reboussin, D. M., D. L. DeMets, K. Kim, and K. K. G. Lan (2000). Computations for group sequential boundaries using the Lan–DeMets spending function method. *Controlled Clinical Trials 21*(3), 190–207.

Rector, T., S. Kubo, and J. Cohn (1993). Validity of the Minnesota Living with Heart Failure questionnaire as a measure of therapeutic response to enalapril of placebo. *American Journal of Cardiology 71*, 1106–1107.

Ridker, P., M. Cushman, M. Stampfer, R. Tracy, and C. Hennekens (1997). Inflammation, aspirin, and the risk of cardiovascular disease in apparently healthy men. *New England Journal of Medicine 336*, 973–979.

Rosner, G. and A. Tsiatis (1988). Exact confidence intervals following a group sequential trial: a comparison of methods. *Biometrika 75*, 723–730.

Rubin, D. (1974). Estimating causal effects of treatment in randomized and non-randomized studies. *Journal of Educational Psychology 66*, 688.

Rubin, D. B. (1987). *Multiple Imputation for Nonresponse in Surveys*. John Wiley & Sons.

Rubin, D. B. (1996). Multiple imputation after 18+ years (Pkg: P473-520). *Journal of the American Statistical Association 91*, 473–489.

Rubin, D. B. (1998). More powerful randomization-based p-values in double-blind trials with non-compliance (Pkg: P251-389). *Statistics in Medicine 17*, 371–385.

Ruffin, J., J. Grizzle, N. Hightower, G. McHardy, H. Shull, and J. Kirsner (1969). A co-operative double-blind evaluation of gastric "freezing" in the treatment of duodenal ulcer. *N Engl J Med 281*, 16–19.

Ryan, L. and K. Soper (2005). Preclinical treatment evaluation. In *Encyclopedia of Biostatistics*. John Wiley & Sons, Ltd.

Sackett, D. L., J. J. Deeks, and D. G. Altman (1996). Down with odds ratios. *Evidence-Based Medicine 1*(6), 164–6.

Samsa, G., D. Edelman, M. Rothman, G. Williams, J. Lipscomb, and D. Matchar (1999). Determining clinically important differences in health status measures: a general approach with illustration to the health utilities index mark II. *Pharmacoeconomics 15*(2), 141–55.

Scandanavian Simvistatin Survival Study (1994). Randomized trial of cholesterol lowering in 4444 patients with coronary heart disease. *The Lancet 344*, 1383–1389.

Scharfstein, D., A. Tsiatis, and J. Robins (1997). Semiparametric efficiency and its implication on the design and analysis of group-sequential studies. *Journal of the American Statistical Association 92*, 1342–1350.

Scharfstein, D. O., A. Rotnitzky, and J. M. Robins (1999). Adjusting for nonignorable drop-out using semiparametric nonresponse models (C/R: P1121-1146). *Journal of the American Statistical Association 94*, 1096–1120.

Schluechter, M. (1992). Methods for the analysis of informatively censored longitudinal data. *Statistics in Medicine 11*, 1861–1870.

Schneiderman, M. (1967). Mouse to man: statistical problems in bringing a drug to clinical trial. In L. LeCam and J. Neyman (Eds.), *Proceedings of the 5th Berkeley Symposium in Mathematical Statistics and Probability, Volume IV*. Berkeley U. Press, Berkeley.

Schoenfeld, D. (1983). Sample-size formula for the proportional-hazards regression model. *Biometrics 39*, 499–503.

Schwartz, D. and J. Lellouch (1967). Explanatory and pragmatic attitudes in therapeutical trials. *J. Chron. Dis. 20*, 637–648.

Senn, S. (1999). Rare Distinction and Common Fallacy [letter]. *eBMJ* http://bmj.com/cgi/eletters/317/7168/1318.

Shen, Y. and L. Fisher (1999). Statistical inference for self-designing clinical trials with a one-sided hypothesis. *Biometrics 55*, 190–197.

Shih, J. H. (1995). Sample size calculation for complex clinical trials with survival endpoints. *Controlled Clinical Trials 16*, 395–407.

Shopland (ed), D. (1982). *The Health Consequences of Smoking: Cancer: A Report of the Surgeon General*. United States. Public Health Service. Office on Smoking and Health.

Sidak, Z. (1967). Rectangular confidence regions for the means of multivariate normal distributions. *Journal of the American Statistical Association 62*, 626–633.

Siegmund, D. (1978). Estimation following sequential tests. *Biometrika 65*, 341–349.

Siegmund, D. (1985). *Sequential Analysis: Tests and Confidence Intervals.* Springer-Verlag Inc.

Silverman, W. (1979). The lesson of retrolental fibroplasia. *Scientific American 236*, 100–107.

Simes, R. J. (1986). An improved Bonferroni procedure for multiple tests of significance. *Biometrika 73*, 751–754.

Simon, R. (1989). Optimal two-stage designs for phase II clinical trials. *Controlled Clinical Trials 10*, 1–10.

Simon, R., B. Freidlin, L. Rubinstein, S. Arbuck, J. Collins, and M. Christian (1997). Accelerated titration designs for phase I clinical trials in oncology. *J National Cancer Inst 89*, 1138–1147.

Simon, R., G. Weiss, and D. Hoel (1975). Sequential analysis of binomial clinical trials. *Biometrika 62*, 195–200.

Simon, R., J. Wittes, and J. Ellenberg (1985). Randomized phase II clinical trials? *Cancer Treatment Reports 69*, 1375–1381.

Sloan, E. P., M. Koenigsberg, D. Gens, et al. (1999). Diaspirin cross-linked hemoglobin (DCLHb) in the treatment of severe traumatic hemorrhagic shock, a randomized controlled efficacy trial. *JAMA 282*(19), 1857–1863.

Sloan, J. and A. Dueck (2004). Issues for statisticians in conducting analyses and translating results for quality of life end points in clinical trials. *Journal of Biopharmaceutical Statistics 14*, 73–96.

Smith, E. L., C. Gilligan, P. E. Smith, and C. T. Sempos (1989). Calcium supplementation and bone in middle-aged women. *Am J Clin Nutr 50*, 833–42.

Speith, L. and C. Harris (1996). Assessment of health-related quality of life in children and adolescents: an integrative review. *Journal of Pediatric Psychology 21*(2), 175–193.

Spiegelhalter, D., L. Freedman, and P. Blackburn (1986). Monitoring clinical trials: conditional or predictive power? *Controlled Clinical Trials 7*, 8–17.

Steering Committee of the Physicians' Health Study Research Group (1989). Final report on the aspirin component of the ongoing Physicians Health Study. *N Engl J Med 321*, 129–135.

Stephens, R. (2004). The analysis, interpretation, and presentation of quality of life data. *Journal of Biopharmaceutical Statistics 14*, 53–71.

Stevens, J., D. Murray, D. Catellier, P. Hannan, L. Lytele, J. Elder, D. Young, D. Simons-Morton, and L. Webber (2005). Design of the trial of activity in adolescent girls (TAAG). *Contemporary Clinical Trials 26*, 223–233.

Storer, B. (1989). Design and analysis of phase I clinical trials. *Biometrics 45*, 925–937.

Storer, B. (1990). A sequential phase II/III trial for binary outcomes. *Statistics in Medicine 9*, 229–235.

Taeger, D., Y. Sun, and K. Straif (1998). On the use, misuse and interpretation of odds ratios. *eBMJ* http://bmj.com/cgi/eletters/316/7136/989.

Taubes, G. (1995). Epidemiology faces its limits. *Science 269*, 164–169.

Taves, D. (1974). A new method of assigning patients to treatment and control groups. *Clin Pharmacol Ther 15*, 443–453.

Taylor, A., S. Ziesche, C. Yancy, et al. (2004). Combination of isosorbide dinitrate and hydralazine in blacks with heart failure. *N Engl J Med 351*, 2049–2057.

Temple, R. and S. Ellenberg (2000). Placebo-controlled trials and active-control trials in the evaluation of new treatments. Part 1: Ethical and scientific issues.

Ann Int Med 133, 455–463.

Temple, R. and G. Pledger (1980). The FDA's critique of the anturane reinfarction trial. *New England Journal of Medicine 303*, 1488.

Thackray, S., K. Witte, A. Clark, and J. Cleland (2000). Clinical trials update: Optime-chf, praise-2, all-hat. *Eur J Heart Fail 2*(2), 209–212.

Thall, P. and R. Simon (1995). Recent developments in the design of phase II clinical trials. In P. Thall (Ed.), *Recent Advances in Clinical Trial Design and Analysis.* Kluwer: New York.

Thall, P. F. and S. C. Vail (1990). Some covariance models for longitudinal count data with overdispersion. *Biometrics 46*, 657–671.

The Alpha-Tocopherol, Beta-Carotene Cancer Prevention Study Group (1994). The effect of vitamin E and beta-carotene on the incidence of lung cancer and other cancers in male smokers. *N Engl J Med 330*, 1029–1035.

The Anturane Reinfarction Trial Research Group (1978). Sulfinpyrazone in the prevention of cardiac death after myocardial infarction. *The New England Journal of Medicine 298*, 289.

The Anturane Reinfarction Trial Research Group (1980). Sulfinpyrazone in the prevention of sudden death after myocardial infarction. *The New England Journal of Medicine 302*, 250.

The Beta-Blocker Evaluation of Survival Trial Investigators (2001). A trial of the beta-blocker bucindolol in patients with advanced chronic heart failure. *The New England Journal of Medicine 344*(22), 1659–1667.

The Cardiac Arrhythmia Suppression Trial (CAST) Investigators (1989). Preliminary report: effect of encainide and flecainide on mortality in a randomized trial of arrhythmia suppression after myocardial infarction. *The New England Journal of Medicine 321*, 129.

The Coronary Drug Project Research Group (1975). Clofibrate and niacin in coronary heart disease. *Journal of American Medical Association 231*, 360.

The Coronary Drug Project Research Group (1980). Influence of adherence to treatment and response of cholesterol on mortality in the coronary drug project. *New England Journal of Medicine 303*, 1038.

The DCCT Research Group: Diabetes Control and Complications Trial (DCCT) (1986). Design and methodologic considerations for the feasibility phase. *Diabetes 35*, 530–545.

The Diabetic Retinopathy Study Research Group (1978). Photocoagulation treatment of proliferative diabetic retinopathy: the second report of the Diabetic Retinopathy Study findings. *Opathalmology 85*, 82–106.

The Global Use of Strategies to Open Occluded Coronary Arteries (GUSTO III) Investigators (1997). A comparison of reteplase with alteplase for acute myocardial infarction. *N Engl J Med 337*, 1118–1123.

The GUSTO Investigators (1993). An international randomized trial comparing four thrombolytic strategies for acute myocardial infarction. *N Engl J Med 329*, 673–82.

The Intermittent Positive Pressure Breathing Trial Group (1983). Intermittent positive pressure breathing therapy of chronic obstructive pulmonary disease. *Annals of Internal Medicine 99*, 612.

The International Steering Committee on Behalf of the MERIT-HF Study Group (1997). Rationale, design, and organization of the metoprolol CR/XL randomized intervention trial in heart failure (MERIT-HF). *Amer J Cardiol 30*, 54J–58J.

The Lipid Research Clinics Program (1979). The coronary primary prevention trial: design and implementation. *J Chronic Dis 32*, 609–631.

The TIMI Research Group (1988). Immediate vs. delayed catheterization and angioplasty following thrombolytic therapy for acute myocardial infarction. *JAMA 260*, 2849–2858.

The Veterans Administration Coronary Artery Bypass Surgery Cooperative Study Group (1984). Eleven-year survival in the veterans administration randomized trial of coronary bypass surgery for stable angina. *N Engl J Med 311*(21), 1333–9.

The Women's Health Initiative Steering Committee (2004). Effects of conjugated equine estrogen in postmenopausal women with hysterectomy: the Women's Health Initiative randomized controlled trial. *JAMA 291*, 1701–1712.

Therneau, T. M. (1993). How many stratification factors are "too many" to use in a randomization plan? *Controlled Clinical Trials 14*, 98–108.

Therneau, T. M., P. M. Grambsch, and T. R. Fleming (1990). Martingale-based residuals for survival models. *Biometrika 77*, 147–160.

Thisted, R. A. (2006). Baseline adjustment: Issues for mixed-effect regression models in clinical trials. In *Proceedings of the American Statistical Association*, pp. 386–391. American Statistical Association.

Tsiatis, A. (1981). The asymptotic joint distribution of the efficient scores test for the proportional hazards model calculated over time. *Biometrika 68*, 311–315.

Tsiatis, A. (1982). Repeated significance testing for a general class of statistics used in censored survival analysis. *Journal of the American Statistical Association 77*, 855–861.

Tsiatis, A., G. Rosner, and C. Mehta (1984). Exact confidence intervals following a group sequential test. *Biometrics 40*, 797–803.

Tsiatis, A. A. and C. Mehta (2003). On the inefficiency of the adaptive design for monitoring clinical trials. *Biometrika 90*(2), 367–378.

Upton, G. J. G. (1982). A comparison of alternative tests for the 2×2 comparative trial. *Journal of the Royal Statistical Society, Series A: General 145*, 86–105.

U.S. Government (1949). *Trials of War Criminals before the Nuremberg Military Tribunals under Control Council Law No. 10*, Volume 2. Washington, D.C.: U.S. Government Printing Office.

Van Elteren, P. (1960). On the combination of independent two-sample tests of Wilcoxon. *Bull Int Stat Inst. 37*, 351–361.

Venables, W. N. and B. D. Ripley (1999). *Modern Applied Statistics with S-PLUS*. Springer-Verlag Inc.

Verbeke, G. and G. Molenberghs (2000). *Linear Mixed Models for Longitudinal Data*. Springer-Verlag Inc.

Verbeke, G., G. Molenberghs, H. Thijs, E. Lesaffre, and M. G. Kenward (2001). Sensitivity analysis for nonrandom dropout: a local influence approach. *Biometrics 57*(1), 7–14.

Veterans Administration Cooperative Urological Research Group (1967). Treatment and survival of patients with cancer of the prostate. *Surg Gynecol Obstet 124*, 1011–1017.

Volberding, P., S. Lagakos, M. Koch, C. Pettinelli, M. Myers, D. Booth, et al., and the AIDS Clinical Trials Group of the National Institute of Allergy and Infectious Diseases (1990). Zidovudine in asymptomatic human immunodeficiency virus infection. A controlled trial in persons with fewer than 500 cd4 positive cells per cubic millimeter. The AIDS Clinical Trials Group of the National Institute of Allergy and Infectious Diseases. *N Engl J Med 322*, 941–949.

Wald, A. (1947). *Sequential Analysis*. New York: Wiley.

Wang, C., J. Douglas, and S. Anderson (2002). Item response models for joint analysis of quality of life and survival. *Statistics in Medicine 21*(1), 129–142.

Wangensteen, O., E. Peter, E. Bernstein, A. Walder, H. Sosin, and A. Madsen (1962). Can physiological gastrectomy be achieved by gastric freezing? *Ann Surg 156*, 579–591.

Ware, J. (2000). SF-36 health survey update. *Spine 25*(24), 3130–3139.

Ware, J. H. (1989). Investigating therapies of potentially great benefit: ECMO (C/R: P306-340). *Statistical Science 4*, 298–306.

Waskow, I. and M. Parloff (1975). *Psychotherapy Change Measures*. U.S. Government Printing Office, Washington, D.C.

Wedel, H., D. DeMets, P. Deedwania, S. G. B Fagerberg, S. Gottlieb, A. Hjalmarson, J. Kjekshus, F. Waagstein, J. Wikstrand, and MERIT-HF Study Group (2001). Challenges of subgroup analyses in multinational clinical trials: experiences from the MERIT-HF trial. *The American Heart Journal 142*(3), 502–511.

Wei, L. (1984). Testing goodness of fit for the proportional hazards model with censored observations. *Journal of the American Statistical Association 79*, 649–652.

Wei, L. and S. Durham (1978). The randomized play-the-winner rule in medical trials. *JASA 73*, 840–843.

Wei, L. and J. Lachin (1988). Properties of the urn randomization in clinical trials. *Controlled Clinical Trials 9*, 345.

Whitehead, J. (1978). Large sample sequential methods with application to the analysis of 2×2 contingency tables. *Biometrika 65*, 351–356.

Whitehead, J. (1983). *The Design and Analysis of Sequential Clinical Trials*. Chichester: Horwood.

Whitehead, J. (1986). On the bias of maximum likelihood estimation following a sequential test. *Biometrika 73*, 573–581.

Whitehead, J. (1997). *The Design and Analysis of Sequential Clinical Trials* (Revised 2nd ed.). Wiley: Chichester.

Whitehead, J. and I. Stratton (1983). Group sequential clinical trials with triangular continuation regions. *Biometrics 39*, 227–236.

Willke, R., L. Burke, and P. Erickson (2004). Measuring treatment impact: a review of patient-reported outcomes and other efficacy endpoints in approved product labels. *Control Clin Trials 25*(6), 535–52.

World Medical Association (1989). *World Medical Association Declaration of Helsinki. Recommendations guiding physicians in biomedical research involving human subjects*. World Health Association.

Writing Group for the Women's Health Initiative Randomized Controlled Trial (2002). Risks and benefits of estrogen plus progestin in healthy postmenopausal women. *JAMA 288*, 321–333.

Wu, M. and R. Carroll (1988). Estimation and comparison of changes in the presence of informative right censoring by modeling the censoring process. *Biometrics 44*, 175–188.

Wu, M., M. Fisher, and D. DeMets (1980). Sample sizes for long-term medical trial with time-dependent dropout and event rates. *Controlled Clinical Trials 1*, 111–121.

Yabroff, K., B. Linas, and K. Shulman (1996). Evaluation of quality of life for diverse patient populations. *Breast Cancer Res Treat* *40*(1), 87–104.

Yusuf, S. and A. Negassa (2002). Choice of clinical outcomes in randomized trials of heart failure therapies: Disease-specific or overall outcomes? *American Heart Journal* *143*(1), 22–28.

Zelen, M. (1969). Play the winner rule and the controlled clinical trial. *JASA* *64*, 131–146.

Zhang, J., H. Quan, J. Ng, and M. Stepanavage (1997). Some statistical methods for multiple endpoints in clinical trials. *Controlled Clinical Trials 18*, 204.

Zhang, J. and K. F. Yu (1998). What's the relative risk? A method of correcting the odds ratio in cohort studies of common outcomes. *JAMA 280*, 1690–1.

Zhao, H. and A. A. Tsiatis (1997). A consistent estimator for the distribution of quality adjusted survival time. *Biometrika 84*, 339–348.

Zhao, H. and A. A. Tsiatis (1999). Efficient estimation of the distribution of quality-adjusted survival time. *Biometrics 55*(4), 1101–1107.

Index